ORAL PATHOLOGY
FOR THE DENTAL HYGIENIST

ORAL PATHOLOGY FOR THE DENTAL HYGIENIST

SIXTH EDITION

OLGA A.C. IBSEN, RDH, MS
Adjunct Professor
Department of Oral and Maxillofacial Pathology,
    Radiology and Medicine
New York University
College of Dentistry
New York, New York
Adjunct Professor
University of Bridgeport
Bridgeport, Connecticut

JOAN ANDERSEN PHELAN, MS, DDS
Professor and Chair
Department of Oral and Maxillofacial Pathology,
    Radiology and Medicine
New York University
College of Dentistry
New York, New York
Diplomate, American Board of Oral and
    Maxillofacial Pathology

ELSEVIER

3251 Riverport Lane
St. Louis, Missouri 63043

ORAL PATHOLOGY FOR THE DENTAL HYGIENIST, SIXTH EDITION   978-1-4557-0370-8

Notices

Knowledge and best practice in this field are constantly changing. As new research and experience broaden our understanding, changes in research methods, professional practices, or medical treatment may become necessary.

Practitioners and researchers must always rely on their own experience and knowledge in evaluating and using any information, methods, compounds, or experiments described herein. In using such information or methods they should be mindful of their own safety and the safety of others, including parties for whom they have a professional responsibility.

With respect to any drug or pharmaceutical products identified, readers are advised to check the most current information provided (i) on procedures featured or (ii) by the manufacturer of each product to be administered, to verify the recommended dose or formula, the method and duration of administration, and contraindications. It is the responsibility of practitioners, relying on their own experience and knowledge of their patients, to make diagnoses, to determine dosages and the best treatment for each individual patient, and to take all appropriate safety precautions.

To the fullest extent of the law, neither the Publisher nor the authors, contributors, or editors, assume any liability for any injury and/or damage to persons or property as a matter of products liability, negligence or otherwise, or from any use or operation of any methods, products, instructions, or ideas contained in the material herein.

Library of Congress Cataloging-in-Publication Data

Ibsen, Olga A. C.
    Oral pathology for the dental hygienist / Olga A.C. Ibsen, Joan Andersen Phelan. – 6th ed.
        p. ; cm.
    Includes bibliographical references and index.
    ISBN 978-1-4557-0370-8 (hardcover : alk. paper)
    I. Phelan, Joan Andersen.   II. Title.
    [DNLM: 1. Mouth Diseases–pathology.   2. Tooth Diseases–pathology.   3. Dental Hygienists. WU 140]
    617.5′22–dc23
                                                                        2012038135

Publisher: Linda Duncan
Executive Content Strategist: Kathy Falk
Content Manager: Kristin Hebberd
Content Development Specialist: Joslyn Dumas
Publishing Services Manager: Pat Joiner-Myers
Senior Project Manager: Joy Moore
Design Direction: Jessica Williams

Printed in China

Last digit is the print number: 9 8 7 6 5 4 3 2 1

Personal Dedication

To
our husbands
Lawrence and **Jerry**

For their years of support and encouragement of all our professional endeavors, especially each and every edition of *Oral Pathology for the Dental Hygienist*. They have assisted us in innumerable ways, and we are most grateful to them. We appreciate their dedication to us and ultimately to the profession.

With our love,
Olga *and* ***Joan***

Professional Dedication

To the faculty who chose this text over the last 20 years to enhance students' knowledge of oral pathology.

To past, present, and future students who have used or will use this text, we welcome you to the profession as clinicians, educators, and colleagues.

Our goal has ultimately been to make a difference. We welcome you to the challenge of providing optimal care to the public we serve.

Olga A.C. Ibsen, RDH, MS
Joan Andersen Phelan, MS, DDS

Contributors

Margaret J. Fehrenbach, RDH, MS
Dental Hygiene Educational Consultant
Dental Science Technical Writer
Seattle, Washington

Kenneth E. Fleisher, DDS
Clinical Associate Professor
Oral and Maxillofacial Surgery
New York University
College of Dentistry
New York, New York
Diplomate, American Board of Oral and
Maxillofacial Surgery

Paul D. Freedman, DDS
Director, Section of Oral Pathology
New York Hospital, Queens
Director, Oral Pathology Laboratory
Flushing, New York
Diplomate, American Board of Oral and
    Maxillofacial Pathology

Olga A.C. Ibsen, RDH, MS
Adjunct Professor
Department of Oral and Maxillofacial Pathology,
    Radiology and Medicine
New York University
College of Dentistry
New York, New York
Adjunct Professor
University of Bridgeport
Bridgeport, Connecticut

Anne Cale Jones, DDS
Distinguished Teaching Professor
Department of Pathology
School of Medicine
The University of Texas Health Science Center at
    San Antonio
San Antonio, Texas
Diplomate, American Board of Oral and
    Maxillofacial Pathology

John E. Kacher, DDS
JKJ Pathology
The Woodlands, Texas
Diplomate, American Board of Oral and
    Maxillofacial Pathology

Joan Andersen Phelan, MS, DDS
Professor and Chair
Department of Oral and Maxillofacial Pathology,
    Radiology and Medicine
New York University
College of Dentistry
New York, New York
Diplomate, American Board of Oral and Maxillofacial
    Pathology

Heddie O. Sedano, DDS, Dr Odont
Professor Emeritus, University of Minnesota;
Lecturer, Section of Pediatric Dentistry
School of Dentistry and Craniofacial Clinic
Department of Pediatrics, School of Medicine
University of California, Los Angeles
Los Angeles, California
Diplomate, American Board of Oral and
    Maxillofacial Pathology

Anthony T. Vernillo, DDS, PhD, MBE
Professor
Oral and Maxillofacial Pathology, Radiology and
    Medicine
New York University
College of Dentistry
New York, New York

Preface

In celebration of the 100th anniversary of the dental hygiene profession in 2013, we welcome you to the sixth edition of *Oral Pathology for the Dental Hygienist!* Times have indeed changed!

Knowledge of oral pathology is an essential component of dental hygiene practice. The sixth edition of *Oral Pathology for the Dental Hygienist* is an optimal resource for achieving success in applying this knowledge to patient care. Our objectives have always been to facilitate both the teaching and learning of oral pathology. It is our goal that the dental hygiene student will learn to recognize lesions and conditions, describe them using professional terminology, and through data collection, assist in the preliminary diagnosis of the lesion/condition identified. The text is supported by full-color illustrations.

Although the intended audience is the dental hygiene student, this text is also an excellent reference for dental students and practicing dental hygiene professionals. It covers those pathologic conditions likely to be encountered in private practice. Furthermore, it can provide an introduction to oral disease for other health professionals, such as nurses and medical technologists.

IMPORTANCE TO THE PROFESSION

Oral pathology is one of the most significant subjects in the dental hygiene curriculum. One person dies every hour of every day from oral cancer; this statistic has not changed in over 40 years. Clinicians need to understand oral pathology to provide thorough extraoral and intraoral examinations that will ensure identification of abnormal conditions as early as possible.

The student's ability to recognize the slightest deviation from normal is the first step in the evaluation process. The diagnostic principles described in this text should be applied to every lesion or condition identified. The application of these principles can begin at the student's very first clinical experience. The student will become more proficient in the data collection process with more clinical experience. In addition to recognizing abnormal findings while doing a clinical examination, students must develop the skills necessary to obtain more information from the patient. This is an important component of the diagnostic process. Besides providing a resource to identify abnormalities clinically, the information in this text will enhance the student's ability to ask appropriate questions.

ABOUT THIS EDITION

The text is divided into ten chapters. Several chapters begin with a general pathology introduction that will assist the student in understanding the pathologic processes discussed within the chapter. The sixth edition includes a variety of **learning features** to help students achieve the best possible outcomes in both the classroom and clinical setting.

- Each chapter begins with a **list of objectives** that provides an overview of the topics covered in the chapter. These objectives clearly define what the student is expected to learn and guide the faculty in test question preparation.
- A **detailed vocabulary list** with definitions and pronunciations is presented at the beginning of each chapter. This list helps students learn essential new dental terminology so that they can more effectively describe lesions and conditions in the classroom and in the clinical setting.
- Useful **synopsis tables** provide the student with a quick review of lesions, conditions, and diseases covered in the chapter. They summarize in outline format the main features of each chapter and include the diagnostic processes used to make the final diagnosis of the lesion. They are also very handy and quick reference guides for the clinical practitioner.
- **Review questions** at the end of each chapter help students test their knowledge of the chapter material and serve as good practice for taking the National Board Dental Hygiene Exam (NBDHE). All questions now have four answer selections, consistent with the national exam. Additional questions have been added to each chapter, and the answers are once again included in this edition.
- A **list of references** appears at the end of each chapter. This provides the student with additional study resources. The references have been updated in each chapter. Some classic references remain. New research is also reflected in the references.
- A **comprehensive glossary** at the end of the text provides easy access to the definitions of all the bolded words in the text.

NEW TO THIS EDITION

In this edition, you will find new information addressing the significance of the human papilloma virus (Chapters 4 and 7); additional vocabulary words, several new illustrations, and additional test questions in each chapter; and new references. Each chapter has been thoroughly reviewed and updated. The glossary has been expanded to include all of the bolded terminology within the chapters, making it an even more valuable reference.

All of the chapter review questions have been revised to offer four answer selections, which more clearly reflect the NBDHE design and format. This format change will assist faculty in preparing students for the NBDHE, course reviews, and curriculum examinations.

ABOUT EVOLVE

An Evolve website offers a variety of additional learning tools and greatly enhances the text for both students and instructors.

FOR THE STUDENT

Evolve Student Resources offer the following:

- **Case Studies.** Over 50 case studies with questions, answers, and rationales, which are set up in the format of the NBDHE. These provide a case-based format that will assist the student with the critical thinking skills necessary for national board examinations as well as for clinical practice.
- **Pathology Identification Exercises.** These interactive identification exercises show photos of a variety of diseases/conditions. Students must identify the disease and move the correct label to the photo it describes. A great visual self-study tool, these exercises allow students to test their ability to identify diseases they may encounter in practice. These exercises are now available as an app that can be downloaded to your mobile device, MP3 player, or tablet.
- **Flashcards.** Interactive, text-only flashcards, created from the text's key terms and glossary, are another excellent visual self-study tool that allows students to test their knowledge of terminology. These exercises are now available as an app that can be downloaded to your mobile device, MP3 player, or tablet.
- **Practice Exam.** A 200-question practice exam, with questions taken from *Mosby's Comprehensive Review of Dental Hygiene*, seventh edition, is designed to help students prepare for the NBDHE as well as for course exams.
- **Dental Hygiene Assessment Forms.** A variety of forms the hygienist may encounter in practice are provided in a printable format. The forms include a health history questionnaire, a head and neck physical examination documentation form, a prevention survey, an oral risk assessment worksheet, and a tobacco use assessment form.
- **Printable Versions of the Synopsis Tables.** The printable versions allow students to print out these helpful tables for inclusion with notes and make it easy to transport them from class to class.
- **Answers to Chapter Review Questions.** Expanded from the answers that appear in the book, the answers include rationales and page number references.
- **WebLinks.** Links to professional organizations, journals, additional image collections, smoking cessation, and meth mouth are provided to supplement the content of the textbook.

FOR THE INSTRUCTOR

Evolve Instructor Resources offer the following:

- **Testbank in ExamView.** A 700-question testbank divided by chapter is included along with rationales for all answer choices. The questions can be sorted by chapter or randomly, making the creation of quizzes and exams much easier for the instructor.
- **Image Collection.** This image collection includes every illustration from the book, making it easy for the instructor to incorporate a photo or drawing into a lecture or quiz.
- **Chapter Review Questions.** The questions that appear at the end of each chapter are provided as Word documents.
- **PowerPoint Presentations.** These presentations provide instructors with ready-made lectures.
- **Synopsis.** The synopses that are included at the end of each chapter are an excellent tool for student discussions, leading to better comprehension of material.

FROM THE AUTHORS

Oral Pathology for the Dental Hygienist has been written specifically for dental hygiene students and dental hygiene practitioners. Our goal for this new edition has been to continue to provide the highest standard oral pathology textbook. We strongly encourage instructors to continue to use the text in other courses, such as radiology, oral histology, and clinical courses. Dental hygienists have earned a reputation for excellence in identifying abnormal oral findings. The integration of oral pathology throughout the dental hygiene curriculum ensures more comprehensive patient care by the student and the dental hygiene practitioner.

Olga A.C. Ibsen, RDH, MS
Joan Andersen Phelan, MS, DDS

Acknowledgments

Through the years, many individuals have contributed to the success of *Oral Pathology for the Dental Hygienist*.

Our former editors at Elsevier have included Shirley Kuhn, who was with us through the first four editions; Publisher Penny Rudolph, who also guided us through the fourth edition; as well as Content Strategist John Dolan who directed us through the fifth edition. We sincerely appreciate their encouragement, support, and direction.

This sixth edition was directed and supported by Kristin Hebberd, Content Manager; Joslyn Dumas, Content Development Specialist; and Joy Moore, Senior Project Manager. They guided us through all the stages of production, and we thank them for their encouragement and attention to this outstanding text, especially their insight into the needs of the Evolve site.

We acknowledge Dr. Neill Serman, Toronto, Canada, who provided suggestions for this edition.

We also appreciate all of the contributions from Dr. Joan M. Iannucci, Ohio State University. Dr. Iannucci contributed to all previous editions of this text.

We will always be grateful to our oral pathology teachers: Drs. Melvin Blake, Ernest Baden, Leon Eisenbud, Paul Freedman, Stanley Kerpel, Harry Lumerman, Michael Marder, James Sciubba, Philip Silverstein, Marshal Solomon, David Zegarelli, and Edward V. Zegarelli. Olga A.C. Ibsen is especially grateful to two individuals who influenced her personal and professional life: her dad, the late Dr. Joseph A. Cuttita, and her godfather, the late Dr. Edward V. Zegarelli. All of these individuals strongly influenced our passion for pathology!

Gloria Turner of the Diagnostic Pathology Laboratory at NYU College of Dentistry prepared most of the slides used for the color photomicrographs that enhanced each edition of *Oral Pathology for the Dental Hygienist*. We extend our sincere appreciation for her outstanding work. Additional color photomicrographs were provided by Oral Pathology Laboratory, Inc., Flushing, New York.

We are proud to present the sixth edition of *Oral Pathology for the Dental Hygienist*.

Olga A.C. Ibsen, **RDH, MS**
Joan Andersen Phelan, **MS, DDS**

Contents

Chapter 1

Introduction to Preliminary Diagnosis of Oral Lesions

Olga A.C. Ibsen

OBJECTIVES

After studying this chapter, the student will be able to:

1. Define each of the terms in the vocabulary list for this chapter.
2. List and define the eight diagnostic categories that contribute to the diagnostic process.
3. Name a diagnostic category and give an example of a lesion, anomaly, or condition for which this category greatly contributes to the diagnosis.
4. Describe the clinical appearance of Fordyce granules (spots), torus palatinus, mandibular tori, and lingual varicosities and identify them in the clinical setting or on a clinical photograph.
5. Describe the radiographic appearance and historical data (including the age, sex, and race of the patient) that are relevant to periapical cemento-osseous dysplasia (cementoma).
6. Define "variant of normal" and give three examples of these lesions involving the tongue.
7. List and describe the clinical characteristics and identify a clinical picture of median rhomboid glossitis, geographic tongue, ectopic geographic tongue, fissured tongue, and hairy tongue.
8. Describe the clinical and histologic differences between leukoedema and linea alba.
9. Define leukoplakia and erythroplakia.
10. Discuss the two risk types of human papillomavirus covered in this chapter.

VOCABULARY

CLINICAL APPEARANCE OF SOFT TISSUE LESIONS

Bulla (adjective, bullous; plural, bullae) A circumscribed, elevated lesion that is more than 5 mm in diameter, usually contains serous fluid, and looks like a blister.

Lobule (adjective, lobulated) A segment or lobe that is a part of the whole; these lobes sometimes appear fused together (Figure 1-1).

Macule An area that is usually distinguished by a color different from that of the surrounding tissue; it is flat and does not protrude above the surface of the normal tissue. A freckle is an example of a macule.

Papule A small, circumscribed lesion usually less than 1 cm in diameter that is elevated or protrudes above the surface of normal surrounding tissue.

Pedunculated Attached by a stemlike or stalklike base similar to that of a mushroom (Figure 1-2).

Pustules Variously sized circumscribed elevations containing pus.

Sessile Describing the base of a lesion that is flat or broad instead of stemlike (Figure 1-3).

Vesicle A small, elevated lesion less than 1 cm in diameter that contains serous fluid.

Continued

VOCABULARY—cont'd

SOFT TISSUE CONSISTENCY

Nodule A palpable solid lesion up to 1 cm in diameter found in soft tissue; it can occur above, level with, or beneath the skin surface.

Palpation The evaluation of a lesion by feeling it with the fingers to determine the texture of the area; the descriptive terms for palpation are soft, firm, semifirm, and fluid filled; these terms also describe the consistency of a lesion.

COLOR OF LESION

Colors Red, pink, salmon, white, blue-black, gray, brown, and black are the words used most frequently to describe the colors of oral lesions; they can be used to identify specific lesions and may also be incorporated into general descriptions.

Erythema An abnormal redness of the mucosa or gingiva.

Erythroplakia A clinical term used to describe an oral mucosal lesion that appears as a smooth red patch or granular red and velvety patch.

Leukoplakia A clinical term for a white plaquelike lesion on the oral mucosa that cannot be rubbed off or diagnosed as a specific disease.

Pallor Paleness of the skin or mucosal tissues.

SIZE OF LESION

Centimeter (cm) One-hundredth of a meter; equivalent to a little less than one-half inch (0.393 inch) (Figure 1-4).

Millimeter (mm) One-thousandth of a meter (a meter is equivalent to 39.3 inches); the periodontal

FIGURE 1-1 ■ Lobulated torus palatinus.

FIGURE 1-2 ■ Fibroma with a pedunculated base. *Arrow* points to the stemlike base.

FIGURE 1-3 ■ Fibroma with a sessile base.

FIGURE 1-4 ■ A ruler measuring centimeters is used to measure all specimens submitted for microscopic examination.

VOCABULARY—cont'd

probe is of great assistance in documenting the size or diameter of a lesion that can be measured in millimeters (general terms such as small, medium, or large are sometimes used, but these terms are not as specific) (Figure 1-5).

SURFACE TEXTURE
Corrugated Wrinkled.
Fissure A cleft or groove, normal or otherwise, showing prominent depth.
Papillary Resembling small, nipple-shaped projections or elevations found in clusters.
Smooth, rough, folded Terms used to describe the surface texture of a lesion.

RADIOGRAPHIC TERMS USED TO DESCRIBE LESIONS IN BONE
Coalescence The process by which parts of a whole join together, or fuse, to make one.
Diffuse Describes a lesion with borders that are not well defined, making it impossible to detect the exact parameters of the lesion; this may make treatment more difficult and, depending on the biopsy results, more radical (Figure 1-6).
Multilocular Describes a lesion that extends beyond the confines of one distinct area and is defined as many lobes or parts that are somewhat fused together, making up the entire lesion; a

FIGURE 1-5 ■ **A,** Probe measuring the diameter of a fibroma with a sessile base. **B,** Gutta-percha point used to explore a radiographic defect. **C,** Periodontal probe placed before a radiograph.

Continued

VOCABULARY—cont'd

multilocular radiolucency is sometimes described as resembling soap bubbles; an odontogenic keratocyst often presents as a multilocular, radiolucent lesion (Figure 1-7).

Radiolucent Describes the black or dark areas on a radiograph; radiant energy can pass through these structures; less dense tissue such as the pulp is seen as a radiolucent structure (Figure 1-8).

Radiolucent and radiopaque Terms used to describe a mixture of light and dark areas within a lesion, usually denoting a stage in the development of the lesion; for example, in a stage I periapical cemento-osseous dysplasia (cementoma) (Figure 1-9, *A*), the lesion is radiolucent; in stage II it is radiolucent and radiopaque (Figure 1-9, *B*).

Radiopaque Describes the light or white area on a radiograph that results from the inability of radiant energy to pass through the structure; the denser the structure, the lighter or whiter it appears on the radiograph; this is illustrated in Figure 1-10.

Root resorption Observed radiographically when the apex of the tooth appears shortened or blunted and irregularly shaped; occurs as a response to stimuli, which can include a cyst, tumor, or trauma; Figure 1-11 illustrates resorption of the roots as a result of a rapid orthodontic procedure

FIGURE 1-6 ■ Squamous cell carcinoma involving the alveolar bone and hard palate showing diffuse borders. (Courtesy Drs. Paul Freedman and Stanley Kerpel.)

FIGURE 1-7 ■ Odontogenic keratocyst *(arrow)*, illustrating a multilocular lesion. (Courtesy Dr. Victor M. Sternberg.)

FIGURE 1-8 ■ Prominent pulp chambers, horns, and canals in mandibular molars.

VOCABULARY—cont'd

(see Figure 1-27); external resorption arises from tissues outside the tooth such as the periodontal ligament, whereas internal resorption is triggered by pulpal tissue reaction from within the tooth; in the latter the pulpal area can be seen as a diffuse radiolucency beyond the confines of the normal pulp area.

Scalloping around the root A radiolucent lesion that extends between the roots, as seen in a traumatic bone cyst; this lesion appears to extend up the periodontal ligament (Figure 1-12).

Unilocular Having one compartment or unit that is well defined or outlined, as in a simple radicular cyst (Figure 1-13).

Well circumscribed Term used to describe a lesion with borders that are specifically defined and in which one can clearly see the exact margins and extent (Figure 1-14).

FIGURE 1-9 ■ **A,** Stage I periapical cemento-osseous dysplasia (cementoma). **B,** Stage II periapical cemento-osseous dysplasia (cementoma).

FIGURE 1-10 ■ Amalgam restorations on the occlusal surfaces of the maxillary and mandibular molars.

Continued

FIGURE 1-11 ■ Resorption of the roots on maxillary anteriors as a result of rapid orthodontic movement.

FIGURE 1-12 ■ Traumatic bone cyst (arrows) around the roots. (Courtesy Drs. Paul Freedman and Stanley Kerpel.)

FIGURE 1-14 ■ Well-circumscribed median palatal cyst (arrow).

FIGURE 1-13 ■ Radicular cyst (arrow) at the apex of the maxillary lateral incisor, illustrating a unilocular lesion.

To understand the material in this text, it is imperative that the reader approach it in a systematic manner. Significant time is spent in the dental hygiene curriculum identifying and describing normal structures. Before one can identify the abnormal condition, it is necessary to have a solid understanding of the basic and dental sciences such as human anatomy and physiology, histology, and dental anatomy. Once one has a solid understanding of normal structures and those that are variants of normal, findings that deviate from normal and pathologic conditions are recognized more easily. The preliminary evaluation and description of these lesions are within the scope of dental hygiene practice and are truly among the most challenging experiences in clinical practice.

In the first part of this chapter the definitions of commonly used terms that describe the clinical and radiographic features of a lesion, including terms used for normal, variants of normal, and pathologic conditions discussed throughout this text, are presented. The reader is encouraged to use these terms in the clinical setting so that they become part of an everyday professional vocabulary, thereby facilitating communication between the hygienist and other dental practitioners in the clinical setting.

The second part of this chapter focuses on the eight diagnostic categories that provide a systematic approach to the preliminary evaluation of oral lesions. Each area is described, and the strength of that area in the diagnostic process is illustrated using specific examples of lesions.

The final part of the chapter includes conditions that are considered variants of normal and those that are benign conditions of unknown cause. Most are diagnosed from their distinct clinical appearance and history.

FIGURE 1-15 ■ Fordyce granules.

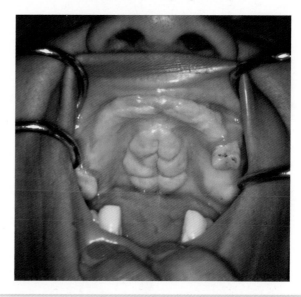

FIGURE 1-16 ■ Lobulated torus palatinus. (Courtesy Dr. Edward V. Zegarelli.)

THE DIAGNOSTIC PROCESS

MAKING A DIAGNOSIS

How is a diagnosis made? What are the essential components? The answers to these questions begin with data collection. The process of diagnosis requires gathering information that is relevant to the patient and the lesion being evaluated; this information comes from various sources.

Certain distinct diagnostic categories should be thought of as pieces in a puzzle, with each piece playing a significant role in the final diagnosis. The eight categories that contribute segments of information leading to the definitive or final diagnosis are (1) clinical, (2) radiographic, (3) historical, (4) laboratory, (5) microscopic, (6) surgical, (7) therapeutic, and (8) differential findings. It is important to note that usually one area alone does not provide sufficient information to make a diagnosis; the strength of the diagnosis is often derived from one or two areas. As the dental hygienist becomes more aware of the diseases and conditions discussed in this text, it will be most helpful to use the diagnostic categories as a guide to evaluating lesions..

CLINICAL DIAGNOSIS

Clinical diagnosis suggests that the strength of the diagnosis comes from the clinical appearance of the lesion. By observing the area in a well-illuminated clinical setting and palpating it if necessary, the clinician can establish a diagnosis for some lesions on the basis of color, shape, location, and history of the lesion. When a diagnosis can be made on the basis of these unique clinical features, biopsy or surgical intervention is not necessary. Examples of lesions that can be clinically diagnosed are Fordyce granules (Figure 1-15), torus palatinus (Figure 1-16), mandibular tori (Figure 1-17), melanin pigmentation (Figure 1-18), retrocuspid papillae (Figure 1-19), and lingual varicosities (see Figure 1-52). These lesions are described later in this chapter.

Other benign conditions of unknown cause that are recognized by their distinct clinical appearance include fissured tongue (Figure 1-20), median rhomboid glossitis (Figure 1-21), geographic tongue (Figure 1-22), and hairy tongue (Figure 1-23). These conditions are also discussed later in this chapter.

FIGURE 1-17 ■ *Arrows* point to mandibular tori.

FIGURE 1-18 ■ Melanin pigmentation.

FIGURE 1-19 ■ *Arrows* point to the retrocuspid papillae on the gingival margin of the lingual aspect of the mandibular cuspids.

FIGURE 1-20 ■ Fissured tongue.

FIGURE 1-21 ■ Median rhomboid glossitis *(top arrow)* and geographic tongue *(bottom arrows)*.

FIGURE 1-22 ■ Geographic tongue. *Arrows* point to areas of depapillation.

FIGURE 1-23 ■ **A,** White hairy tongue. **B,** White hairy tongue showing a circumvallate papilla *(arrow)*. **C,** Black hairy tongue.

Sometimes the diagnostic process requires historical information in addition to the clinical findings. For example, an amalgam tattoo (focal argyrosis) can be observed as a blue-to-gray patch on the gingiva or mucosa where an amalgam restoration is or has been located (Figure 1-24). Although this condition is usually easily observed and a clinical diagnosis made, any history involving the area can still be very helpful in confirming the clinical impression. The patient in Figure 1-24 had root canal therapy and a retrograde amalgam on a deciduous tooth. The amalgam tattoo is observed in the apical area of the permanent central incisor; no evidence of an amalgam restoration exists in the entire anterior area. The history helped confirm the clinical diagnosis.

FIGURE 1-24 ■ *Arrow* points to an amalgam tattoo at the apical area of the patient's maxillary right central incisor. This patient had a root canal procedure on a deciduous tooth. No other amalgam restoration is in the area; therefore it was helpful to know the patient's past dental history to confirm this diagnosis.

RADIOGRAPHIC DIAGNOSIS

In a radiographic diagnosis the radiograph provides sufficient information to establish the diagnosis. Although additional clinical and historical information may contribute, the diagnosis is obtained from the radiograph. Conditions for which the radiograph provides the most significant information include periapical pathosis (Figure 1-25), internal resorption (Figure 1-26), external resorption (Figure 1-27), heavy interproximal calculus (Figure 1-28), dental caries (Figure 1-29), compound odontoma (Figure 1-30), complex odontoma (Figure 1-31), supernumerary teeth (Figure 1-32), impacted or unerupted teeth (Figure 1-33), and

Text continued on page 13

FIGURE 1-25 ■ **A,** Periapical pathosis (PAP); a radiolucency is seen at the apex of the mandibular second premolar *(arrow).* **B,** In another patient a fistula is seen on the maxillary lateral incisor. A fistula is usually an indication of PAP. When a fistula is observed clinically, a radiograph is necessary for diagnostic and treatment purposes.

FIGURE 1-27 ■ *Arrow* points to external resorption on a mandibular central incisor. (Courtesy Dr. Gerald P. Curatola.)

FIGURE 1-26 ■ *Arrow* points to the area of internal resorption on the maxillary first molar.

FIGURE 1-28 ■ *Arrows* point to heavy interproximal calculus.

FIGURE 1-29 ■ **A,** Dental caries. The reader should observe the interproximal radiolucencies. Clinical examination is necessary to confirm the involvement of some of the areas. **B,** Periapical radiograph showing a subtle carious area on the distal aspect of the mandibular second premolar. **C,** The patient in **(B)** was seen a year later. During the scaling procedure a defect on the distal aspect of the mandibular second premolar was detected. This vertical bitewing radiograph was taken. The reader should note the definite radiolucent, carious area on the distal aspect of the mandibular second premolar. This example emphasizes the need for careful clinical and radiographic evaluation. (**B** and **C,** Courtesy Dr. Victor M. Sternberg.)

FIGURE 1-30 ■ *Arrow* points to compound odontoma.

FIGURE 1-31 ■ **A,** Compound odontoma rather easily diagnosed from the radiograph alone. **B,** Complex odontoma *(arrow)* not diagnosed from the radiograph alone. (**B,** Courtesy Drs. Paul Freedman and Stanley Kerpel.)

FIGURE 1-32 ■ **A,** Mesiodens *(arrow).* A supernumerary tooth is located between the maxillary central incisors. **B,** A radiograph showing a supernumerary mandibular premolar *(arrow)* surrounded by a radiolucent area diagnosed as a dentigerous cyst. Clinically this area was thought to be a mandibular torus (until the radiograph was taken).

FIGURE 1-33 ■ **A,** Impacted mandibular cuspid. **B,** Impacted maxillary cuspid.

FIGURE 1-34 ■ Calcified pulp in the mandibular first molar.

calcified pulp (Figure 1-34). Normal anatomic landmarks are also easily observed radiographically. In some cases the radiograph may show very distinct and well-defined structures such as the nutrient canals seen in Figure 1-35, *A* and *B* and the mixed dentition seen in Figure 1-35, *C*. Unusual radiographic findings are illustrated in Figure 1-36.

HISTORICAL DIAGNOSIS

Historical data constitute an important component in every diagnosis; occasionally when historical data are combined with observation of the clinical appearance of the lesion, the historical information constitutes the most important contribution to the diagnostic process. Personal history, family

FIGURE 1-36, cont'd ■ G, *Arrow* points to a retained deciduous tooth with an amalgam restoration. **H,** *Arrow* points to a radiopaque area that identifies a retained shotgun pellet on the distal aspect of the mandibular third molar. **I,** *Arrow* points to a radiopaque circular area that is a nose ring. **J,** Periapical radiograph showing a radiopaque area at the apex of the mesial root of the mandibular second molar. This object was a retained piece of shrapnel. **K,** Panoramic radiograph of the same patient showing the same object *(arrow).* This radiograph gives a more accurate view of the location of the object. It was found to be in the soft tissue in the area and not within bone.

history, past and present medical and dental histories, history of drug ingestion, and history of the presenting disease or lesion can provide information necessary for the final diagnosis. Thorough medical and dental histories must be a part of every patient's permanent record. The clinician should review these documents carefully and update them with the patient at each visit.

Pathologic conditions in which the family history contributes a significant role in the diagnosis include amelogenesis imperfecta (Figure 1-37), dentinogenesis imperfecta (Figure 1-38), and many other genetic disorders. In addition, clinical findings and radiographs also provide significant assistance to the diagnostic process of these conditions.

FIGURE 1-37 ■ **A,** One of the clinical appearances of amelogenesis imperfecta. **B,** The radiographic aspect of amelogenesis imperfecta. (Courtesy Dr. Edward V. Zegarelli.)

FIGURE 1-38 ■ **A,** Clinical appearance of dentinogenesis imperfecta. **B,** Radiographic appearance of dentinogenesis imperfecta. (Courtesy Dr. Edward V. Zegarelli.)

A patient's medical or dental status, including drug history, can also contribute significant information to a diagnosis. For example, a history of ulcerative colitis may contribute to the diagnosis of oral ulcers (Figure 1-39, *A*), which could be related to this medical condition. Another example of the value of this type of information is the patient in Figure 1-39, *B,* who experienced gingival enlargement; drug history revealed that the patient was taking a calcium channel blocker. Allergic reactions may also be a part of the patient's medical history. Urticaria (hives) (see Chapter 3) is an immediate response to an allergen. Ingested allergens are often the cause of urticaria but other causes include insect venom, drugs, topical agents, or systemic disease. Although the cause cannot always be identified, urticaria appears as well-demarcated areas of swelling on the skin, often erythematous (Figure 1-39, *C* and *D*). Sometimes hypersensitivity reactions may be delayed. However, in any case, each time the patient comes in contact with the allergen, their reaction may be more severe.

A history of a skin graft from the hip to the ridge and mucobuccal fold area in the anterior mandible in a patient can provide significant information relevant to the diagnosis of a white- or brown-pigmented area on the mandibular anterior ridge and vestibule (Figure 1-40).

Periapical cemento-osseous dysplasia (cementoma) is another lesion in which the patient's personal history contributes significantly. It is found most frequently in black women in the third decade of life. Other characteristics of the lesion reveal that it is asymptomatic and that the teeth involved are vital (see Figure 1-9).

LABORATORY DIAGNOSIS

Clinical laboratory tests, including blood chemistries and urinalysis, can provide information that contributes to a diagnosis. An elevated serum alkaline phosphatase level is significant in the diagnosis of Paget disease. This feature, in addition to a distinctive radiographic appearance that includes a "cotton-wool effect" (Figure 1-41) and hypercementosis, provides conclusive information for a definitive diagnosis.

Laboratory cultures are also helpful in determining the diagnosis of oral infections.

Erythroplakia is a clinical term for a red lesion that cannot be diagnosed on the basis of clinical features alone (Figure 1-42, C). Most erythroplakias (90%) are microscopically diagnosed as severe epithelial dysplasia (premalignant) or squamous cell carcinoma (see Chapter 7).

There are more than 150 types of the human papillomavirus (HPV). Some are very low risk, and others are high risk. Those associated with squamous cell carcinoma are high-risk types. Others, such as those causing verruca vulgaris (the common wart), are low-risk types. Verruca vulgaris exhibits microscopic features that are characteristic of HPV infection (see Chapter 4).

SURGICAL DIAGNOSIS

The strength of a surgical diagnosis comes from surgical intervention. For example, diagnosis is made using the information gained during the surgical procedure for the traumatic bone cyst shown in Figure 1-43. A traumatic or simple bone cyst will appear as a radiolucency that scallops around the roots. Surgical intervention provides conclusive evidence when the lesion is opened and an empty void within the bone is found. The void usually fills with bone and heals after the surgical procedure. Lingual mandibular bone concavity, also referred to as a static bone cyst or Stafne bone cyst (Figure 1-44), is a developmental anomaly that is often bilateral. The radiolucent area is oval or elliptical in shape and is found anterior to the angle of the ramus and inferior to the mandibular canal. A computed tomography scan would further confirm the diagnosis, showing the invagination of the lingual aspect of the mandible. However, if the radiolucency is not in the classic location, surgical examination and biopsy would be necessary to confirm the diagnosis. There is no treatment necessary for lingual mandibular bone concavity.

THERAPEUTIC DIAGNOSIS

Nutritional deficiencies are common conditions to be diagnosed by therapeutic means. Although angular cheilitis (Figure 1-45) may be associated with a deficiency of the B-complex vitamins, it is most commonly a fungal condition and responds to topical application of an antifungal cream or ointment such as nystatin. A thorough patient history should be obtained to rule out a contributory nutritional deficiency.

Necrotizing ulcerative gingivitis (NUG) has distinct clinical features (Figure 1-46) and constitutional signs. It responds to hydrogen peroxide rinses because the anaerobic bacteria that cause NUG cannot survive in an oxygenated environment. Prescribing hydrogen peroxide rinses and observing the results without culturing the bacteria applies the principle of therapeutic diagnosis because it is based solely on clinical and historical information with confirmation by the response of the condition to therapy. Antibiotic therapy can also be used in the treatment of NUG.

DIFFERENTIAL DIAGNOSIS

The differential diagnosis is that point in the diagnostic process when the practitioner decides which test or

FIGURE 1-43 ■ Traumatic bone cyst. (Courtesy Dr. Edward V. Zegarelli.)

FIGURE 1-44 ■ *Arrow* points to a static (Stafne) bone cyst. (Courtesy Dr. Edward V. Zegarelli.)

FIGURE 1-45 ■ Angular cheilitis.

FIGURE 1-46 ▪ **A,** Necrotizing ulcerative gingivitis (NUG). **B,** Another example of NUG. The clinician should note the gingival contours and punched-out, blunted papillae.

procedure is required to rule out the conditions originally suspected and to establish the definitive or final diagnosis. All the previously discussed components are applied to the differential diagnosis. The final diagnosis emerges from a thorough evaluation of the suspected lesions (Box 1-1).

To arrive at a diagnosis, the data collection included the patient's medical and dental health histories, the history of the lesion in question, a clinical description and evaluation, and biopsy and microscopy reports. Box 1-1 illustrates the fact that arriving at a diagnosis involves a process. As stated previously, the diagnostic process can be thought of as a puzzle because the information from each diagnostic category becomes part of it. In Box 1-1 the microscopic examination contributed most significantly to the definitive or final diagnosis. The differential diagnosis included three possible diagnoses; the biopsy and microscopic examinations provided conclusive information in the diagnostic process.

The hygienist can be effective in the preliminary evaluation of the lesion by calling it to the attention of the dentist and then gathering and preparing all the data for the clinician who will perform the biopsy. In addition, it is both challenging and stimulating to discuss diagnostic impressions with other professionals on the basis of the data available at the time.

BOX 1-1

CASE STUDY

The following case study illustrates how the diagnostic processes work together and how the differential diagnosis is used.

An 11-year-old white girl came to the dental office with her mother. The mother was concerned about the interdental papilla on the child's labial aspect between the maxillary right central and lateral incisors (Figure 1-47). Nothing in the medical history explained the condition; the child had been wearing orthodontic appliances for about 1 year.

Clinically, the interdental papilla was enlarged and had a papillary surface that bled easily when probed. The sessile lesion measured 5 mm cervicoincisally by 3 mm mesiodistally. No pain was felt in the area. Information pertinent to the history of the lesion was secured from the mother. The lesion had been there for about 1 year and was first noticed around the time the child began wearing braces. At times tags of the lesion or pieces of it "fell off" during brushing. The orthodontist "pulled most of it off" at one point, but it was never surgically removed or submitted for microscopic examination and seemed to grow back. Additional questioning revealed that the child had a wart on her foot within the last year. A biopsy was performed, and the tissue sample was placed in formalin and sent to an oral pathology laboratory with the following differential diagnosis:

- **Pyogenic granuloma:** The spongy inflammatory tissue was possibly caused by mechanical irritation from the orthodontic bands, thereby causing pyogenic granuloma.
- **Papilloma:** On the basis of the papillary surface texture of the lesion, it was thought to be a papilloma.
- **Verruca vulgaris:** Because the child had a wart and could have spread the virus, verruca vulgaris was suggested. In addition, histologically a wart has lateral lipping, and it was thought that this could explain why pieces of the lesion fell off periodically during brushing. However, the surface of a verruca vulgaris is usually keratinized and therefore whiter than the lesion illustrated in Figure 1-47.

The microscopic examination revealed stratified squamous epithelium covering a core of loose and edematous fibrous connective tissue. The stroma contained numerous endothelium-lined, blood-filled capillaries and a dense infiltrate of lymphocytes, plasma cells, and neutrophils.

The definitive or final diagnosis was pyogenic granuloma.

FIGURE 1-47 ▪ *Arrow* points to a pyogenic granuloma between the patient's right maxillary central and lateral incisors. (Courtesy Dr. Victor M. Sternberg.)

FIGURE 1-52 ■ Lingual varices. (Courtesy Dr. David Zegarelli.)

FIGURE 1-53 ■ *Arrow* points to linea alba on the buccal mucosa.

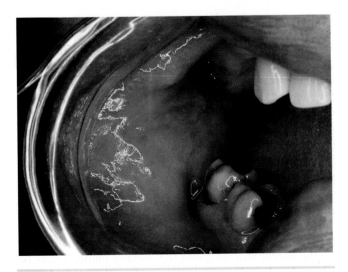

FIGURE 1-54 ■ Leukoedema of the buccal mucosa, showing an opalescent, velvety texture.

LEUKOEDEMA

A generalized opalescence is imparted to the buccal mucosa by **leukoedema.** It is most commonly observed in black adults (up to 85%), suggesting an ethnic predisposition. Leukoedema can also be seen in white individuals. Clinically, a gray-white film is diffused throughout the buccal mucosa, giving the mucosa an opaque quality. If the mucosa is stretched, the opalescence becomes less prominent. The condition becomes more pronounced in smokers. The opalescence is an integral part of the buccal tissue and cannot be removed. Histologically significant intracellular edema in the spinous cells and acanthosis of the epithelium are seen. It is a benign anomaly that requires no treatment (Figure 1-54).

BENIGN CONDITIONS OF UNKNOWN CAUSE

LINGUAL THYROID NODULE

The thyroid gland begins to develop during the first month of fetal life and is located initially in the area of the foramen cecum on the posterior tongue. In normal development the thyroid gland descends to its normal location in the neck. When thyroid tissue either does not descend or remnants become entrapped in the tissue that makes up the tongue, a developmental anomaly called a **lingual thyroid nodule** results. Research has indicated a high predilection in females, and studies have linked the emergence of a lingual thyroid nodule with hormonal changes because it appears to be associated with puberty, pregnancy, and menopause. Clinically, a lingual thyroid nodule is observed as a mass in the midline of the dorsal surface of the tongue posterior to the circumvallate papillae in the area of the foramen cecum. The lesion usually has a sessile base and is 2 to 3 cm in width. On histologic examination normal thyroid tissue is found. Treatment requires careful evaluation of the patient to determine whether the thyroid gland is present in its normal location. Surgical intervention is generally not required and is contraindicated if the nodule is the patient's functioning thyroid tissue.

MEDIAN RHOMBOID GLOSSITIS

The cause of **median rhomboid glossitis** is not clear. Research has suggested that it may be associated with a chronic fungal infection by *Candida albicans.* Clinically, median rhomboid glossitis appears as a flat or slightly raised oval or rectangular erythematous area in the midline of the dorsal surface of the tongue, beginning at the junction of the anterior and middle thirds and extending posterior to the circumvallate papillae. It is devoid of filiform papillae; therefore its texture is smooth. If the remaining surface of the tongue is coated, the area appears more prominent. No specific treatment exists; however, sometimes an antifungal agent is applied, and the lesion resolves, but this is not always the case. On occasion the condition resolves with no specific treatment at all (Figure 1-55).

GEOGRAPHIC TONGUE

The cause of **geographic tongue** (erythema migrans, benign migratory glossitis) is not clear. The familial occurrence of geographic tongue suggests that genetic factors play a role. Some investigators suggest that it is exacerbated by stress, and studies exist that associate the histologic findings with those found in psoriasis. The clinical appearance involves the dorsal and lateral borders of the tongue. Diffuse areas devoid of filiform papillae can be observed. These areas appear as erythematous patches that are surrounded by a white or yellow perimeter. The fungiform papillae appear distinct within the erythematous patch. The condition does not remain static; remission and changes in the depapillated areas appear to occur. On occasion a patient complains of a burning discomfort associated with geographic tongue. Usually no treatment is indicated (Figure 1-56, *A*).

Ectopic geographic tongue is the term used to describe the condition when it is found on mucosal surfaces other than the tongue. In Figure 1-56, *B* it is seen in the mandibular anterior mucobuccal fold.

FISSURED TONGUE

The cause of **fissured tongue** is unknown. It is seen in about 5% of the population. Familial patterns of occurrence suggest that genetic factors are probably involved. Clinically, the dorsal surface of the tongue appears to have deep fissures or grooves that may become irritated if food debris collects in them. No treatment is indicated for the condition. However, a patient with a fissured tongue may be advised to brush the tongue gently with a soft toothbrush to keep the fissures clean of debris and irritants (Figure 1-57; and see Figure 1-20).

HAIRY TONGUE

Hairy tongue is a condition in which the patient has an increased accumulation of keratin on the filiform papillae that results in a white, "hairy" appearance. This may be the

FIGURE 1-55 ■ Median rhomboid glossitis. (Courtesy Dr. Edward V. Zegarelli.)

FIGURE 1-57 ■ Fissured tongue and attrition.

FIGURE 1-56 ■ **A,** Geographic tongue. **B,** Ectopic geographic tongue observed in the mandibular anterior mucosa.

FIGURE 1-58 ■ White hairy tongue.

FIGURE 1-59 ■ Black hairy tongue.

result of either an increase in keratin production or a decrease in normal desquamation. Unless otherwise pigmented, the elongated filiform papillae are white (Figure 1-58). In the condition known as black hairy tongue, the papillae are a brown-to-black color because of chromogenic bacteria (Figure 1-59). Tobacco and certain foods may also discolor the papillae. Although the cause is unknown, hydrogen peroxide, alcohol, or chemical rinses have been suggested to stimulate the elongation of the filiform papillae that results in the appearance of hairy tongue.

Treatment involves directing the patient to brush the tongue gently with a toothbrush (wet with water only) to remove debris. The condition usually clears completely but may recur.

SELECTED REFERENCES

Books

Darby ML: *Mosby's comprehensive review of dental hygiene*, ed 7, St. Louis, 2012, Mosby.
Neville BW, Damm DD, White DH: *Color atlas of clinical oral pathology*, Philadelphia, 1991, Lea & Febiger.
Neville BW, Damm DD, Allen CM, et al: *Oral and maxillofacial pathology*, ed 3, Philadelphia, 2009, Saunders.
Regezi JA, Sciubba JJ, Jordan RCK: *Oral pathology: clinical pathologic correlations*, ed 6, St. Louis, 2012, Saunders.
Stedman's Medical Dictionary for the Dental Professions, Illustrated, ed 1, 2007, Lippincott, Williams & Wilkins.

Journal Articles

Bouquot JE, Gundlach KKH: Odd tongues: the prevalence of common tongue lesions in 23,616 white Americans over 35 years of age, *Quintessence Int* 17:719, 1986.
Brannon RB, Pousson RR: The retrocuspid papillae: a clinical evaluation of 51 cases, *J Dent Hyg* 77:180, 2003.
Chapnick L: External root resorption: an experimental radiographic evaluation, *Oral Surg Oral Med Oral Pathol* 67:578, 1989.
Comfort M, Wu PC: The reliability of personal and family medical histories in the identification of hepatitis B carriers, *Oral Surg Oral Med Oral Pathol* 67:531, 1989.
Daley TD: Pathology of intraoral sebaceous glands, *J Oral Pathol Med* 22:241, 1993.
Ibsen OAC: Diagnosing smoking-related lesions, *Dimens Dent Hyg* 2:32-35, 2004.
Ibsen OAC: Putting the pieces together, *Dimens Dent Hyg* 2:3-10, 2004.
Ibsen OAC: Oral cancer: incidence, the diagnostic process, and screening techniques, *Dimens Dent Hyg* 4:4, 2006.
Ibsen OAC: The missing link, *Dimens Dent Hyg* 6:28-31, 2008.
Kalan A, Tarig M: Lingual thyroid gland: clinical evaluation and comprehensive management, *Ear Nose Throat J* 78:340, 1999.
Kaugars GE, Miller ME, Abbey LM: Odontomas, *Oral Surg Oral Med Oral Pathol* 67:2172, 1989.
Lydiatt DD, Hollins RR, Peterson GP: Multiple idiopathic root resorption: diagnostic considerations, *Oral Surg Oral Med Oral Pathol* 67:208, 1989.
McCann AL, Wesley RK: A method for describing soft tissue lesions of the oral cavity, *J Dent Hyg* 60:304, 1986.
Neupert EA, Wright JM: Regional odontodysplasia presenting as a soft tissue swelling, *Oral Surg Oral Med Oral Pathol* 67:193, 1989.
Pogrel MA, Cram D: Intraoral findings in patients with psoriasis with a special reference to ectopic geographic tongue (erythema circinata), *Oral Surg Oral Med Oral Pathol* 66:184, 1988.
Rosen DJ, Ardekian L, Machtei EE, et al: Traumatic bone cyst resembling apical periodontitis, *J Periodontol* 68:1019, 1997.
Suzuki M, Sakae T: A familial study of torus palatinus and torus mandibularis, *Am J Phys Anthropol* 18:263, 1960.

Review Questions

1. After arriving at a differential diagnosis, information from which one of the following categories will best establish a final or definitive diagnosis?
   A. Clinical
   B. Historical
   C. Microscopic
   D. Radiographic

2. The descriptive term that would best be used for a freckle is a:
   A. Bulla
   B. Vesicle
   C. Lobule
   D. Macule

3. Which one of the following terms describes the base of a lesion that is stalklike?
   A. Sessile
   B. Lobule
   C. Pedunculated
   D. Macule

4. Clinical diagnosis can be used to determine the final or definitive diagnosis of all of the following *except*:
   A. Fordyce granules
   B. Unerupted supernumerary teeth
   C. Mandibular tori
   D. Geographic tongue

5. Radiographic diagnosis would contribute to the definitive diagnosis of all of the following *except*:
   A. Internal resorptions
   B. Periapical cemento-osseous dysplasia
   C. Odontomas
   D. A retained deciduous tooth

6. To determine the presence of blood dyscrasias, which one of the following would provide the most definitive information?
   A. Laboratory blood tests
   B. Bleeding during probing
   C. Pallor of the gingiva and mucosa
   D. Patient complaint of weakness

7. When an antifungal ointment or cream is used to treat suspected angular cheilitis, which one of the following diagnostic categories is being used?
   A. Clinical
   B. Therapeutic
   C. Laboratory
   D. Differential

8. Yellow clusters of ectopic sebaceous glands commonly observed on the buccal mucosa and evaluated through clinical diagnosis are most likely:
   A. Lipomas
   B. Fibromas
   C. Fordyce granules
   D. Linea alba

9. A slow-growing, bony hard exophytic growth on the midline of the hard palate is developmental and hereditary in origin. The diagnosis is determined through clinical evaluation. You suspect:
   A. Torus palatinus
   B. Mixed tumor
   C. Palatal cyst
   D. Nasopalatine cyst

10. The "white line" observed clinically on the buccal mucosa that extends from anterior to posterior along the occlusal plane is:
    A. Leukoedema
    B. Leukoplakia
    C. Linea alba
    D. Lichen planus

11. Which one of the following occurs as an erythematous area, is devoid of filiform papillae, is oval to rectangular in shape, and is on the midline of the dorsal surface of the tongue?
    A. Median rhomboid glossitis
    B. Geographic tongue
    C. Fissured tongue
    D. Lingual thyroid

Continued

Review Questions—cont'd

12. Which one of the following diagnostic categories would the dental hygienist most easily apply to the preliminary evaluation of oral lesions?
    A. Microscopic
    B. Clinical
    C. Therapeutic
    D. Differential

13. These examples of exostoses are found on the lingual aspect of the mandible in the area of the premolars. They are benign, bony hard, and require no treatment. Radiographically they appear as radiopaque areas and are often bilateral. You suspect:
    A. Retrocuspid papilla
    B. Lingual mandibular bone concavity
    C. Genial tubercles
    D. Mandibular tori

14. Which one of the following terms is most often used when describing mandibular tori?
    A. Bullous
    B. Lobulated
    C. Sessile
    D. Pedunculated

15. Which of the following conditions is a benign anomaly, has a diffuse gray-to-white opaque appearance on the buccal mucosa, and is most commonly seen in adult black individuals?
    A. Leukoedema
    B. Linea alba
    C. Ectopic geographic tongue
    D. Lichen planus

16. A patient has the clinical signs of necrotizing ulcerative gingivitis. The hygienist has the patient begin hydrogen peroxide rinses without culturing the bacterial flora. This action applies to which one of the following diagnostic categories?
    A. Therapeutic
    B. Microscopic
    C. Clinical
    D. Final or definitive

17. A small circumscribed lesion usually less than 1 cm in diameter that is elevated and protrudes above the surface of normal surrounding tissue is called a:
    A. Bulla
    B. Macule
    C. Vesicle
    D. Papule

18. The base of a sessile lesion is:
    A. Broad and flat
    B. Stemlike
    C. Corrugated
    D. Lobulated

19. The identification of which one of the following is *not* determined by clinical diagnosis?
    A. Fordyce granules
    B. Tori
    C. Compound odontoma
    D. Retrocuspid papilla

20. Another term for geographic tongue is:
    A. Allergic tongue
    B. Median rhomboid glossitis
    C. Migratory glossitis
    D. White hairy tongue

21. The cause of supernumerary teeth is most likely:
    A. Genetic
    B. Traumatic
    C. Cystic
    D. Systemic

22. Historical diagnosis can include the patient's:
    A. Age and sex
    B. Family history
    C. Medical history
    D. All of the above

23. Which condition is most often seen on the buccal mucosa?
    A. Melanin pigmentation
    B. Fordyce granules
    C. Nicotine stomatitis
    D. Angular cheilitis

24. Which one of the following is *not* considered a variant of normal?
    A. Migratory glossitis
    B. White hairy tongue
    C. Fissured tongue
    D. Hairy leukoplakia

25. Which cyst is often described as a radiolucency that scallops around the roots of the teeth involved?
    A. Stafne bone
    B. Traumatic bone
    C. Radicular
    D. Residual

26. What percentage of erythroplakias is diagnosed as severe epithelial dysplasia or squamous cell carcinoma?
    A. 10%
    B. 25%
    C. 60%
    D. 90%

27. Which of the following best describes the number of types of HIV? More than:
    A. 35
    B. 75
    C. 100
    D. 150

28. Which one of the following terms best describes leukoplakia?
    A. Clinical
    B. Histologic
    C. Historical
    D. Microscopic

Chapter 2

Inflammation and Repair

Margaret J. Fehrenbach, Joan Andersen Phelan

OBJECTIVES

After studying this chapter, the student will be able to:

1. Define and pronounce each of the words in the vocabulary list for this chapter.
2. List the classic signs of inflammation that occur locally at the site of inflammation.
3. List and describe the major systemic signs of inflammation.
4. List and describe the microscopic events of the inflammatory process.
5. Describe the microscopic events associated with each of the local signs of inflammation.
6. List the white blood cells that are involved in acute inflammation and describe how each is involved.
7. Describe the differences between acute and chronic inflammation.
8. Define and contrast hyperplasia, hypertrophy, and atrophy.
9. Describe the microscopic events that occur during mucosal tissue repair
10. Describe the microscopic events that occur during healing in bone.
11. Describe and contrast healing by primary intention, healing by secondary intention, and healing by tertiary intention.
12. List local and systemic factors that can impair healing.
13. Describe and contrast internal and external tooth resorption.
14. Describe and contrast attrition, abrasion, and erosion.
15. Describe the pattern of erosion seen in bulimia.
16. Describe the relationship between bruxism and abrasion.
17. Describe the cause, clinical features, and treatment of each of the following: aspirin and phenol burns, electric burn, traumatic ulcer, frictional keratosis, linea alba, and nicotine stomatitis.
18. Describe the clinical features, cause (when known), treatment, and microscopic appearance of each of the following: traumatic neuroma, postinflammatory melanosis, oral and labial melanotic macule, solar cheilitis, mucocele, ranula, necrotizing sialometaplasia, pyogenic granuloma, peripheral giant cell granuloma, chronic hyperplastic pulpitis, and irritation fibroma.
19. Describe the difference between a mucocele and a ranula.
20. Define sialolithiasis.
21. Describe the difference between acute and chronic sialadenitis.
22. Describe the clinical features, radiographic appearance, and microscopic appearance of a periapical abscess, a periapical granuloma, and a radicular (periapical) cyst.

VOCABULARY

Abscess (ab'ses) A collection of purulent exudate that has accumulated in a cavity formed by the tissue.

Actinic (ak-tin'ic) Relating to or exhibiting chemical changes produced by radiant energy, especially the visible and ultraviolet parts of the spectrum; relating to exposure to the ultraviolet rays of sunlight.

Acute (ah-kūt') A course of disease that is either of short duration or one that is both short and relatively severe.

Angiogenesis (an″je-o-jen'ə-sis) The formation and differentiation of blood vessels.

Atrophy (at'rə-fe) The decrease in size and function of a cell, tissue, organ, or whole body.

Central (sen'trəl) Describes a lesion that is at the center of an involved area; in the context of oral lesions, it indicates that the lesion is within bone.

Chemotaxis (ke″mo-tak'sis) The movement of white blood cells, as directed by biochemical mediators, to an area of injury.

Chronic (kron'ik) Course of disease persisting for a long time.

C-reactive protein A nonspecific protein, produced in the liver, that becomes elevated during episodes of acute inflammation or infection.

Cyst (sist) An abnormal sac or cavity lined by epithelium and surrounded by fibrous connective tissue.

Cytolysis (si-tol'ə-sis) The dissolution or destruction of a cell.

Edema (ə-dē'mə) Excess plasma or exudate in the interstitial space that results in tissue swelling.

Emigration (em″ĭ-gra'shən) The passage of white blood cells through the walls of small blood vessels and into injured tissue.

Epithelialization (ep″ĭ-the″le-əl-ĭ-za'shən) The process of being covered with epithelium.

Erythema (er″ə-the'mə) Redness of the skin or mucosa.

Exudate (eks'u-dāt) Fluid with a high protein content that leaves the microcirculation during an inflammatory response. An exudate consists of serum that contains white blood cells, fibrin, and other protein molecules.

Fever (fe'vər) An elevation of body temperature to greater than the normal level of 37° C (98.6° F).

Fibroplasia (fi″bro-pla'shə) The formation of fibrous tissue, as normally occurs in healing.

Fistula (fis'tu-lə) An abnormal passage that leads from an abscess to the body surface.

Granulation tissue (gran″u-la'shən) The initial connective tissue formed in healing.

Granuloma (gran″u-lo'mə) A collection of macrophages usually surrounded by a rim of lymphocytes.

Hyperemia (hi″pər-e'me-ə) An excess of blood within blood vessels in a part of the body.

Hyperplasia (hi″pər-pla'zhə) An enlargement of a tissue or organ resulting from an increase in the number of normal cells; the result of increased cell division.

Hypertrophy (hi″pər'tro-fe) An enlargement of a tissue or organ resulting from an increase in the size of its individual cells, but not in the number of cells.

Inflammation (in″flə-ma'shən) A nonspecific response to injury that involves the microcirculation and its blood cells.

Leukocytosis (loo″ko-si-to'sis) A temporary increase in the number of white blood cells circulating in blood.

Local (lo'kəl) A disease process that is confined to a limited location in the body; not general or systemic.

Lymphadenopathy (lim-fad″ĕ-no-p'ə-the) Abnormal enlargement of lymph nodes.

Macrophage (mak'ro-fāj) The second type of white blood cell to arrive at a site of injury; it participates in phagocytosis during inflammation and continues to be active in the immune response.

Margination (mahr″jĭ-na'shən) A process during inflammation in which white blood cells tend to move to the periphery of the blood vessel at the site of injury.

Microcirculation (mi″kro-sur″ku-la'shən) Small blood vessels, including arterioles, capillaries, and venules.

Myofibroblast (mi″o-fi′bro-blast) A fibroblast that has some of the characteristics of smooth muscle cells, such as the ability to contract.

Necrosis (nə-kro'sis) The pathologic death of one or more cells, or a portion of tissue, or an organ that results from irreversible damage to cells.

Neutrophil (noo'tro-fil) The first white blood cell to arrive at a site of injury; the primary cell involved in acute inflammation; also called a *polymorphonuclear leuko*cyte.

Opacification (o-pas″ĭ-fĭ-ka'shən) The process of becoming opaque.

Opsonization (op″sə-nĭ-za'shən) The enhancement of phagocytosis by a process in which a pathogen is marked, with opsonins, for destruction by phagocytes.

Pavementing (pāv'mənt-ing) The adherence of white blood cells to blood vessel walls during inflammation.

Peripheral (pə-rif'ər-əl) Located away from the center; in the context of oral lesions, peripheral indicates that the lesion is within the gingival tissue or alveolar mucosa.

Phagocytosis (fag″o-si-to'sis) The ingestion and digestion of particulate material by cells.

Continued

VOCABULARY—cont'd

Purulent (pu'roo-lənt) A secretion containing or forming pus.

Radicular (rə-dik'u-lər) Pertaining to the root of a tooth.

Regeneration (re-jən″ər-a'shən) The process by which injured tissue is replaced with tissue identical to that present before the injury.

Repair (re-pār') The restoration of damaged or diseased tissues by cellular change and growth.

Serous (sēr'əs) A secretion having a watery consistency; relating to serum.

Systemic (sis-tem'ik) Pertaining to or affecting the body as a whole; a disease process pertaining to or affecting the body as a whole.

Transudate (trans'u-dāt) The fluid component of blood that normally passes through the endothelial cell walls of the microcirculation.

Traumatic injury (trə-mat'ik) A disease process that results from injury that causes tissue damage.

Waldeyer's ring The ring of lymphatic tissue formed by the two palatine tonsils, the pharyngeal tonsil, the lingual tonsil, and intervening lymphoid tissue.

Inflammation, immunity, and repair are the body's responses to injury. Inflammation allows the human body to eliminate tissue injured by trauma or infection, to contain injuries, and to begin the process of healing. This chapter begins with a description of the inflammatory response, tissue regeneration, and repair, and continues with a description of oral lesions that occur in response to injury. Many of these lesions are quite common and are likely to be encountered when the dental hygienist examines the hard and soft tissues of the oral cavity. Lesions that occur as a result of destruction through activity of the immune responses are described in Chapter 3. Lesions that occur as a result of infection are included in Chapter 4.

INJURY

Injury is the result of an alteration in the environment that causes tissue damage. Severe injury may result in **necrosis,** the pathologic death of one or more cells or a portion of tissue or an organ that results from irreversible damage to cells. Less severe injury may result in reversible cellular responses such as hyperplasia, hypertrophy, and atrophy, which are described later in this chapter. Injury to oral tissues may have different causes. These include physical injury, chemical injury, infection, and nutritional toxicities and deficiencies. Physical injury can affect teeth, soft tissue, and bone. Chemical injury can occur from the application of caustic substances to oral tissues. Microorganisms can cause injury by invading orofacial tissues. causing infections. Nutritional deficiencies can render oral tissues more susceptible to injury from other sources, and overdoses of some nutrients can cause tissue damage.

INNATE DEFENSES

The body has a number of innate defenses to protect against injury. These are inborn defenses that are present from birth. Intact skin or mucosa acts as a physical barrier to injury. Cilia and mucus in the respiratory system serve as a mechanical defense system. Stomach acid kills most of the microorganisms that are taken into the body through the mouth. The flushing action of tears, saliva, urine, and diarrhea also removes foreign substances. Components of saliva and tears have antimicrobial activity. The resident microflora on skin and mucosa prevents colonization by pathogenic bacteria. The process of inflammation and its white blood cells that are brought to the area of injury are innate or inborn responses to injury.

INFLAMMATION

Inflammation is a nonspecific response to injury and occurs in the same manner, regardless of the nature of the injury. The extent and duration of the injury determine the extent and duration of the inflammatory response. The inflammatory response may be **local** and limited to the area of injury, or it may become **systemic** if the injury is extensive. Inflammation of a specific tissue is denoted by the suffix -itis combined with the name of the tissue, such as in *tonsillitis, pulpitis,* and *gingivitis.*

The inflammatory response may be **acute** or **chronic.** If the injury is minimal and brief and its source is removed from the tissue, it is considered **acute** and the duration of the acute inflammatory response is short, lasting only a few days. The tissue may return to its original state (regeneration), or repair of the tissue may begin immediately. If injury to the tissue continues and the inflammatory response is longer lasting, it is referred to as **chronic inflammation.** Thus, chronic inflammation may last weeks, months, or even indefinitely. The inflammatory response is a dynamic process, continually changing in response to injury and repair.

Thus transitional stages exist during which the response is changing from one type of inflammation to the next and from an innate inflammatory response to an immune response (see Chapter 3). In addition, an acute inflammatory response may be superimposed over a chronic inflammatory response. On occasion, an overwhelming inflammatory response may lead to further injury. Repair of the tissue occurs only if the persistent source of injury is removed.

Current research is demonstrating that chronic inflammation is a major component of the pathogenesis of common disorders such as atherosclerosis, insulin resistance, colon cancer, and Alzheimer's disease.

MICROSCOPIC EVENTS OF INFLAMMATION AND CLINICAL SIGNS

Microscopic events occur within the injured tissues during both acute and chronic inflammation. These events cause changes that can be observed clinically. The local clinical changes at the site of injury are called the classic (cardinal) signs of inflammation: redness, heat, swelling, pain, and loss of normal tissue function (Table 2-1). In addition, systemic signs of inflammation may be present when the response is more extensive; these signs are discussed later in this chapter.

The microscopic events of inflammation involve the small blood vessels or **microcirculation.** These include arterioles, capillaries, and venules in the area of injury as well as red blood cells, white blood cells, and chemicals in the body called biochemical mediators (Figure 2-1). Normally, blood, and the cells it contains, flows through the microcirculation. Exchange of oxygen and nutrients needed for the health of the surrounding tissue occurs as plasma fluid passes between the endothelium lining the vessel walls of the arterioles and capillaries. Plasma is the fluid component of blood in which the blood cells are suspended; it is composed mainly of water and proteins. Normally most of the plasma that leaves the microcirculation reenters the circulation through the venules. The lymphatic vessels carry away any excess plasma that does not reenter the blood vessels.

During inflammation these normal events undergo a change, with underlying microscopic events proceeding faster than the visible clinical changes. The sequence of events is shown in Box 2-1.

The first microscopic event of the inflammatory response is a brief, immediate reflex constriction of the microcirculation in the area of the injury. This is followed, within seconds, by a dilation of the same small blood vessels. *Dilation* is an increase in the diameter of the vessels and is caused by biochemical mediators that are released at the time of the injury. Dilation of the microcirculation results in increased blood flow through the vessels. The increased blood flow that fills the capillary beds in the injured tissue is called **hyperemia.** Hyperemia is responsible for two clinical signs of inflammation: **erythema** and heat. Erythema, or redness, is easily visible in most inflamed orofacial tissues. However, local temperature changes may be more difficult to recognize.

While hyperemia is occurring, the permeability of the vessels of the microcirculation also increases; the blood vessels become "leaky." The endothelial cells contract and spaces form between the cells. As a result, plasma fluid with a low protein content that contains no cells passes between the endothelial cells and enters the tissue. This fluid is called a **transudate** and is the same type of fluid that normally moves from the microcirculation to the tissues to supply oxygen and nutrients. The loss of fluid within the microcirculation leads to increased blood viscosity. The blood becomes thicker and cannot flow as easily. This eventually results in decreased flow through the microcirculation. As the blood flow slows down, the red blood cells begin to pile up in the center of the blood vessels, and the white blood cells are displaced to the periphery of the blood vessels. This movement of the white blood cells to the periphery is called **margination.** The white blood cells are now in position to adhere themselves to the inner walls of the injured blood vessels, which have become "sticky" because of specific factors on the surfaces of the cells. This lining of the walls by white blood cells is called **pavementing** (Figure 2-2).

After pavementing the vessel walls, the white blood cells begin to escape from the blood vessels, along with more fluid, and enter the injured tissue. This process by which the white blood cells escape from the blood vessels is called **emigration.** Emigration occurs as a result of opening of the cellular junctions of the endothelial cells lining the blood vessels; these cells contract in size in response to biochemical mediators. As the white blood cells (primarily neutrophils) emigrate through the blood vessel walls and surrounding basement membrane, they further increase the permeability of the microcirculation and allow larger molecules and other cells to escape. The fluid that now flows into the injured tissues is called an **exudate.** This fluid contains cells and a higher concentration of protein molecules than in a transudate. The presence of transudate and exudate in the injured tissue helps to dilute injurious agents that may be

TABLE 2-1

Local and Systemic Clinical Signs of Inflammation and Associated Microscopic Events

CLINICAL FEATURE	ASSOCIATED MICROSCOPIC EVENTS
Localized Signs of Inflammation	
Redness (erythema) and heat	Hyperemia resulting from dilation of the microcirculation
Swelling	Permeability of the microcirculation leads to exudate formation in the tissues
Pain	Pressure on nerves by exudate formation and release of biochemical mediators
Loss of normal tissue function	Events associated with swelling and pain
Systemic Signs of Inflammation	
Fever	Production of pyrogens affects the hypothalamus, which influences body temperature
Leukocytosis	An increase in the number of white blood cells circulating in the blood
Lymphadenopathy	Hyperplasia and hypertrophy of lymphocytes
Elevated C-reactive protein	A protein produced in the liver and elevated in the circulating blood when inflammation is present somewhere in the body

FIGURE 2-5 ■ An intraoral abscess has been incised, and a drain (*arrow*) placed to allow the escape of purulent exudate from the tissue. (Courtesy Dr. Sidney Eisig.)

Lysosomes containing lysosomal enzymes

Phagocytosis of bacterium

FIGURE 2-6 ■ Phagocytosis of a foreign substance (bacterium) by a white blood cell. The foreign substance will later be destroyed by digestion within the cell by lysosomal enzymes that are contained within lysosomes.

cause a loss of normal tissue function, another clinical sign of inflammation.

This directed movement of white blood cells toward the site of the injury is called **chemotaxis;** biochemical mediators that enhance this directed movement are *chemotactic factors.* Emigration and chemotaxis of white blood cells to the area of injury allow these cells to be mobilized in the defense against the injury.

At first these cells try to wall off the site of the injury from the surrounding healthy tissue. Later, in the injured tissue, the white blood cells also try to remove foreign substances from the site by ingesting and then digesting them, thus undergoing **phagocytosis** (Figure 2-6). The foreign substances may include pathogenic microorganisms or tissue debris. The presence of these substances interferes with the repair process; therefore they must be removed for the inflammation to resolve and any necessary tissue repair to proceed.

WHITE BLOOD CELLS IN THE INFLAMMATORY RESPONSE

Emigration of white blood cells (leukocytes) from the blood vessels into the site of injury and subsequent chemotaxis and phagocytosis are important components of the process of inflammation. Two types of white blood cells are initially involved in the inflammatory response: (1) **neutrophils** and (2) monocytes circulating in the blood, which become **macrophages** in tissue. Neutrophils are also called **polymorphonuclear leukocytes** because they are the most prevalent of the white blood cells that contain a multilobed nucleus. However, this term also includes other white blood cells; therefore *neutrophil* is a more specific name for this cell. Other cells within the blood and tissue, such as lymphocytes and plasma cells, eosinophils, and mast cells, participate in both inflammatory and immune responses. The immune response and the involvement of these cells are discussed in Chapter 3.

As inflammation begins and continues over the 2 weeks after an injury, changes take place in the relative numbers of white blood cell populations present in the tissue (Figure 2-7).

The neutrophil is the first type of white blood cell to arrive at the site of injury and is the most common inflammatory cell present during acute inflammation (Figure 2-8). The second type of white blood cell to arrive at the site of injury within the tissue is the **macrophage.** This cell, when circulating in the blood, was called a *monocyte.* When it leaves the microcirculation and enters the tissue it becomes a macrophage. As inflammation continues, the number of neutrophils decreases. If the injury persists and chronic inflammation occurs, macrophages, lymphocytes, and plasma cells replace the neutrophils and become the most prevalent white blood cells present in the tissue (Figure 2-9).

NEUTROPHILS

As discussed, the neutrophil is the first type of white blood cell recruited into the area of injury in response to

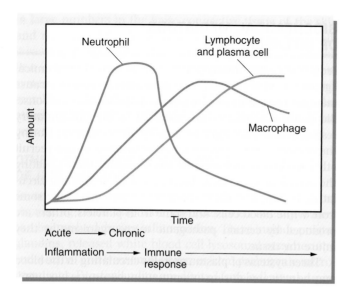

FIGURE 2-7 ■ Changes in the white blood cell population of injured tissue over time, starting with acute inflammation, continuing to chronic inflammation, and extending to the beginning of the immune response.

FIGURE 2-9 ■ Microscopic view of chronic inflammation and the beginning of the immune response, mainly showing macrophages, lymphocytes, and plasma cells (medium magnification).

FIGURE 2-8 ■ Microscopic view of acute inflammation, showing an increase in the number of neutrophils. Macrophages are also present (medium magnification).

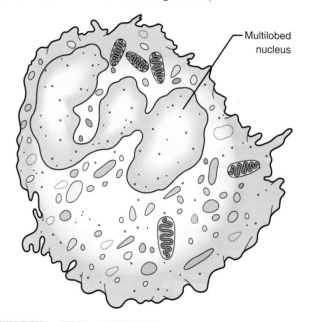

FIGURE 2-10 ■ A neutrophil has a multilobed nucleus and granular cytoplasm.

chemotactic factors. The main function of the neutrophil is phagocytosis of substances such as pathogenic micro-organisms and tissue debris. Microscopically, neutrophils possess a multilobed nucleus, which is why they are called **polymorphonuclear leukocytes,** and a granular cytoplasm that contains **lysosomal enzymes** (Figure 2-10). Lysosomal enzymes contained within vacuoles in the cell cytoplasm destroy substances after the cell has engulfed them. Removal of these substances from the site of injury is necessary to allow the process of repair. Neutrophils die shortly after phagocytosis; as a result, lysosomal enzymes and other damaging cellular substances that were meant only for intracellular destruction of foreign substances are released from the cells. This can cause further tissue damage to the site when large numbers of neutrophils die.

Normally, neutrophils constitute 60 to 70 percent of the entire white blood cell population. Like all white blood cells, neutrophils are derived from stem cells in the bone marrow (Figure 2-11). Stem cells are undifferentiated cells in the spongy tissue that is found in the center of certain long and flat bones, such as the bones of the pelvis and sternum. Neutrophils are produced throughout life and are mobile cells.

MACROPHAGES

The monocyte is the second type of white blood cell to emigrate from the blood vessels into the injured tissue, where it becomes a macrophage. Like neutrophils, monocytes are derived from stem cells in the bone marrow (see Figure 2-11). As a macrophage, it responds to chemotactic factors, diseases that do not allow mobility and thus function of the body ("use it or lose it"). It can also happen with changes in cellular growth, malnutrition, *ischemia* (disruption of blood supply), or hormonal changes.

REGENERATION AND REPAIR

With resolution of the inflammatory response, the injured tissue undergoes healing as either regeneration or repair. When tissue damage has been slight, the inflamed area may return completely to its normal structure and function. This is called **regeneration.** Regeneration is the most favorable resolution of acute inflammation and involves complete removal of all cells, by-products, and inflammatory exudate that entered the tissue during inflammation and return of the microcirculation to its preinflammatory state.

In contrast, the process of repair takes place when complete return of the tissue to normal is not possible because the damage has been too great. Some tissue types such as epithelium, fibrous connective tissue, and bone have the ability to undergo repair. Other tissue types such as enamel do not.

Repair is the final defense mechanism of the body in its attempt to restore injured tissue to its original state. During the repair process cells and tissues that have undergone necrosis are replaced with live cells and new tissue components. However, the repair process cannot be completed until the source of injury is removed or the injurious agents are destroyed. Repair is not always a perfect process. Functioning cells and tissue components are often replaced by nonfunctioning scar tissue. Research studies are currently investigating ways to enhance the repair process.

MICROSCOPIC EVENTS DURING REPAIR

After an injury occurs microscopic events occur in both the epithelium and connective tissue (Figure 2-16). These events are different for each of these tissue types, but occur almost simultaneously and are dependent on each other for optimal healing. If the source of the injury is removed, the repair process for both types of tissues is usually completed within 2 weeks. The repair process is slightly different in the oral cavity than in skin because mucosal tissues are moist and a scab does not form. There are three phases to the repair process that occur during these 2 weeks: (1) inflammation, (2) proliferation, and (3) maturation.

DAY OF INJURY

Immediately after the injury, a clot forms as blood flows into the injured tissue. The clot is produced in the area of injury as a result of activation of the clotting mechanism. The clot consists of a meshwork structure composed of locally produced fibrin, aggregated red blood cells, and platelets. Platelets are cellular fragments found in the blood and are extremely important in the formation of a clot. There are 250,000 to 400,000 platelets/ml³ within the blood. The number of platelets is measured within the panel of the complete blood count (CBC). Hereditary factors, drugs,

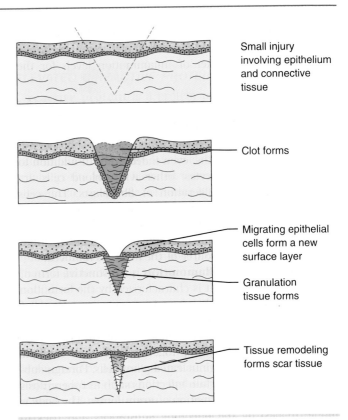

Small injury involving epithelium and connective tissue

Clot forms

Migrating epithelial cells form a new surface layer

Granulation tissue forms

Tissue remodeling forms scar tissue

FIGURE 2-16 ■ Underlying microscopic events of the repair process from the day of injury to 2 weeks later.

extensive injury, or certain diseases may affect red blood cells, platelets, and other factors involved in the formation of the clot and thus prevent or delay tissue repair.

DAY AFTER INJURY

The day after the injury, acute inflammation is taking place in the area of future repair. Neutrophils emigrate from the microcirculation into the injured tissue, and phagocytosis of foreign substances and necrotic tissue with its dead cells occurs as part of the inflammatory response.

TWO DAYS AFTER INJURY

Within 2 days of the injury, monocytes begin to emigrate from the microcirculation into the injured area as macrophages. Macrophages continue phagocytosis in a manner similar to that of the neutrophils. Neutrophils are reduced in number as the chronic inflammatory process proceeds. Fibroblasts proliferate within the injured connective tissue in response to biochemical mediators from macrophages. Fibroblasts become the most important cells during healing as they begin to produce and secrete new collagen fibers, using the fibrinous meshwork of the clot as a scaffold. This process is called **fibroplasia.**

Because an ample blood supply is necessary to sustain new tissue growth, the microcirculation begins to establish itself in the immature connective tissue (type 1 collagen). Macrophages, while removing tissue debris by phagocytosis and promoting fibroblast levels, also secrete growth factors to stimulate the growth of new blood vessels. This process is called **angiogenesis.**

The initial connective tissue formed is called **granulation tissue.** It is an immature tissue, with many more capillaries and fibroblasts than the usual connective tissue so that it clinically appears a vivid pink or red. It consists of immature collagen (type 1 collagen) that is laid down in a haphazard disorganized fashion. In some cases, the growth of this tissue is excessive (exuberant) and may interfere with the repair process until it is removed surgically.

If the surface epithelium has been destroyed by the injury, the epithelial cells create a new surface tissue at the same time that granulation tissue forms in the injured connective tissue. The epithelial cells from the borders of the healing injured area lose their cellular junctions and become mobile. They then divide and migrate across the injured tissue, using the fibrinous meshwork of the clot as a guide to form a new surface layer. This process is called **epithelialization.**

In addition to serving as a guide for migrating epithelial cells and as a scaffold for forming connective tissue, the fibrinous meshwork of the clot serves to protect these two newly formed deeper tissue types from further injury. Thus it is important for the clot to remain in place during this healing time to allow optimal repair in the tissues. In some injuries, dressings placed over the clot may prove beneficial to the healing process (e.g., periodontal pack).

At the end of 2 days, lymphocytes and plasma cells begin to emigrate from the surrounding blood vessels into the injured area as chronic inflammation and an immune response begin. The macrophages already present in the area now assist the lymphocytes in the immune response occurring at the site of injury.

SEVEN DAYS AFTER INJURY

If the source of the injury has been completely removed, the inflammatory and immune responses in the tissue are completed 1 week after the injury. The fibrinous meshwork of the clot is digested by tissue enzymes and sloughs off, and the initial repair of the tissue is completed. Clinically the surface of the repaired injury remains redder than normal because of the thinness of the new surface epithelium and the increased vascularity of the new underlying connective tissue. The immature type of collagen fibers found in granulation tissue is still present and remains fragile and at risk of reinjury. During this time fibroblasts differentiate into **myofibroblasts,** cells that are similar to smooth muscle cells,

and the tissue in the site begins to contract. This contracting peaks 5 to 15 days after the injury and continues until the site is completely reepithelialized.

TWO WEEKS AFTER INJURY

Two weeks after the injury, the initial granulation tissue and its fibers have been remodeled, giving the tissue its full strength. This matured fibrous connective tissue is now called *scar tissue*; it clinically appears whiter or paler at the surface of the repaired injury because of the increased number of collagen fibers and decreased vascularity. A stronger type of collagen (type 3 collagen) has replaced the immature collagen (type 1 collagen) and the collagen overall becomes more organized.

TYPES OF REPAIR

The amount of scar tissue remaining after an injury depends on many factors such as heredity, the strength and flexibility needed in the tissue, the tissue type involved, and the type of repair that has occurred. The oral mucosa is less prone to scar formation than skin. There are three types of repair that can occur: (1) healing by primary intention, (2) healing by secondary intention, and (3) healing by tertiary intention.

HEALING BY PRIMARY INTENTION

Healing by primary intention refers to the healing of an injury in which little loss of tissue takes place, such as in a surgical incision. In this type of healing the clean edges of the incision are joined with sutures to form only a small clot, and very little granulation tissue forms (Figure 2-17). Thus less scar tissue forms, and more normal tissue is retained. The use of sutures is an attempt to try to join the edges of the injury surgically so that healing by primary intention occurs and scarring is minimized.

HEALING BY SECONDARY INTENTION

Healing by secondary intention involves injury in which tissue is lost; thus the edges of the injury cannot be joined during healing. A large clot slowly forms, resulting in increased formation of granulation tissue (Figure 2-18). Healing of a tooth extraction site is an example of healing by secondary intention. After healing, scar tissue increases, and normal tissue function is greatly reduced. This scar

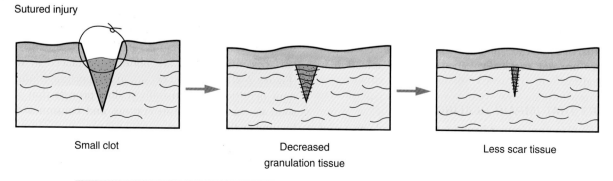

Sutured injury

Small clot

Decreased granulation tissue

Less scar tissue

FIGURE 2-17 ■ Use of sutures to encourage healing by primary intention.

commonly seen on exposed root surfaces because the cementum and dentin are not as hard as enamel; however, abrasion also occurs on enamel surfaces. The process of abrasion is usually slow, and the dentin responds by laying down an inner protective layer of secondary dentin. Therefore pulpal exposure does not usually result.

Abrasion most frequently presents as a notching of the root surface in areas of gingival recession and may occur from an improper toothbrushing technique, most commonly a back-and-forth scrubbing motion using excessive pressure. The use of an abrasive toothpaste or a hard toothbrush may accelerate abrasion (Figure 2-23). However, most dentifrices manufactured in the United States have a very low abrasive index, and toothbrushes with soft bristles are now recommended. Other causes of abrasion include habits such as opening bobby pins with the teeth or holding needles or pins in the teeth. These practices result in a notching of the maxillary incisors. Musicians who play wind instruments may also exhibit forms of abrasion of the teeth in the area of the mouth where the instrument is placed, and pipe smokers may show evidence of abrasion in the area of pipe placement. Abrasion may also result from porcelain crowns, bridges, or denture materials on surfaces of opposing teeth (unrestored, amalgam, resins, etc.) as well as the sand in smokeless tobacco. Abrasion may lead to exposed dentin resulting in hypersensitivity and an increased risk of caries.

The diagnosis of abrasion can often be made by correlating the clinical appearance of the lesions with information gained from questioning the patient about possible factors that may be causing the lesions. The patient should be informed of the cause of the abrasion, and corrective measures should be taken to prevent further destruction of tooth structure. Restorative dental treatment to repair the defect may be appropriate.

ABFRACTION

Abfraction typically appears as a wedge-shaped defect at the cervical area of teeth, especially premolars (Figure 2-24). These lesions occur in adults; the cause is related to microfracture of tooth structure in areas of concentration of stress. This may be related to fatigue, flexure, fracture, and deformation of tooth structure as the result of biomechanical forces on the teeth. The weakened tooth structure is more susceptible to abrasion, particularly toothbrush abrasion. The lesions may be treated with composite or glass ionomer materials, but the forces on the teeth may result in dislodging of the restorations or cause additional damage to the abfracted area. Prevention may involve fabricating an acrylic splint.

EROSION

Erosion is the loss of tooth structure resulting from chemical action without bacterial involvement. The loss may occur on the smooth facial or lingual surfaces of the teeth and on the proximal and occlusal surfaces (Figure 2-25, *A*). The area of erosion appears smooth and polished and is usually extensive, involving several teeth. If erosion occurs in an area where restorations exist, the tooth structure is lost around the restoration, making the restoration appear raised from the surrounding demineralized tooth structure. This phenomenon is not seen in abrasion or attrition because in those cases the restoration is worn down along with the tooth surface.

Erosion may be seen in individuals who work in industries in which acid is used, such as battery manufacturing, plating companies, and soft-drink manufacturing, because the workers breathe the acid in the air. Erosion of teeth associated with intraorally applied cocaine hydrochloride drug abuse has been reported. Because of their low pH, overuse of soft drinks, especially diet formulations, is also strongly implicated in dental erosion and can be noted in some cases of early childhood caries when these drinks are placed in the baby bottle. In addition, erosion of the facial surfaces of the

FIGURE 2-23 ■ Abrasion at the cervical area of mandibular bicuspids caused by toothbrushing.

FIGURE 2-24 ■ Abfraction. (Courtesy Dr. Mark Wolff.)

FIGURE 2-25 ■ **A,** Erosion of buccal and labial surfaces of teeth that occurred as a result of accidental exposure to sulfuric acid. Erosion caused by bulimia: **B,** Decreased tooth size. **C,** Erosion of maxillary lingual surfaces.

teeth may occur as a result of frequent sucking on lemons. Erosion of the lingual surfaces of the teeth may occur as a result of chronic vomiting.

The location of erosion and abrasion cannot reliably identify the cause. The patient's history must be correlated with the location and cause.

Bulimia is an eating disorder characterized by food binges, usually of very high caloric intake, followed by self-induced vomiting. The frequent vomiting in an individual with bulimia results in generalized erosion of the lingual surfaces of teeth (Figure 2-25, *B* and *C*). The dental hygienist may be the first health care professional to identify a patient with bulimia and may assist in encouraging the patient to seek treatment. Bulimia differs from **anorexia nervosa,** another eating disorder, which is characterized by intense fear of gaining weight, and self-imposed starvation. Vomiting after eating is a component of bulimia, but not of anorexia nervosa. The patient with bulimia maintains a normal body weight but is secretive about eating habits. Electrolyte imbalance and signs of malnutrition may be present. Irritation of the oral mucosa and lips may occur,

and there may be traumatic lesions on the back of the fingers caused by their continual use to induce vomiting.

Dental management of patients who vomit frequently includes an effort to minimize the effects of acid on tooth enamel by encouraging the daily use of fluoride rinse and toothpaste containing fluoride. Rinsing the mouth with water after vomiting episodes also lessens the effects of acid. Brushing immediately after vomiting should be avoided and patients with this disorder should be encouraged to use a toothbrush with very soft bristles: the mineralized tooth structure has been affected by acid and the friction of brushing may increase the loss of tooth structure. Patients with severe bulimia–associated erosion may require full-coverage restorative dental treatment for esthetics and function.

Recently, the oral manifestations of **methamphetamine** abuse have been described. The acid content of methamphetamine, decreased salivary flow, and craving for high sugar–containing beverages combined with lack of oral hygiene care results in the extensive and rapid destruction of teeth that is called **"meth mouth"** (Figure 2-26).

HEMATOMA

A **hematoma** is a lesion that results from the accumulation of blood within tissue as a result of trauma. In the oral cavity a hematoma appears as a red to purple to bluish-gray mass and is most frequently seen on the labial or buccal mucosa (Figure 2-29). The size may vary from small to large, depending on the extent of the trauma. The trauma may be due to extensive biting or chewing of the oral tissue, from the administration of a local anesthetic, or surgical trauma. No treatment is required if the lesion is small because the lesion will spontaneously resolve; however, the patient should be advised of its presence. Larger lesions may require pressure on the site and the placement of ice on the site immediately after the trauma.

TRAUMATIC ULCER

A **traumatic ulcer** occurs as a result of some form of trauma (Figure 2-30). Sources of trauma vary. Biting

FIGURE 2-29 ■ Hematoma on the buccal mucosa.

FIGURE 2-30 ■ **A,** Traumatic ulceration caused by irritation of gingiva by fingernails. **B,** Traumatic ulcer caused by denture. **C,** Traumatic ulcer on lateral tongue caused by chronic trauma to tongue by teeth. **D,** Traumatic ulcer (traumatic granuloma) of buccal mucosa.

FIGURE 2-31 ■ Frictional keratosis (indicated by *arrow*) caused by an opposing third molar **(A)**, and chronic tongue chewing **(B). C,** Microscopic appearance of hyperkeratosis (low magnification) showing an increase in surface keratin *(K)*.

the cheek, lip, or tongue may result in a traumatic ulcer, as can irritation from a complete or partial denture or mucosal injury from sharp edges of food. The rapid removal of a dry cotton roll from the oral tissue after a dental procedure can cause a traumatic ulcer, and it is not uncommon to see a patient present for a dental hygiene appointment with a traumatic injury to the gingival tissues or vestibular mucosa that results from overzealous brushing before the appointment.

Traumatic ulcers are usually diagnosed on the basis of the relationship of the history to the lesion. Healing is usually uneventful and occurs in 7 to 14 days unless the trauma persists. If trauma persists, ulcers may last for weeks to months. The patient is monitored until healing is ensured. If an ulcer does not heal in 7 to 14 days, a biopsy is usually indicated to rule out a more serious lesion such as neoplasia. Persistent trauma may result in a hard (indurated), raised lesion called a **traumatic granuloma** (see Figure 2-30, *D*). A traumatic ulcerative granuloma

with stromal eosinophilia (TUGSE) is a type of traumatic ulceration with a unique microscopic appearance. This lesion appears microscopically as an ulcer with an underlying inflammatory infiltrate that contains numerous eosinophils. Persistent traumatic granulomas often heal rapidly after biopsy.

FRICTIONAL KERATOSIS

Chronic rubbing or friction against an oral mucosal surface may result in hyperkeratosis, a thickening of the keratin on the surface. This results in an opaque, white appearance of the tissue and represents a protective response, analogous to a callus on the skin. An example of frictional keratosis is an increase in surface keratin that results from chronic cheek and tongue chewing (Figure 2-31) and chewing on edentulous alveolar ridges. There may be areas of ulceration or hematomas present. Frictional keratosis is not associated with malignancy.

FIGURE 2-32 ■ Linea alba.

FIGURE 2-33 ■ Nicotine stomatitis.

The diagnosis of frictional keratosis is made by identification of the trauma causing the lesion, elimination of the cause, and observing resolution of the lesion. The keratosis may take a while to disappear on keratinized surfaces such as the hard palate and attached gingiva. Those on the buccal mucosa may resolve more rapidly.

Frictional keratosis must be distinguished from other white lesions. White lesions that are not caused by trauma and arise spontaneously are called **leukoplakia** or **idiopathic leukoplakia.** Leukoplakia may be a premalignant lesion (see Chapter 7). Scalpel biopsy is necessary to establish the diagnosis of any white lesion for which a specific cause cannot be identified.

LINEA ALBA

Linea alba is a white raised line that forms most commonly on the buccal mucosa at the occlusal plane (Figure 2-32). In some patients the line becomes prominent as a result of a teeth-clenching habit. The line follows the pattern of the teeth at the level of the occlusal plane. Although it is most commonly seen on the buccal mucosa, linea alba may form on the labial mucosa as well. Microscopically the white raised line is caused by epithelial hyperplasia and hyperkeratosis. No treatment is indicated. The prominence of linea alba may be helpful in evaluating the severity of a clenching habit.

NICOTINE STOMATITIS

Nicotine stomatitis is a benign lesion on the hard palate most typically associated with heavy, long-term pipe and cigar smoking, and is due to the effect of heat on the palatal mucosa; it may also be associated with cigarette smoking The initial response of the palatal mucosa to the heat from these substances is an erythematous appearance, with keratinization and **opacification** increasing over time. After the

increase in keratinization, raised red dots are seen at the openings of the ducts of the minor salivary glands on the palatal surface (Figure 2-33). The minor salivary glands become inflamed as a result of obstruction by keratin at the mucosal opening of the ducts. The palate may develop a very similar clinical appearance as a result of the chronic intake of very hot liquids.

SMOKELESS TOBACCO–ASSOCIATED KERATOSIS

Individuals who use smokeless tobacco in any of its many forms may develop a white lesion, **smokeless tobacco keratosis,** which is also called **tobacco pouch keratosis,** in the area where the tobacco is habitually placed. The mucobuccal fold is the most common location. The epithelium usually has a granular or wrinkled appearance in early lesions. Long-standing lesions may be more opaquely white and have a corrugated surface (Figure 2-34). Microscopically the epithelium may show changes that vary from hyperplasia and hyperkeratosis to atypical premalignant changes that are called **epithelial dysplasia** (see Chapter 7).

The lesion caused by smokeless tobacco often disappears when the tobacco is no longer placed in the area. Long-term exposure to smokeless tobacco has been associated with an increased risk of squamous cell carcinoma. Biopsy and microscopic examination of these lesions is indicated if the habit and lesion persists. In addition, the patient with this habit has an increased risk of caries, periodontal disease, attrition, and staining.

TRAUMATIC NEUROMA

A **traumatic neuroma** is a lesion caused by injury to a peripheral nerve. Nerve tissue is encased in a sheath composed of Schwann cells and their fibers. When this sheath is disrupted, the nerve loses its framework. When a nerve and its sheath are damaged, the proximal end of the damaged nerve proliferates into a mass of nerve and Schwann cells mixed with dense fibrous scar tissue. In the oral cavity injury to a nerve may occur from injection of local anesthesia, surgery, or other sources of trauma.

Traumatic neuromas are often painful. The pain may range from pain on palpation to severe and constant pain. Most traumatic neuromas occur in adults, and the mental foramen is the most common location. However, a traumatic neuroma may occur in other locations as well. Although the clinical features, particularly the pain that is characteristic, may suggest that a lesion is a traumatic neuroma, the diagnosis is made on the basis of a biopsy and microscopic examination. Traumatic neuromas are treated by surgical excision, and recurrence is rare.

The **palisaded encapsulated neuroma (PEN)** is a benign lesion that has microscopic features similar to those of a traumatic neuroma. The PEN presents clinically as a mucosal nodule and has a distinct microscopic appearance. Unlike the traumatic neuroma, which exhibits a proliferation of small nerves, the PEN is a well-circumscribed lesion composed of nerve tissue partially surrounded by fibrous connective tissue. Although the pathogenesis of the PEN is not clear, it has been considered a reactive, hyperplastic lesion. A history of trauma is usually not identified. However, these do not recur even if not completely removed.

AMALGAM TATTOO

An **amalgam tattoo** is a flat, bluish-gray lesion of the oral mucosa that results from the introduction of amalgam into the oral tissues (Figure 2-35, *A*). This may occur at the time of placement or removal of an amalgam restoration or at the time of tooth extraction if fragments of amalgam fracture off a restoration and remain in the tissue. The metallic particles disperse in the connective tissue and result in a permanent area of pigmentation. Over time the mercury-silver-tin amalgam changes, and it is mainly silver that remains in the tissue.

Amalgam tattoos may be seen in any location in the oral cavity but are most commonly found on the gingiva or eden-

FIGURE 2-34 ■ Smokeless tobacco–associated keratosis. Note the rough texture of the surface. **A,** Labial mucosa. **B,** Anterior buccal mucosa.

FIGURE 2-35 ■ **A,** This bluish-gray pigmentation of the gingiva is an amalgam tattoo. **B,** Periapical radiograph showing amalgam particles in the gingival tissue.

tulous alveolar ridge. The posterior region of the mandible is the most common location.

An amalgam tattoo is usually diagnosed on the basis of clinical appearance of the pigmented area. If the amalgam fragments are large enough, they may be seen as radiopacities on a periapical or panoramic radiograph (Figure 2-35, B). As amalgam particles diffuse in the tissue over time, the size of the amalgam tattoo may increase. Biopsy may be necessary to distinguish an amalgam tattoo from a melanocytic lesion, particularly if it is located in an area other than the gingiva or alveolar ridge. Once the diagnosis of amalgam tattoo has been established, treatment is generally not indicated. Surgical removal of the lesion may be considered if there are esthetic concerns.

MELANOSIS

Normal physiologic pigmentation of the oral mucosa is common, particularly in dark-skinned individuals (see Figures 1-18 and 1-51). Melanin pigmentation that occurs after an inflammatory response is called **postinflammatory melanosis** (Figure 2-36, A). The **oral melanotic macule** is a flat, well-circumscribed brown lesion of unknown cause. These are usually small (<1 cm in diameter) and may require biopsy and microscopic examination for diagnosis (Figure 2-36, B). The **labial melanotic macule** is a similar lesion that occurs on the vermilion of the lips. When occurring on the lips, the lesion characteristically darkens with exposure to sunlight.

Another type of melanosis is called **smoker's melanosis** or **smoking-associated melanosis.** In this type of melanosis the melanin pigmentation is associated with smoking, and the intensity is related to the amount and duration of smoking. The pigmentation fades when smoking is discontinued. However, this may take months to years. The anterior labial gingiva is the most commonly affected site. Women are affected more frequently than men. A relationship to female hormones and birth control pills has been suggested. Oral mucosal melanin pigmentation may also be associated with genetic, bone, and systemic diseases.

SOLAR CHEILITIS

Sun exposure, particularly in fair-skinned individuals, can result in degeneration of the tissue of the vermilion of the lips, called **solar** or **actinic cheilitis** (Figure 2-37). The development of this condition is related to the total cumulative exposure to sunlight and the amount of skin pigmentation; it may be seen in individuals of various ages, but usually increases with age. The lower lip is usually more severely involved than the upper lip.

The lips appear dry and cracked. The color of the vermilion of the lips appears pale pink and mottled. The interface between the lips and the skin is indistinct, with fissures appearing at right angles to the skin and vermilion junction. Microscopically, the epithelium is thinner than normal and often exhibits abnormal maturational changes that are called *epithelial dysplasia.* Epithelial dysplasia is described in detail in Chapter 7. Degenerative changes are seen in the connective tissue.

No specific treatment is indicated. However, a strong relationship exists between these epithelial and connective tissue changes and the development of squamous cell carcinoma of the vermilion of the lip. The risk is greater for the lower lip than the upper lip. Smoking and alcohol consumption may increase this risk. Biopsy is indicated for persistent scaling or ulceration. Identification of patients at high risk and with early indications of sun damage can be helpful in preventing future lesions. Patients at risk should be advised to avoid sun exposure, to use sun-blocking agents for protection, and that they are at increased risk for basal cell carcinoma and squamous cell carcinoma of skin.

FIGURE 2-36 ■ **A,** Posttraumatic melanin pigmentation: area of melanin pigmentation on the gingiva after healing of a traumatic injury. **B,** Oral melanotic macules on the buccal mucosa. (**B,** Courtesy Dr. A. Ross Kerr.)

FIGURE 2-37 ■ Solar cheilitis. The color of the vermilion appears mottled and the interface between the vermilion and skin is indistinct.

MUCOUS RETENTION LESIONS

Mucous retention lesions include the mucocele, ranula, and mucous cyst.

A **mucocele** is a lesion that forms when a salivary gland duct is severed and the mucous salivary gland secretion spills into the adjacent connective tissue. An inflammatory response occurs, granulation tissue forms, and the mucus is walled off to form a cystlike structure lined with compressed granulation tissue. This is not a true cyst because the cystic space is not lined with epithelium.

A mucocele presents as a swelling in the tissue that often increases and decreases in size over time. The lower labial mucosa is the most common site of occurrence (Figure 2-38). However, mucoceles may form in any area of the oral mucosa in which minor salivary glands are found. On the lower labial mucosa, they are usually lateral to the midline. If a mucocele is near the surface, it may appear bluish. The color of the mucosa may appear normal if the mucocele is deeper in the tissue. Most mucoceles occur in children and adolescents. However, they may occur in adults as well. Some mucoceles resolve spontaneously with no treatment. If they are chronic or persistent, treatment is by surgical excision with removal of the adjacent minor salivary glands. A mucoepidermoid carcinoma may clinically resemble a mucocele and should be considered in the differential diagnosis for lesions that are indurated or persist.

On occasion, an epithelium-lined cystic structure occurs in association with a salivary gland duct. This is also called a **mucocele, mucous cyst,** or **mucous retention cyst.** These occur much less frequently than the type described previously. They are not true cysts, but are dilated salivary gland ducts that are believed to develop as a result of salivary duct obstruction. A ballooning of the duct occurs, which appears microscopically as an epithelium-lined cystlike structure. Mucous cysts usually occur in adults older

FIGURE 2-38 ■ Mucocele of the lower lip. **A,** Fluid-filled lesion is seen on the lower lip. **B,** Microscopic appearance of a mucocele, showing a cystlike space lined by granulation tissue (low magnification). **(A,** Courtesy Dr. A. Ross Kerr.)

FIGURE 2-39 ■ Ranula.

than 50 years of age. They may occur anywhere in the oral cavity where minor salivary glands are found and are treated by removal of the affected minor salivary glands.

Ranula is a term used for a larger mucocele-like lesion that forms unilaterally on the floor of the mouth ((Figure 2-39). The ranula may increase in size during meals. It is

FIGURE 2-41 ■ **A,** Occlusal radiograph showing a sialolith *(arrow)* in Wharton's duct. **B,** A panoramic radiograph showing a sialolith *(arrow).* (**A,** Courtesy Dr. Barry Wolinsky. **B,** Courtesy Dr. K.C. Chan.)

FIGURE 2-40 ■ Sialoliths. **A,** Sialolith *(arrow)* in a minor salivary gland on the floor of the mouth. **B,** Microscopic appearance of a sialolith, showing concentric rings.

associated with the ducts of the sublingual and submandibular glands. The name *ranula* is derived from *rana,* the Latin word for frog (the clinical appearance of the ranula resembles the outpouching that occurs under the jaw of the frog when croaking). Obstruction of a salivary duct is considered to be the most likely cause for the development of a ranula. Microscopically, a ranula may resemble either a mucocele or a mucous cyst. Ranulas are treated by surgery; the cause of obstruction, often a salivary gland stone, must be removed.

SIALOLITH

A **sialolith** is a salivary gland stone. Sialoliths occur in both major and minor salivary glands and form by precipitation of calcium salts around a central core (Figure 2-40). When they occur in minor glands, a hard "pea sized" nodule may be palpated in soft tissue (Figure 2-40, *A*). They may cause obstruction of the involved salivary gland. When they occur in the floor of the mouth, they can often be seen as a radiopaque structure on an occlusal or panoramic radiograph (Figure 2-41, *A* and *B*).

FIGURE 2-42 ■ Necrotizing sialometaplasia.

NECROTIZING SIALOMETAPLASIA

Necrotizing sialometaplasia is a benign condition of the salivary glands characterized by moderately painful swelling and ulceration in the affected area (Figure 2-42). It characteristically affects the tissue at the junction of the hard and soft palate and is thought to result from blockage of the blood supply to the area of the lesion, resulting in tissue necrosis.

Microscopically, necrosis of the salivary glands is seen. The salivary gland duct epithelium is replaced by squamous epithelium (metaplasia) and appears microscopically as islands of squamous epithelium deep in the connective tissue. If the duration of the ulcer is prolonged, a biopsy is needed to establish the diagnosis. However, the ulcer heals spontaneously by secondary intention, usually within a few weeks.

SIALADENITIS

Inflammation of salivary gland tissue is called **sialadenitis.** Sialadenitis may be acute or chronic and may be a result of infectious or noninfectious causes. Acute sialadenitis is characterized by an infiltrate of primarily neutrophils, whereas lymphocytes and plasma cells are present in chronic sialadenitis. Sialadenitis may occur as a result of obstruction of a salivary gland caused by constriction of a duct or the presence of a sialolith. Sialadenitis may also be a result of decreased salivary flow. In some cases the cause cannot be identified. Sialadenitis presents as a painful swelling of the involved salivary gland, usually one of the major glands. Diagnosis may require injection of a radiopaque dye into the gland, followed by taking a radiograph of the gland (a sialogram). Antibiotics may be necessary in cases of infection.

REACTIVE CONNECTIVE TISSUE HYPERPLASIA

Reactive connective tissue hyperplasia consists of proliferating, exuberant granulation tissue and hyperplastic fibrous connective tissue. These lesions result from overzealous repair. They may occur as a response to a single event or as a chronic low-grade injury. The reason for the exuberant overgrowth of reparative tissue is not known.

PYOGENIC GRANULOMA

A **pyogenic granuloma** is a commonly occurring intraoral lesion that is characterized by a proliferation of connective tissue containing numerous blood vessels and inflammatory cells that resembles granulation tissue. It occurs as a response to injury. The term *pyogenic granuloma* is a misnomer because the lesion does not produce purulent exudate and is not a true granuloma.

The pyogenic granuloma (Figure 2-43) usually exhibits an ulcerated surface, is soft to palpation, and bleeds easily. It is deep red to purple because of the vascularity of the proliferating tissue. It is generally elevated and may be either sessile or pedunculated. When ulcerated, the fibrin membrane on the surface appears yellowish white. The gingiva is the most common location of occurrence, but the lesion also occurs in other areas such as the lips, tongue, and buccal mucosa. Pyogenic granulomas may vary

FIGURE 2-43 ▪ Pyogenic granuloma.

FIGURE 2-44 ▪ Pyogenic granuloma of pregnancy (pregnancy tumor).

considerably in size, from a few millimeters to several centimeters. They usually develop rapidly and then remain static.

Pyogenic granulomas are most common in teenagers and young adults. They may occur at any age and are more common in women than men. Pyogenic granulomas often occur in pregnant women and have been called **pregnancy tumors** (Figure 2-44). The lesions are microscopically identical to the pyogenic granuloma seen in men and nonpregnant women and may be caused by changing hormonal levels and increased response to oral biofilm. They often regress after delivery. Similar gingival lesions occur during puberty.

The pyogenic granuloma is treated by surgical excision if it does not resolve spontaneously. On occasion, the lesion may recur if the injurious agent (e.g., calculus) remains.

PERIPHERAL GIANT CELL GRANULOMA

A **giant cell granuloma** is a lesion composed of well-vascularized connective tissue with multinucleated giant cells. Red blood cells and chronic inflammatory cells are commonly seen in this lesion. The cause of giant cell granulomas is not clear. They occur only in the jaws, possibly arising from the periodontal ligament or the periosteum, and are thought to be a response to injury. Giant cell granulomas occur both on the gingiva (peripheral giant cell granuloma) and within bone (central giant cell granuloma). The term **peripheral** pertains here to lesions occurring outside the bone, generally on the gingiva or alveolar mucosa, and the term **central** refers to a lesion occurring within the maxilla and mandible. A description of central giant cell granulomas is included in Chapter 8.

The **peripheral giant cell granuloma** always occurs on the gingiva or alveolar process, usually anterior to the molars. It is considered a reactive lesion, usually occurring as a result of local irritating factors such as dental biofilm or calculus, periodontal disease, fracture restorations, ill-fitting dental appliances, or dental extractions. Peripheral giant cell granulomas associated with dental implants have been reported. The peripheral giant cell granuloma may resemble the pyogenic granuloma in clinical appearance (Figure 2-45). As with the pyogenic granuloma, surface ulceration is often present. Peripheral giant cell granulomas may vary in size from 0.5 to 1.5 cm in diameter and are usually dark red because of the numerous blood vessels and extravasated red blood cells present. The peripheral giant cell granuloma may occur at any age but has been reported to be more frequent in people between 40 and 60 years of age and more common in women than men. Peripheral giant cell granulomas may cause superficial destruction of the alveolar bone and radiographs may show a cupping or saucerization of bone in the area. They are treated by surgical excision of the lesion and generally do not recur if completely removed.

IRRITATION FIBROMA, FOCAL FIBROUS HYPERPLASIA

The irritation fibroma **(focal fibrous hyperplasia, fibroma, traumatic fibroma)** is a broad-based, persistent exophytic lesion composed of dense, scarlike connective tissue containing few blood vessels (Figure 2-46). It occurs as a result of chronic trauma or an episode of trauma. Many irritation fibromas likely result from fibrosis of a pyogenic granuloma. As in the normal healing process, the granulation tissue that forms the pyogenic granuloma is replaced by mature fibrous connective tissue. The irritation fibroma is usually a small lesion. Most are less than 1 cm in diameter; fibromas greater than 2 cm in diameter are rare. The fibroma occurs most frequently on the buccal mucosa. It also occurs on the gingiva, tongue, lips, and palate. The color of the irritation fibroma is usually lighter than that of the surrounding mucosa because the connective tissue contains so few blood vessels. The surface is covered by

FIGURE 2-45 ■ **A,** Peripheral giant cell granuloma. **B** and **C,** Microscopic appearance of a peripheral giant cell granuloma. Low magnification **(A)** shows the surface epithelium. Higher magnification **(C)** shows multinucleated giant cells *(M)*, capillaries, and fibroblasts.

stratified squamous epithelium and may appear opaque and white if it has a thick keratin surface, or it may be ulcerated because of local secondary trauma.

An irritation fibroma is removed surgically. Many benign soft tissue neoplasms resemble the irritation fibroma in clinical appearance. Excision and microscopic examination

FIGURE 2-47 ■ Denture-induced fibrous hyperplasia (epulis fissuratum; *arrows*). **A,** With denture; **B,** without denture.

FIGURE 2-46 ■ Irritation fibroma. **A,** Development of fibroma followed by the healing of a periodontal abscess. **B,** Irritation fibroma of the buccal mucosa. **C,** Microscopic appearance of a fibroma. (**A,** Courtesy Dr. Murray Schwartz.)

of the tissue are important for diagnosis if the clinician is unsure about the nature of the lesion. Irritation fibromas usually do not recur at the same site, but additional lesions may occur as a response to additional trauma.

The **peripheral ossifying fibroma** is a common exophytic gingival lesion that can clinically resemble an irritation fibroma. The cause is not known. It is thought to originate from the cells forming the periodontal ligament. However, it is not clear whether this lesion is a reactive or neoplastic lesion. The peripheral ossifying fibroma is described in Chapter 7.

DENTURE-INDUCED FIBROUS HYPERPLASIA

Denture-induced fibrous hyperplasia is commonly called **epulis fissuratum** or **denture-associated inflammatory hyperplasia.** This lesion is caused by an ill-fitting denture and is generally located in the vestibule along the denture flange. The lesion is usually somewhat larger than an irritation fibroma. It is arranged in elongated folds of tissue into which the denture flange fits (Figure 2-47). It is composed of dense, fibrous connective tissue surfaced by stratified squamous epithelium, the same type of tissue seen in an irritation fibroma. The surface of the lesion is often ulcerated. Because this lesion does not resolve even with prolonged removal of the denture, treatment involves surgical removal of the excess tissue, relining of the prosthesis, and possibly construction of a new denture.

INFLAMMATORY PAPILLARY HYPERPLASIA OF THE PALATE

Papillary hyperplasia of the palate, or **palatal papillomatosis,** is a form of denture-induced hyperplasia. It is also considered a form of denture stomatitis. It is almost always associated with a maxillary removable full or partial denture or an orthodontic appliance. The palatal mucosa, most commonly the vault area, is covered by multiple erythematous papillary projections that give the area a granular or "cobblestone" appearance (Figure 2-48).

Each of the papillary projections consists of fibrous connective tissue, usually chronically inflamed and surfaced by stratified squamous epithelium. The erythematous appearance is generally due to a superficial infection with the fungus *Candida albicans*. Oral mucosal infections with this fungus are described in Chapter 4. The precise cause of this type of hyperplasia is not known. It is usually related to an ill-fitting upper denture or other removable prosthetic device that is worn continuously, 24 hours a day. Surgical removal of the hyperplastic papillary tissue may be necessary before construction of a new denture.

GINGIVAL ENLARGEMENT

Gingival enlargement is characterized by an increase in the size of the marginal and attached gingiva usually involving the interdental papillae (Figure 2-49). No stippling is seen, and the gingival margins are bulbous and rounded. The tissue consistency may vary from soft to firm, and the appearance may vary from erythematous to a normal pink color, depending on the degree of inflammation and vascularity. Gingival enlargement may be generalized or localized and may vary from mild focal enlargement of interdental papillae to severe generalized gingival enlargement that may cover the crowns of the teeth. Although generally considered to be **gingival hyperplasia,** enlargement of the gingiva may also be the result of hypertrophy.

Most cases are the result of an unusual tissue response to chronic inflammation associated with local irritants such as dental biofilm or calculus. Hormonal changes such as those occurring in pregnancy and puberty and certain drugs such as phenytoin, calcium channel blockers, and cyclosporine can increase the tissue response to local

FIGURE 2-48 ■ Papillary hyperplasia of the palate. **A,** Full denture. **B,** Partial denture. (Courtesy Dr. Edward V. Zegarelli.)

FIGURE 2-49 ■ Gingival enlargement. **A,** Fibrous. **B,** Inflamed.

factors. Hereditary forms of gingival fibromatosis occur, beginning in early childhood. In some cases the cause of gingival enlargement cannot be identified. Gingival enlargement may occur in some patients with leukemia because of an infiltration of abnormal white blood cells into the gingival tissue. If the tissue is inflamed and bleeds easily, laboratory testing may be appropriate to rule out the gingival enlargement that may occur with leukemia.

Gingivoplasty (reshaping the gingiva) or *gingivectomy* (removing gingival tissue) may be necessary to recontour the gingival tissue and may have to be done periodically if the cause cannot be eliminated and gingival enlargement persists. Meticulous oral hygiene is helpful in reducing enlargement.

CHRONIC HYPERPLASTIC PULPITIS

Chronic hyperplastic pulpitis, or **pulp polyp,** is an excessive proliferation of chronically inflamed dental pulp tissue. In children and young adults it occurs in teeth with large, open carious lesions; both primary and permanent molars may be affected. Chronic hyperplastic pulpitis appears as a red or pink nodule of tissue that often fills the entire cavity in the tooth, with tissue protruding from the pulp chamber (Figure 2-50). It is usually asymptomatic; because the hyperplastic tissue contains so few nerves, it is usually insensitive to manipulation. The proliferation of pulp tissue rather than pulpal necrosis, which can also result from caries, may be related to the large root opening and blood supply of the tooth involved.

The hyperplastic tissue consists of granulation tissue with inflammatory cells, primarily lymphocytes and plasma cells. Neutrophils may also be present. The tissue is generally surfaced by stratified squamous epithelium. Because no

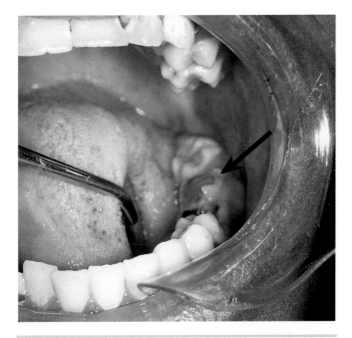

FIGURE 2-50 ■ Chronic hyperplastic pulpitis (pulp polyp) *(arrow).*

epithelium exists in normal pulp tissue, this epithelium is thought to result from desquamation of the surface oral mucosa. Chronic hyperplastic pulpitis is treated by either extraction or endodontic treatment of the involved tooth.

INFLAMMATORY PERIAPICAL LESIONS

Caries or traumatic injury to a tooth may result in a variety of responses: inflammation, infection, chronic hyperplastic pulpitis, and necrosis of the dental pulp. The inflammatory process begins in the dental pulp and then extends into the periapical area, which is the area surrounding the apical portion of the tooth root at the site of the apical foramen. This condition occurs because, once the inflammatory process has been established in the dental pulp, the only route it can follow is through the root canal into the periapical area. The presence of accessory (lateral) canals may lead to areas of inflammation located on the lateral portion of the tooth root.

PERIAPICAL ABSCESS

An acute **periapical abscess** is composed of a purulent exudate (pus or suppuration), surrounded by connective tissue containing neutrophils and lymphocytes. The patient complains of severe pain, which is the result of inflammation. The inflammatory exudate puts pressure on nerves, and chemical mediators can also cause pain. The periapical abscess may develop directly from the inflammation in the pulp, or develop in an area of previously existing chronic inflammation. The purulent exudate seeks a path of least resistance and finds either a channel or a fistula (fistulous tract) out of the tissue, or it spreads to contiguous areas through oral and facial tissue spaces (see Figure 2-3). The tooth associated with the abscess is usually quite painful and may be slightly extruded from its socket. If the acute abscess develops directly from pulpal inflammation, there may initially be no radiographic changes except for a slight thickening of the apical periodontal ligament space. If the abscess develops in a preexisting area of periapical chronic inflammation, a distinct radiolucent area is seen at the apex. The tooth may or may not test positive by electric pulp testing with a vitalometer.

The clinician treats a periapical abscess by establishing drainage, by opening the pulp chamber or by extracting the tooth. If the abscess has extended into adjacent tissue, an incision may be necessary to establish drainage. In some cases, the tooth is extracted. The patient may also be given antibiotic therapy.

PERIAPICAL GRANULOMA

A periapical granuloma, dental granuloma, or **chronic apical periodontitis** is a localized mass of chronically inflamed granulation tissue that forms at the opening of the pulp canal, generally at the apex of a nonvital tooth root (Figure 2-51). This is a chronic process from the outset and

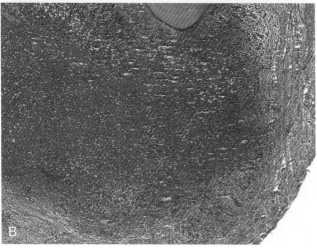

FIGURE 2-51 ■ **A,** Radiograph of a periapical granuloma. **B,** Microscopic appearance of a periapical granuloma, showing a collection of inflammatory cells at the apex of a tooth (low magnification). (**A,** Courtesy Dr. Herbert Frommer.)

most cases are completely asymptomatic. In some cases, the tooth is sensitive to pressure and percussion because of the inflammation in the apical area. The tooth may also appear slightly extruded from its socket. The radiographic change may vary from a slight thickening of the periodontal ligament space in the area of inflammation to a diffuse radiolucency to a distinct, well-circumscribed radiolucency surrounding the root apex.

The periapical granuloma is composed of granulation tissue containing lymphocytes, plasma cells, and macrophages. Neutrophils may also be present, and areas of dense fibrous connective tissue are often seen. The periapical granuloma differs from granulomatous inflammation, which is a distinctive type of inflammation characteristic of certain diseases (e.g., tuberculosis). Epithelial rests of Malassez, which are remnants of tooth-forming tissue of the Hertwig epithelial root sheath, are often present in the periapical granuloma. The periapical granuloma is treated by endodontic therapy (root canal therapy) or extraction of the tooth.

RADICULAR CYST (PERIAPICAL CYST)

A **radicular cyst,** or **periapical cyst,** is a true cyst consisting of a pathologic cavity lined by epithelium. It occurs in association with the root of a nonvital tooth (Figure 2-52). A true cyst is an abnormal closed, epithelium-lined cavity in the body. The radicular cyst is the most commonly occurring cyst in the oral region. The epithelial lining of the cyst develops in a periapical granuloma as a result of proliferation of the epithelial rests of Malassez, remnants of the Hertwig epithelial root sheath after tooth development.

A radicular cyst develops when the epithelium within the inflamed connective tissue of the periapical granuloma proliferates, forming an epithelial mass that increases in size through division of the peripheral cells. The peripheral cells are the equivalent of the basal cell layer of the epithelium. As the cells in the central portion of the mass become increasingly separated from the source of nutrition in the connective tissue, they undergo necrosis centrally, forming a cavity that is lined by epithelium and filled with fluid. Microscopically, the tissue surrounding this epithelium-lined cystic cavity is similar to that seen in the periapical granuloma.

Most radicular cysts are asymptomatic and discovered on radiographic examination. The radiographic appearance of the radicular cyst is the same as that of the periapical granuloma. It appears as a radiolucency, usually well circumscribed, that surrounds the apex of a tooth root. It is not possible to differentiate reliably a periapical granuloma from a radicular cyst on the basis of the radiographic appearance alone. A radicular cyst may form in association with any tooth. The cyst may occur lateral to the tooth root rather than at the apex if it is associated with a lateral pulp canal. Other types of cysts can resemble a radicular cyst radiographically; therefore removal of the cyst and microscopic examination of the tissue are necessary.

The radicular cyst is treated by endodontic therapy (root canal therapy), apicoectomy, or extraction and curettage of the periapical tissues. A **residual cyst** forms when the tooth is removed and all or part of a radicular cyst is left behind (Figure 2-53). Radiographically, a residual cyst is a well-circumscribed radiolucency located at the site of tooth extraction. It is treated by surgical removal of the cyst.

TOOTH RESORPTION

Tooth structure can be resorbed in the same manner as bone. This occurs normally in the process of exfoliation of deciduous teeth and may also occur in other situations. Resorption of the tooth structure beginning at the outside of the tooth is called *external resorption.* This usually involves the root of a tooth but can occasionally involve the crown of an impacted tooth.

Like bone resorption, tooth resorption can occur when inflammatory tissue is present. Resorption of the root of a tooth can occur when a periapical granuloma is present. Bone resorption as a response to pressure allows orthodontic tooth movement to occur. Pressure can also cause

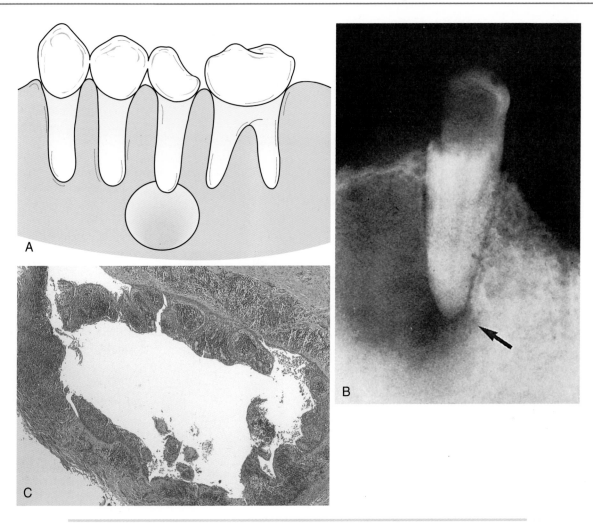

FIGURE 2-52 ■ Radicular cyst. **A,** Diagram of a radicular cyst located around the root of an erupted tooth. **B,** Radiograph showing a well-circumscribed radiolucency *(arrow)* around the root of a tooth. **C,** Microscopic features of a radicular cyst.

resorption of tooth structure. This can occur from excessive occlusal or orthodontic forces and with benign and malignant neoplasms. When a tooth that has been avulsed is reimplanted, the root is usually resorbed and then replaced by bone. External root resorption first appears as a slight raggedness or blunting of the root apex and can proceed to severe loss of tooth substance (Figure 2-54). The condition is not reversible, but progression of the process can be avoided if the cause can be identified and removed. Resorption of impacted teeth can also occur. Generalized root resorption may also occur after orthodontic tooth movement and root resorption may be associated with certain neoplasms of the jaws (see Chapter 7). On occasion, resorption may involve the crown of an impacted tooth or the roots of teeth, and the cause cannot be identified. This is called **idiopathic tooth resorption.**

Internal tooth resorption (see Chapter 1, Figure 1-26) can occur in any tooth. Usually only a single tooth is involved. In some cases no cause can be identified. However, it is usually associated with an inflammatory response in the pulp. If the process occurs in the coronal part of the tooth, it may be seen clinically as a pinkish area in the crown. The

dental hard tissue has resorbed and is thinner than normal, and the pink color results from the vascular, inflamed connective tissue that can be seen through the remaining enamel and dentin. When the process involves the root, it can be seen only radiographically. A round-to-ovoid radiolucent area associated with the pulp is seen in the central portion of the tooth.

Endodontic therapy can be performed successfully if internal resorption is discovered early. If not treated, the process can extend through the dental hard tissue and cause a perforation. After this perforation occurs, the tooth must be extracted.

FOCAL SCLEROSING OSTEOMYELITIS

Focal sclerosing osteomyelitis, also called **condensing osteitis,** is a change in bone near the apices of teeth that may be a reaction to low-grade infection. The tooth most commonly associated with focal sclerosing osteomyelitis is the mandibular first molar. On occasion, the mandibular second molar and the mandibular premolars may also be involved.

FIGURE 2-53 ■ **A,** Diagram of a residual cyst. **B,** Radiograph of a residual cyst, showing radiolucency at the site of a previously extracted tooth. (Courtesy Drs. Paul Freedman and Stanley Kerpel.)

Radiographically, focal sclerosing osteomyelitis appears as a radiopaque area in the periapical area of teeth (Figure 2-55). The borders may be diffuse or well defined. On occasion, the periphery of the area is radiolucent; in other cases a central radiolucency surrounded by radiopacity is seen. Microscopically, it is dense bone with little marrow or connective tissue, and little inflammation is present. Focal sclerosing osteomyelitis is often associated with a carious or restored tooth. It is generally asymptomatic. However, pain may be associated if pulpal inflammatory disease is present. Focal sclerosing osteomyelitis may be present at any age, but it is usually first seen in young adults.

Diagnosis of focal sclerosing osteomyelitis usually can be made on the basis of the characteristic radiographic appearance. Idiopathic osteosclerosis can appear radiographically similar to sclerosing osteomyelitis. This lesion is not associated with inflammation and, as with sclerosing osteomyelitis, generally does not require biopsy and microscopic examination for diagnosis. Idiopathic osteosclerosis is described in Chapter 8. On occasion, biopsy may be necessary to rule out other radiopaque lesions such as osteoma, complex odontoma, or central ossifying fibroma. Treatment of

FIGURE 2-54 ■ Tooth resorption. **A,** Root resorption of a mandibular anterior tooth associated with chronic inflammation. **B,** Resorption of tooth structure and bone because of chronic inflammation. **C,** Idiopathic resorption of an impacted tooth. **D,** Generalized root resorption associated with orthodontic tooth movement. (**A,** Courtesy Dr. Gerald P. Curatola.)

sclerosing osteomyelitis is not necessary. The sclerotic bone remains even after treatment of the involved tooth.

ALVEOLAR OSTEITIS

Alveolar osteitis or **"dry socket"** is a postoperative complication of tooth extraction. The most frequently affected

FIGURE 2-55 ■ Focal sclerosing osteomyelitis (condensing osteitis).

area is the socket of an extracted mandibular third molar. After the extraction of the tooth, the blood clot is lost before healing has taken place. Pain develops several days after the extraction. On examination the tooth socket appears empty, and the bone surfaces are exposed. The patient complains of pain, bad odor, and bad taste. Because no infection exists, fever, swelling, and erythema are not present. Risk factors for the development of alveolar osteitis include a dissolution of the clot at the surgical site, traumatic extraction, the presence of infection prior to the extraction, and tobacco smoking after the extraction. Treatment of alveolar osteitis is directed at relief of pain and includes gentle irrigation and insertion of a medicated dressing.

SELECTED REFERENCES

Books

Cawson RA: *Essentials of oral pathology and oral medicine,* ed 8, Philadelphia, Churchill Livingstone, 2008.

Bath-Balogh M, Fehrenbach MJ: *Illustrated dental embryology, histology, and anatomy,* ed 3, St. Louis, 2011, Saunders.

Fehrenbach MJ, Herring SW: *Illustrated anatomy of the head and neck,* ed 4, St. Louis, 2012, Saunders.

Fehrenbach MJ, Weiner J: *Saunders review of dental hygiene,* ed 2, St. Louis, 2009, Saunders.

Kumar V, Cotran RS, Robbins SL: *Robbins basic pathology,* ed 9, Philadelphia, 2013, Saunders.

McCance K, Huether S: *Pathophysiology,* ed 6, St. Louis, 2010, Mosby.

Nelson S: *Wheeler's dental anatomy, physiology, and occlusions,* ed 9, Philadelphia, 2010, Saunders.

Neville BW, Damm DD, Allen CM, et al: *Oral and maxillofacial pathology,* ed 3, St. Louis, 2009, Saunders.

Regezi JA, Sciubba JJ, Jordan R: *Oral pathology: clinical-pathologic correlations,* ed 6, St. Louis, 2012, Saunders.

Journal Articles
Inflammation and Repair

Broughton G II, Janis JE, Attinger CE: Wound healing: an overview, *Plast Reconstr Surg* 117(7 Suppl):S1e, 2006.

Eming SA, Krieg T, Davidson JM: Inflammation in wound repair: molecular and cellular mechanisms, *J Invest Dermatol* 127:514, 2007.

Kobayashi SD, Voyich JM, Burlak C, et al: Neutrophils in the innate immune response, *Arch Immunol Ther Exp (Warsz)* 53:505, 2005.

Krishnamoorthy S, Honn KV: Inflammation and disease progression, *Cancer Metastasis Rev* 25:481, 2006.

Krishnaswamy G, Ajitawi O, Chi DS: The human mast cell: an overview, *Methods Mol Biol* 315:13, 2006.

Moore K: An anatomy of an infection: overview of the infectious process, *Crit Care Nurs Clin North Am* 19:9, 2007.

Rankin JA: Biological mediators of acute inflammation, *AACN Clin Issues* 15:3, 2004.

Semiali A, Chakir J, Goulet JP, et al: Whole cigarette smoke promotes human gingival epithelial cell apoptosis and inhibits cell repair processes, *J Periodontal Res* 46:533, 2011.

Lesions from Physical and Chemical Injuries to the Oral Tissues

Bouquot JE, Seime RJ: Bulimia nervosa: dental perspectives, *Pract Periodontics Aesthet Dent* 9:655, 1997.

Ferguson MM, Dunbar RJ, Smith JA, et al: Enamel erosion related to winemaking, *Occup Med* 46:159, 1996.

Gandara BK, Truelove EL: Diagnosis and management of dental erosion, *J Contemp Dent Pract* 1:16, 1999.

Geurtsen W: Rapid general dental erosion by gas-chlorinated swimming pool water: review of the literature and case report, *Am J Dent* 13:291, 2000.

Grippo JO, Simring M, Coleman TA: Abfraction, abrasion, biocorrosion, and the enigma of noncarious cervical lesions: a 20-year perspective, *J Esthet Restor Dent* 24:10, 2012.

Hague AL: Eating disorders: screening in the dental office, *J Am Dent Assoc* 141:675, 2010.

Hanamura H, Houston F, Rylander H, et al: Periodontal status and bruxism: a comparative study of patients with periodontal disease and occlusal parafunctions, *J Periodontol* 58:173, 1987.

Harpenau LA, Noble WH, Kao RT: Diagnosis and management of dental wear, *J Calif Dent Assoc* 39:225, 2011.

Imbery TA, Edwards P: Necrotizing sialometaplasia: literature review and case reports, *J Am Dent Assoc* 127:1087, 1996.

Järvinen V, Meurman JH, Hwärinen H, et al: Dental erosion and upper gastrointestinal disorders, *Oral Surg Oral Med Oral Pathol* 65:298, 1988.

Kapila YL, Kashani H: Cocaine-associated rapid gingival recession and dental erosion: a case report, *J Periodontol* 68:485, 1997.

Lineberry TW, Bostwick JM: Methamphetamine abuse: a perfect storm of complications, *Mayo Clin Proc* 81:77, 2006.

Little JW: Eating disorders: dental implications, *Oral Surg Oral Med Oral Pathol Oral Radiol Endod* 93:138, 2002.

Maron FS: Enamel erosion resulting from hydrochloric acid tablets, *J Am Dent Assoc* 127:781, 1996.

Mitchell-Lewis DA, Phelan JA, Kelly RB, et al: Identifying oral lesions associated with crack cocaine use, *J Am Dent Assoc* 125:1104, 1994.

Owens BM, Johnson WW, Schuman NJ: Oral amalgam pigmentation (tattoos): a retrospective study, *Quintessence Int* 23:805, 1992.

Owens BM, Schuman NJ, Johnson WW: Oral amalgam tattoos: a diagnostic study, *Compendium* 14:210, 1993.

Ozelik O, Haytac MC, Akkaya M: Iatrogenic trauma to oral tissues, *J Periodontol* 76:1793, 2005.

Piotrowski BT, Gillette WB, Handcock EB: Examining the prevalence and characteristics of abfraction-like cervical lesions in a population of US veterans, *J Am Dent Assoc* 132:1694, 2001.

Pullinger AG, Seligman DA: The degree to which attrition characterizes differentiated patient groups of temporomandibular disorders, *J Orofac Pain* 7:196, 1990.

Rawlinson A: Case report: labial cervical abrasion caused by misuse of dental floss, *Dent Health (London)* 26:3, 1987.

Roberts MW, Li SH: Oral findings in anorexia nervosa and bulimia nervosa: a study of 47 cases, *J Am Dent Assoc* 115:497, 1987.

Rossie KM, Guggenheimer J: Thermally induced "nicotine" stomatitis: a case report, *Oral Surg Oral Med Oral Pathol* 70:597, 1990.

Rugh JD, Harlan J: Nocturnal bruxism and temporomandibular disorders, *Adv Neurol* 49:329, 1988.

Rytömaa I, Järvinen V, Kanerva R, et al: Bulimia and tooth erosion, *Acta Odontol Scand* 56:36, 1998.

Silvestre FJ, Perez-Herbera Af, Puente-Sandoval A, et al: Hard palate perforation in cocaine abusers: a systematic review, *Clin Oral Investig* 14:621, 2010.

Simmons MS, Thompson DC: Dental erosion secondary to ethanol-induced emesis, *Oral Surg Oral Med Oral Pathol* 64:731, 1987.

Witton R, Brennan PA: Severe tissue damage and neurological deficit following extravasation of sodium hypochlorite solution during routine endodontic treatment, *Br Dent J* 198:749, 2005.

Wray A, McGuirt F: Smokeless tobacco usage associated with oral carcinoma, *Arch Otolaryngol Head Neck Surg* 119:929, 1993.

Zimmers PL, Gobetti JP: Head and neck lesions commonly found in musicians, *J Am Dent Assoc* 125:1487, 1994.

Reactive Connective Tissue Hyperplasia

Bodner L, Peist M, Gatot A, et al: Growth potential of peripheral giant cell granuloma, *Oral Surg Oral Med Oral Pathol Oral Radiol Endod* 83:548, 1997.

Bonetti F, Pelosi G, Martignoni G, et al: Peripheral giant cell granuloma: evidence for osteoclastic differentiation, *Oral Surg Oral Med Oral Pathol* 70:471, 1990.

Brown RS, Sein P, Corio R, et al: Nitrendipine-induced gingival hyperplasia: first case report, *Oral Surg Oral Med Oral Pathol* 70:593, 1990.

Brunet L, Miranda J, Roset P, et al: Prevalence and risk of gingival enlargement in patients treated with anticonvulsant drugs, *Eur J Clin Invest* 31:781, 2001.

Cloutier M, Charles M, Carmichael RP, et al: An analysis of peripheral giant cell granuloma associated with dental implant treatment, *Oral Surg Oral Med Oral Pathol Oral Radiol Endod* 103:618, 2007.

Daley T, Wysocki G, Day C: Clinical and pharmacologic correlations in cyclosporine-induced gingival hyperplasia, *Oral Surg Oral Med Oral Pathol* 62:417, 1986.

Daley TD, Nartey NO, Wysocki GP: Pregnancy tumor: an analysis, *Oral Surg Oral Med Oral Pathol* 72:196, 1991.

Fay AA, Satheesh K, Gapski R: Felodipine-influenced gingival enlargement in an uncontrolled type 2 diabetic patient, *J Periodontol* 76:1217, 2005.

Gould A, Escobar V: Symmetrical gingival fibromatosis, *Oral Surg Oral Med Oral Pathol* 51:62, 1981.

Koutlas IG, Scheithauer BW: Palisaded encapsulated ("solitary circumscribed") neuroma of the oral cavity: a review of 55 cases, *Head and Neck Pathol* 4:15, 2010.

Miranda J, Brunet L, Roset P, et al: Prevalence and risk of gingival enlargement in patients treated with nifedipine, *J Periodontol* 72:605, 2001.

Proia NK, Paszkiewicz GM, Nasca MA, et al: Smoking and smokeless tobacco-associated human buccal cell mutations and their association with oral cancer—a review, *Cancer Epidemiol Biomarkers Prev* 15:1061, 2006.

Roberson JB, Crocker DJ, Schiller T: The diagnosis and treatment of central giant cell granuloma, *J Am Dent Assoc* 128:81, 1997.

Silverstein LH, Burton CH Jr, Garnick JJ, et al: The late development of oral pyogenic granuloma as a complication of pregnancy: a case report, *Compendium* 17:192, 1996.

Zain RB, Fei YJ: Fibrous lesions of the gingiva: a histopathologic analysis of 204 cases, *Oral Surg Oral Med Oral Pathol* 70:466, 1990.

Inflammatory Periapical Lesions

Gunraj MN: Dental root resorption, *Oral Surg Oral Med Oral Pathol Oral Radiol Endod* 88:647, 1999.

Halabi D, Escobar J, Muñoz C, et al: Logistic regression analysis of risk factors for the development of alveolar osteitis, *J Oral Maxillofac Surg* 70:1040, 2012.

Harris EF, Butler MI: Patterns of incisor root resorption before and after orthodontic correction in cases with anterior open bites, *Am J Orthod Dentofacial Orthop* 101:112, 1992.

Harris EF, Robinson QC, Woods MA: An analysis of causes of apical root resorption in patients not treated orthodontically, *Quintessence Int* 24:417, 1993.

Websites

American Dental Hygienists' Association. Inflammation: the relationship between oral health and systemic disease. Available at http://www.adha.org/CE_courses/course13/indexpg.htm

Estrela C, Aguirre Guedes O, Almeida Silva J, et al: Diagnostic and clinical factors associated with pulpal and periapical pain (in *Brazilian Dental Journal*). Available at http://www.scielo.br/scielo.php?script=sci_arttext&pid=S0103-64402011000400008&lng=en&nrm=iso&tlng=en

Kao RT, Harpenau LA: Dental erosion and tooth wear (in *Journal of the California Dental Association*). Available at http://www.cda.org/library/cda_member/pubs/journal/journal_0411.pdf

Medscape. The biological mechanisms behind injury and inflammation. Available to members at http://www.medscape.com/viewarticle/557490

National Institute of Dental and Craniofacial Research. Dry mouth. Available at http://www.nidcr.nih.gov/OralHealth/Topics/DryMouth/DryMouth.htm

Review Questions

1. Which of the following is the body's initial response to injury?
   A. The immune response
   B. The inflammatory response
   C. Repair
   D. Hyperplasia

2. What type of inflammation occurs if the injury is minimal and brief and the source is removed from the tissue?
   A. Fatal
   B. Acute
   C. Chronic
   D. Life-threatening

3. During the inflammatory response, the first microscopic event is:
   A. Dilation of the microcirculation
   B. Increased permeability of the microcirculation
   C. Formation of exudate
   D. Constriction of the microcirculation

4. Which one of the following conditions is considered a chronic inflammatory lesion?
   A. Necrotizing sialometaplasia
   B. Periapical granuloma
   C. Aphthous ulcer
   D. Aspirin burn

5. The directed movement of white blood cells to the area of injury is called:
   A. Pavementing
   B. Margination
   C. Chemotaxis
   D. Hyperemia

6. Which of the following cells are the most prevalent cells seen in chronic inflammation?
   A. Neutrophils
   B. Macrophages and lymphocytes
   C. Lymphocytes and plasma cells
   D. Neutrophils and lymphocytes

7. The macrophage has many functions. Which of the following is *not* a function of the macrophage?
   A. Phagocytosis
   B. Removal of large foreign matter
   C. Removal of inhaled particles
   D. Formation of antibodies

8. Which of the following is the term used to describe blood plasma with cells and proteins that leaves the blood vessels and enters the surrounding tissues during inflammation?
   A. Hyperemia
   B. Hypertrophy
   C. Margination
   D. Exudate

9. The process of phagocytosis during inflammation directly involves the:
   A. Ingestion of foreign substances by white blood cells
   B. Escape of plasma fluids and proteins from the microcirculation into the surrounding tissues
   C. Displacement of white blood cells to the blood vessel walls
   D. Attachment of white blood cells to the blood vessel walls

10. Which of the following statements is *incorrect* concerning the neutrophil? The neutrophil:
    A. Makes up 30% of white blood cells
    B. Contains lysosomal enzymes
    C. Is a cell whose main function is phagocytosis
    D. Has a multilobed nucleus

11. During the process of inflammation, the second type of white blood cell to emigrate from the blood vessel into the injured tissue is the:
    A. Neutrophil
    B. Red blood cell
    C. Lymphocyte
    D. Macrophage

12. Components of the complement system mediate the inflammatory process by:
    A. Decreasing vascular permeability
    B. Releasing histamine granules from neutrophils
    C. Causing cytolysis of cells
    D. Decreasing phagocytosis

13. Two days after injury, granulation tissue can be described as:
    A. Immature vascular connective tissue
    B. Fluid in the form of exudate
    C. Dense avascular connective tissue
    D. Ulcerated tissue

14. The enlargement of superficial lymph nodes that occurs as a systemic sign of inflammation is:
    A. Called leukocytosis
    B. Regulated by the hypothalamus
    C. Caused by changes in their lymphocytes
    D. A process that involves only the lymph nodes in the submental area

15. Which statement concerning repair in the body is *true*?
    A. Repair can be completed with the injurious agents present.
    B. Functioning cells and tissue components are always replaced by functioning scar tissue.
    C. Repair always results in regeneration.
    D. The process of repair is initiated by the inflammatory response.

Continued

Review Questions—cont'd

16. The clot that forms during repair after injury:
    A. Consists of fibrous connective tissue
    B. Serves as a guide for migrating epithelial cells
    C. Forms after skin injury, but not after mucosal injury
    D. Occurs only with healing by secondary intention

17. Healing by secondary intention refers to healing of an injury when:
    A. The incision has clean edges joined by sutures
    B. Only a small clot forms
    C. An infection forms in the injured area
    D. There is increased formation of granulation tissue

18. Which of the following is the term used to describe an increase in the size of an organ or tissue resulting from an increase in the number of its cells?
    A. Hyperemia
    B. Hyperplasia
    C. Inflammation
    D. Hypertrophy

19. Normal bone tissue repair in the body can be delayed by:
    A. Maintenance of osteoblast-producing tissues
    B. Inadequate movement of bone tissue
    C. Drainage of an area of edema
    D. Reduction in the amount of tissue infection

20. Which one of the following lesions would clinically appear as a pigmented lesion?
    A. Amalgam tattoo
    B. Traumatic ulcer
    C. Frictional keratosis
    D. Aspirin burn

21. Which of the following statements is *false*?
    A. Attrition is the wearing away of tooth structure during mastication.
    B. Bruxism is the same process as mastication.
    C. Erosion is the loss of tooth structure resulting from chemical action.
    D. Abrasion is caused by mechanical, repetitive habits.

22. Loss of tooth structure associated with bulimia is caused by:
    A. Attrition
    B. Erosion
    C. Bruxism
    D. Abrasion

23. An aspirin burn in the oral cavity:
    A. Occurs as a result of an overdose of aspirin
    B. Is usually painless
    C. Results from a misuse of aspirin
    D. Usually takes several weeks to heal

24. A patient has a generalized white appearance of the palate. Tiny erythematous dots can be seen, surrounded by a thickened, raised, white-to-gray area. Overall the palate appears wrinkled. This condition is most likely:
    A. Papillary hyperplasia of the palate
    B. Nicotine stomatitis
    C. An aspirin burn
    D. Necrotizing sialometaplasia

25. Which of the following is the most common cause of a mucocele?
    A. Acute inflammation
    B. Tumor formation
    C. Minor salivary gland duct trauma
    D. A sialolith

26. A ranula is located on the:
    A. Lower lip
    B. Buccal mucosa
    C. Retromolar area
    D. Floor of the mouth

27. Which one of the following lesions would *not* occur on the gingiva?
    A. Irritation fibroma
    B. Pyogenic granuloma
    C. Giant cell granuloma
    D. Epulis fissuratum

28. Generalized loss of tooth structure primarily on the lingual surfaces of maxillary anterior teeth is associated with:
    A. Erosion
    B. Attrition
    C. Abrasion
    D. Abfraction

29. Which of the following may be a cause of external tooth resorption?
    A. Caries
    B. Salivary gland dysfunction
    C. Chronic inflammation
    D. Medication

30. Which one of the following is considered to be the most likely cause of necrotizing sialometaplasia?
    A. Loss of blood supply
    B. Radiation therapy
    C. Smoking
    D. A sialolith

31. The most common site for a mucocele to occur is the:
    A. Floor of the mouth
    B. Tongue
    C. Buccal mucosa
    D. Lower lip

Review Questions—cont'd

32. The peripheral giant cell granuloma occurs only on the:
    A. Gingiva or alveolar mucosa
    B. Hard palate
    C. Buccal mucosa
    D. Floor of the mouth

33. A sialolith is:
    A. Chronic inflammation of a salivary gland
    B. Acute inflammation of a salivary gland
    C. A pooling of saliva in the connective tissue
    D. A salivary gland stone

34. Which of the following statements is *false*?
    A. A periapical cyst develops from a periapical granuloma.
    B. A periapical abscess always causes radiographic periapical changes.
    C. A periapical granuloma is a circumscribed area of chronically inflamed tissue.
    D. A periapical cyst is also called a radicular cyst.

35. Epulis fissuratum results from irritation caused by:
    A. A denture flange
    B. Denture adhesive
    C. Poor suction from the denture in the palatal vault
    D. An allergic reaction to the acrylic in the denture

36. Which of the following statements is *true*?
    A. A traumatic neuroma is never painful.
    B. Necrotizing sialometaplasia is considered a denture-related lesion.
    C. Chronic hyperplastic pulpitis is similar to gingival hyperplasia.
    D. Gingival enlargement may be caused by medication.

37. Loss of tooth structure caused by chemical action describes:
    A. Abrasion
    B. Internal resorption
    C. Erosion
    D. Attrition

38. Which of the following cysts is characteristically associated with a tooth that is nonvital on pulp testing?
    A. Residual
    B. Radicular
    C. Dentigerous
    D. Dermoid

39. Which of the following cysts results when a tooth is extracted without removing the periapical cystic sac?
    A. Radicular
    B. Primordial
    C. Residual
    D. Periodontal

40. The most common cause of a radicular cyst is:
    A. Deep restorations without a base
    B. Caries
    C. Occlusal trauma
    D. Toothbrush abrasion at the cemento-enamel junction

41. The wearing away of tooth structure through an abnormal mechanical action defines:
    A. Attrition
    B. Abrasion
    C. Erosion
    D. Resorption

42. Which one of the following is *not* associated with attrition?
    A. Toothpaste
    B. Bruxism
    C. Mastication
    D. Age

43. Heavy plaque and calculus deposits, mouth breathing, orthodontic appliances, and overhanging restorations best describe some of the causative factors for:
    A. Phenytoin (Dilantin) hyperplasia
    B. A reaction from nifedipine (Procardia)
    C. Irritation fibromatosis
    D. Chemical fibromatosis

44. A pink, granular or "cobblestone"-like appearance of the hard palate under a denture is most likely:
    A. Nicotine stomatitis
    B. Necrotizing sialometaplasia
    C. Papillary hyperplasia of the palate
    D. Multiple fibromas

45. During examination of the dentition, the dental hygienist notes the presence of active wear facets. This indicates that the patient is:
    A. Chewing too vigorously
    B. A bruxer
    C. A vegetarian
    D. Lip biting

46. A patient has a loss of tooth structure on the labial surfaces of the anterior teeth and reports a high intake of citrus fruit juices. The dental hygienist would most likely suspect:
    A. Abrasion
    B. Bulimia
    C. Bruxism
    D. Erosion

Continued

CHAPTER 2 *Synopsis—cont'd*

CONDITION/DISEASE	CAUSE	AGE/RACE/SEX	LOCATION
Traumatic ulcer	Trauma to mucosa	*	Site of trauma
Frictional keratosis	Chronic friction against mucosal surface	*	Site of friction
Linea alba	Teeth clenching/habit	*	Buccal mucosa at occlusal plane
Nicotine stomatitis	Smoking	*	Hard palate
Smokeless tobacco associated keratosis	Chewing tobacco	*	Site where tobacco is habitually placed
Traumatic neuroma	Injury to a peripheral nerve	*	Site of injured nerve
Amalgam tattoo	Particles of amalgam in connective tissue	*	Most common on gingiva and edentulous alveolar ridge
Melanosis	Smoking (smoker's melanosis), trauma, postinflammatory melanosis, oral and labial melanotic macule, unknown	†	Depends on cause
Solar (actinic) cheilitis	Sun exposure	Adults	Vermilion of lips
Mucocele	Severed salivary gland duct	Any age	Most common: lower lip
Ranula	Obstruction/severing of salivary gland duct	*	Floor of mouth
Sialolith	Precipitation of calcified material around a central core	*	Major and minor salivary glands
Necrotizing sialometaplasia	Compromised blood supply to area	*	Most common: junction of the hard and soft palate
Sialadenitis	Infection Obstruction of salivary gland duct	*	Symptomatic when involving major salivary glands
Reactive Connective Tissue Hyperplasia			
Pyogenic granuloma	Response to injury Puberty Pregnancy	*	Most common: gingiva Also other areas
Peripheral giant cell granuloma	Unknown	Any age More frequent between 40 and 60 yr of age More common in women than men	Gingiva
Irritation fibroma	Trauma	*	Common on the gingiva Many other oral locations

N/A, Not applicable.
*No significant information.
†Not covered in this text.

CLINICAL FEATURES	RADIOGRAPHIC FEATURES	MICROSCOPIC FEATURES	TREATMENT/ MANAGEMENT	DIAGNOSTIC PROCESS
Painful, mucosal ulceration	N/A	Ulcer with eosinophils present in inflammatory infiltrate	Elimination of cause	Clinical
White mucosal surface	N/A	Hyperkeratosis	Elimination of cause	Clinical
Anterior-to-posterior white line	N/A	Epithelial hyperplasia and hyperkeratosis	None	Clinical
White, opacification of the palatal mucosa with raised red dots	N/A	Hyperkeratosis with inflamed minor salivary glands	Elimination of cause	Clinical
Granular to white, wrinkled appearance	N/A	Hyperkeratosis and epithelial hyperplasia Can have epithelial atypia	Elimination of cause	Clinical Microscopic
Painful, submucosal nodule	N/A	Mass of nerve cells	Surgical excision	Microscopic
Bluish-gray macule	Fine opaque granules	Black granular material in connective tissue	No treatment after identification	Clinical Microscopic Radiographic
Diffuse grayish-brown color of areas on the gingiva; localized macular pigmentation	N/A	Melanin pigment in basal layer of epithelium and in underlying connective tissue	Fades with decreased smoking None	Clinical Microscopic
Indistinct, fissured skin–mucosal interface	N/A	Degenerative changes in connective tissue	Protect lips and skin from sun exposure	Clinical
Localized tissue swelling that increases/decreases in size	N/A	Extravasated mucus in tissue surrounded by granulation tissue	Excision May spontaneously resolve	Clinical Microscopic
Fluid-filled swelling that increases/decreases in size	N/A	Resembles mucocele or mucous cyst	Surgery	Clinical
Obstruction of the gland Hard nodule in soft tissue	Floor of the mouth: radiopaque structure(seen in occlusal or panoramic radiograph)	Calcified structure arranged in concentric rings	Surgical removal of stone	Clinical Radiographic Microscopic
Moderately painful swelling and ulceration Acute onset	N/A	Necrosis of the salivary glands Replacement of salivary duct epithelium with squamous epithelium	Spontaneous resolution	Microscopic
Painful swelling of gland	N/A	Acute or chronic inflammatory infiltrate in salivary gland	Antibiotic if infection	Clinical Laboratory Microscopic
Deep red-purple exophytic lesion, usually ulcerated	N/A	Ulcerated granulation tissue	Surgical excision	Microscopic
Deep red exophytic lesion	N/A	Many multinucleated giant cells in well-vascularized connective tissue	Surgical excision	Microscopic
Broad-based, pink exophytic lesion	N/A	Dense fibrous connective tissue usually surfaced by normal epithelium	Surgical excision	Microscopic

Continued

CHAPTER 2 *Synopsis—cont'd*

CONDITION/DISEASE	CAUSE	AGE/RACE/SEX	LOCATION
Denture-induced fibrous hyperplasia (epulis fissuratum)	Ill-fitting denture Continuous wearing of denture	*	Vestibule along a denture border
Papillary hyperplasia of the palate	Constant wearing of maxillary removable prosthesis	*	Hard palate
Gingival enlargement	Response to chronic inflammation Idiopathic Drug reaction Hormonal changes Genetic	*	Gingiva: generalized or localized
Chronic hyperplastic pulpitis	Caries	Children and young adults	Primary or permanent molars
Inflammatory Periapical Lesions			
Periapical abscess	Inflammation of the dental pulp Preexisting periapical chronic inflammation	*	Roots of primary or permanent teeth
Periapical granuloma	Pulpal inflammation and necrosis	*	Roots of primary or permanent teeth
Radicular cyst (periapical cyst)	Nonvital tooth	*	Roots of primary or permanent teeth
Residual cyst	Radicular cyst not removed with extracted tooth		Site of tooth extraction
Resorption of teeth (external resorption, internal resorption)	Chronic inflammation Chronic pulpal inflammation		Roots of primary or permanent teeth Dental hard tissue within root or crowns
Focal sclerosing osteomyelitis	Low-grade chronic infection	*	Bone adjacent to any tooth Mandibular first molar most common
Alveolar osteitis ("dry socket")	Postoperative complication of tooth extraction	*	Extraction site

N/A, Not applicable.
*No significant information.
†Not covered in this text.

CLINICAL FEATURES	RADIOGRAPHIC FEATURES	MICROSCOPIC FEATURES	TREATMENT/ MANAGEMENT	DIAGNOSTIC PROCESS
Elongated folds of exophytic tissue surrounding denture flange	N/A	Dense fibrous connective tissue surfaced by epithelium that may be hyperplastic and ulcerated	Surgical excision Fabrication of new denture	Clinical Microscopic
Mucosa surfaced by multiple, erythematous papillary projections	N/A	Papillary projections composed of fibrous connective tissue (usually inflamed) surfaced by squamous epithelium	Surgical removal of papillary tissue Fabrication of new denture	Clinical
Increase in the bulk of the free and attached gingiva No stippling Erythematous to normal color	N/A	Connective tissue (usually inflamed) surfaced by squamous epithelium	Gingivectomy Meticulous oral hygiene	Clinical Microscopic
Red or pink nodule protruding from the pulp chamber of a tooth with a large, open carious lesion	N/A	Granulation tissue surfaced by squamous epithelium	Extraction of tooth or endodontic treatment	Clinical
Pain, swelling, fistula, slight extrusion of tooth	None Thickening of periodontal ligament space Periapical radiolucency	Acute inflammatory infiltrate	Establish drainage	Clinical
Asymptomatic Tooth sensitive to percussion Slight extrusion of tooth	Slight thickening of periodontal ligament space Periodontal radiolucency	Chronic inflammatory infiltrate	Endodontic therapy Extraction	Radiographic Microscopic
Most are asymptomatic	Radiolucency associated with the root of a nonvital tooth	Space lined by epithelium surrounded by an infiltrate of chronic inflammatory cells	Endodontic therapy Apicoectomy Extraction and curettage of the extraction site	Radiographic Microscopic
	Radiolucency at the site of tooth extraction		Surgical removal	
Asymptomatic May see pinkish color if crown involved	Blunting of root apex to severe loss of root substance Round to ovoid radiolucency in the central part of the tooth	N/A	Identify and remove cause Root canal therapy Extraction	Radiographic
Asymptomatic	Radiopaque area below roots of the tooth	Dense bone	None	Radiographic
Pain develops several days after extraction	N/A	N/A	Gentle irrigation Insertion of medicated dressing	Clinical

Chapter 3

Immunity and Immunologic Oral Lesions

Margaret J. Fehrenbach, Joan Andersen Phelan, Olga A.C. Ibsen

OBJECTIVES

After studying this chapter, the student will be able to:

1. Define and pronounce each of the words in the vocabulary list for this chapter.
2. Describe the differences between an immune response and an inflammatory response.
3. List and describe the two main types of lymphocytes, including their origins and activities.
4. List and describe the different types of T-cell lymphocytes and their functions.
5. Describe the origin of macrophages and list their activities in the immune response.
6. Describe the differences between humoral immunity and cell-mediated immunity and include the cells involved in each.
7. Describe the differences between passive and active immunity and give an example for each type of immunity.
8. List and describe four types of hypersensitivity reactions and give an example for each type of hypersensitivity.
9. Describe the process of autoimmunity and how it results in disease.
10. Describe the process of immunodeficiency and how it results in disease.
11. Describe and contrast the clinical features of each of the three types of aphthous ulcers.
12. List systemic diseases associated with aphthous ulcers.
13. Describe and compare the clinical features of urticaria, angioedema, contact mucositis, and fixed drug eruption.
14. Describe the clinical features of erythema multiforme and Stevens-Johnson syndrome.
15. Describe the clinical and microscopic features of lichen planus.
16. List the triad of systemic signs that comprise reactive arthritis (Reiter syndrome) and describe the oral lesions that occur in this condition.
17. Name the two cells that characterize Langerhans cell disease microscopically. Describe the acute disseminated form, chronic disseminated form, and chronic localized form and state the names that traditionally have been used for each of these conditions.
18. Describe the oral manifestations of each of the following autoimmune diseases: lupus erythematosus, pemphigus vulgaris, mucous membrane pemphigoid, and Behçet syndrome.
19. Define desquamative gingivitis, describe the clinical features, and list three diseases in which desquamative gingivitis may occur.
20. Describe the clinical features of Behçet syndrome.

VOCABULARY

Acantholysis (akan″-thol′ĭ-sis) Dissolution of the intercellular bridges of the prickle cell layer of the epithelium.

Acquired immune response Immune response to a foreign substance, based on the specific memory of a past exposure to that same foreign substance; the second, acquired immune response is quicker than the initial response.

Active immunity Type of immunity based on antibodies developed in response to an antigen. There are two types of active immunity: natural and acquired.

Allergen (al′ər-jen) Antigen producing a hypersensitivity, or allergic, reaction.

Allergy (al′ər-je) Hypersensitivity acquired through exposure to a particular allergen that elicits an exaggerated reaction on reexposure to the same allergen.

Anaphylaxis (an″ə-fə-lak′sis) Severe, immediate type of hypersensitivity or allergy in which an exaggerated immunologic reaction occurs on reexposure to a foreign protein or other substance after sensitization, resulting in hives, itching, swelling, vascular collapse, and shock. Also called *anaphylactic shock.*

Antibody (an′tĭ-bod″e) Protein molecule, an immunoglobulin, that is secreted by plasma cells and reacts with a specific antigen. There are five classes of antibodies: IgA, IgD, IgE, IgG, and IgM.

Antibody titer Level of a specific antibody in the blood.

Antigen (an′tĭ-jən) Any substance able to induce a specific immune response.

Attenuate (ə-ten′u-āt) To reduce the severity of a disease or the virulence of a pathogenic agent, as is done in the development of certain vaccines.

Autoantibody (aw″to-an′tĭ-bod″e) Antibody that reacts against a normal tissue constituent of one's own body.

Autoimmune disease Disease characterized by tissue trauma caused by an immune response against tissue constituents of one's own body.

B-cell lymphocyte Type of lymphocyte that develops in lymphoid tissue other than the thymus, and that can later develop into a plasma cell that produces antibody, the main initiator of humoral immunity.

Cell-mediated immunity Type of immunity in which the major role is played by T-cell lymphocytes.

Cytokines (si′to-kīns) Proteins produced by various cell types for the purpose of intercellular communication; immunological cytokines are involved in the immune response.

Dendritic cell A type of white blood cell that acts as an antigen-presenting cell in the skin and mucosa.

Humoral immunity Type of immunity in which both B-cell lymphocytes and the antibodies they produce as plasma cells play the predominant role.

Hyposalivation (hi″po-sal′ĭ-va′shən) Decreased salivary flow that may result in xerostomia (dry mouth).

Hypersensitivity (hi″pər-sen″sĭ-tiv′ĭ-te) Altered state of reactivity in which the body reacts to a foreign agent, or allergen, with an exaggerated immune response. There are four types of hypersensitivity: types I through IV.

Immune complex Combination of an antibody and antigen, producing a complex that can initiate a hypersensitivity reaction.

Immunization (im″u-nĭ-za′shən) Induction of active immunity. When the pathogenic microorganism used to induce active immunity is encountered after vaccination, a stronger, faster immune response is produced, which prevents disease development.

Immunodeficiency (im″u-no-də-fish′ən-se) Reduced immune response resulting from hypoactivity or decreased numbers of lymphoid cells.

Immunoglobulins (im″u-no-glob′u-lins) Proteins that, when secreted by plasma cells, serve as antibodies designed to respond to a specific antigen. Surface immunoglobulins remain attached to the surface of certain B cells and function as receptors.

Immunomodulator (im″u-no-mod′u-la″tor) A substance that alters the immune response by augmenting or reducing the ability of the immune system to produce antibodies or sensitized cells that recognize and react with the antigen that initiated their production.

Langerhans cell (lahng′ər-hahnz) Specialized dendritic cell, found in the skin and mucosa, that is involved in the immune response.

LE cell Mature neutrophil with a phagocytized spherical inclusion derived from another neutrophil; it is used as a marker of autoimmune diseases.

Lymphoid tissue (lim′foid) Tissue composed of lymphocytes supported by a meshwork of connective tissue; includes tonsillar tissue, lymph nodes, and lymphatic organs.

Lymphokines (lim′fo-kīns) Cytokines produced by B-cell or T-cell lymphocytes in contact with antigens; mediators in an immune response.

Macrophage (mak′ro-fāj) Large tissue-bound mononuclear phagocyte derived from monocytes circulating in the blood, which can become mobile when stimulated by inflammation and interact with lymphocytes in an immune response.

Continued

VOCABULARY—cont'd

Monokines (mon'o-kīns) Cytokines produced by monocytes or macrophages; mediators in an immune response.

Mucositis (mu″ko-si′tis) Mucosal inflammation due to a disease process.

Natural killer cell Type of lymphocyte that is part of the initial innate immune response, which by unknown mechanisms is able to directly destroy cells recognized as foreign.

Nikolsky sign Diagnostic sign whereby the superficial epithelium separates easily from the basal layer on exertion of firm, sliding manual pressure with the fingers.

Passive immunity Type of immunity that uses antibodies produced by another person to protect an individual against infectious disease. There are two types of passive immunity: natural and acquired.

Plasma cell Cell derived from B-cell lymphocytes that produces antibodies in response to the presence of antigen.

Pruritus (proo-ri′təs) Itching.

Rheumatoid factor (roo′mə-toid) Antibody that binds to certain antibodies found in the serum of patients with rheumatoid arthritis and connective tissue diseases such as Sjögren syndrome. Current assays test for IgM class rheumatoid factor.

Syndrome (sin'drōm) Group of signs and symptoms that occur together.

T-cell lymphocyte Lymphocyte that matures in the thymus and is mainly responsible for initiating cell-mediated immunity, as well as also modulating humoral immunity.

Thymus (thi'məs) Organ consisting of lymphoid tissue located high in the chest, which is large in an infant and gradually shrinks in size in adulthood; site of T-cell lymphocyte maturation.

Xerostomia (zēr″o-sto′me-ə) Dryness of the mucus membranes, including the oral cavity; usually caused by hyposalivation or decreased salivary flow.

The inflammatory response, as described in Chapter 2, is a rapid first line of defense against injury. The immune response, described in this chapter, follows the inflammatory response and is necessary for complete recovery. This chapter begins with a description of the acquired immune response and then includes a discussion of the most commonly encountered oral diseases that may result from harmful effects of such a response. Surveillance against neoplastic cells also involves the immune response and is described, along with the neoplastic process and neoplastic oral lesions, in Chapter 7.

ACQUIRED IMMUNE RESPONSE

Like the inflammatory response, the **acquired immune response** defends the body against injury, particularly from foreign substances such as microorganisms. The immune response differs from the inflammatory response in that it has the capacity for memory and responds more quickly to a foreign substance if encountered again. It works amid the background of an already activated inflammatory response and innate immune response, as well as a working repair process. The innate immune response does not involve memory and is described, along with inflammation, in Chapter 2. In contrast, the acquired immune response involves a complex network of white blood cells. Similar to the inflammatory response, the immune response may also result in an increased level of tissue damage and disease as it fights against what it considers foreign.

ANTIGENS

Antigens, or *immunogens,* are foreign substances against which the immune system defends the body. These substances are mainly proteins and are often microorganisms and their toxins. The immune system tolerates the normal components of the body, or *self,* with their normal diversity. In contrast, antigens are substances that the immune system recognizes as foreign, or *nonself.* Transformed human cells such as neoplasm cells or cells infected with viruses can become antigens. Human tissue, as in the case of an organ transplant, tissue graft, or incompatible blood transfusion, can also become an antigen.

In one type of disease, an *autoimmune disease,* parts of an individual's own body become antigens. In another type of disease, an *immunodeficiency,* the body no longer recognizes certain antigens as foreign. In another type of reaction involving *hypersensitivity,* the body overreacts to what it sees as foreign, creating a multitude of complications. Thus disease can occur when the immune response identifies components of self as antigen, does not recognize foreign material as antigen, or overreacts to antigens.

CELLULAR INVOLVEMENT IN THE IMMUNE RESPONSE

A complex network of white blood cells is involved in the immune response. These cells can produce cell products, or *cytokines,* that are active during the immune response. The primary white blood cells involved in the immune response are lymphocytes. These cells are able to recognize and respond to an antigen when it is in contact with receptor sites located on the cell surface. Lymphocytes, like other white blood cells, are derived from stem cells in the bone marrow. Lymphocytes constitute 20 to 25% of the white blood cell population. They are mobile antigen-sensitive cells with a long life. They have a round nucleus and only a small amount of cytoplasm. Different types of lymphocytes have differing functions. There are three main types of lymphocytes: (1) the B-cell lymphocyte, (2) the T-cell lymphocyte, and (3) the natural killer cell. The macrophage and the dendritic cell are also part of the immune response.

B-CELL LYMPHOCYTE

The **B-cell lymphocyte** (B cell) develops from a stem cell in the bone marrow and then resides and matures in **lymphoid tissue** (Figure 3-1). When antigen stimulates a B cell, the B cell travels to the site of the injury. Two main types of B cells develop when stimulated by an antigen: (1) the B-memory cell and (2) the plasma cell.

The B-memory cell retains a memory of the antigen. In the presence of an antigen recognized by the B-memory cell, this cell reacts by duplicating itself many times over in a process called *clonal selection*. All of these newly formed B cells retain the capacity to recognize the previously encountered antigen.

The **plasma cell** has a round, pinwheel-shaped nucleus and visible cytoplasm. The plasma cell produces and releases many copies of a particular protein **(antibody)** in response to the presence of antigen. Antibodies circulating within the blood serum are considered **immunoglobulins.** Five different general types of immunoglobulins exist: (1) IgA, (2) IgD, (3) IgE, (4) IgG, and (5) IgM (Table 3-1). They all are

variations of the same basic structure (Figures 3-2 and 3-3). Each immune response involves specific antibodies produced in response to a specific antigen by a specific plasma cell. This specificity is a characteristic function of the immune response. The level of a specific antibody in the blood is called the **antibody titer.** This can be measured by

TABLE 3-1

Immunoglobulins (Antibodies)

IMMUNOGLOBULIN (IG)	DESCRIPTION
IgA	Has two subgroups: serous in the blood and secretory in the saliva and other secretions such as tears and breast milk; aids in defense against proliferation of microorganisms in body fluids as well as protecting mucosal sites (e.g., gastrointestinal and genitourinary tracts)
IgD	Functions in the activation of B-cell lymphocytes, because it is found on their surface, but full role is unclear
IgE	Involved in hypersensitivity or allergic reactions because it can bind to mast cells and basophils to bring about the release of biochemical mediators such as histamine; and also attacks parasites
IgG	Major antibody in blood serum (about 75%); can pass the placental barrier, produced in secondary immune response, and serves as the first passive immunity for the newborn
IgM	Involved in early immune responses because of its involvement with IgD in the activation of B-cell lymphocytes, activates complement, and reacts to blood group antigens

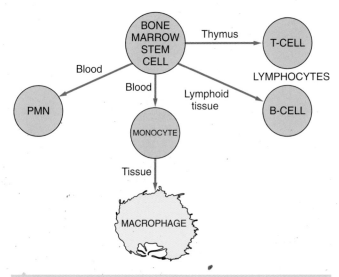

FIGURE 3-1 ■ Primary cells of the immune response include the lymphocytes, both B-cell lymphocytes and T-cell lymphocytes. Lymphocytes, polymorphonuclear neutrophils *(PMN)* and, macrophages are derived from stem cells in the bone marrow.

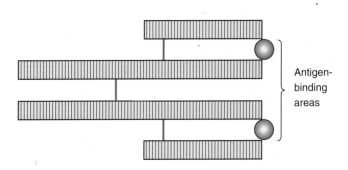

FIGURE 3-2 ■ Antibody or immunoglobulin (Ig) basic structure, with four protein chains with two identical heavy polypeptide chains and two identical light chains, forming a Y-shape. The tips of the arms are called the *variable region* because they vary greatly, creating a pocket uniquely shaped to enfold or "bind" a specific antigen (Fab). The stem or base, called the *constant region,* is identical in all antibodies of the same class and serves to link the antibody to other cells and products in the immune response (Fc).

diagnostic laboratory tests and is useful in the diagnosis and evaluation of infectious disease.

The combination of an specific antibody with a specific antigen is an **immune complex.** The formation of an immune complex usually renders the antigen inactive. Immune complexes may also be involved in certain disease states. Some of these are discussed later in this chapter.

IMMUNOGLOBULINS
G(IgG), E(IgE), D(IgD)

IMMUNOGLOBULIN A
(IgA)

IMMUNOGLOBULIN M
(IgM)

FIGURE 3-3 ■ Five general types of antibodies or immunoglobulins in serum include the same basic structure arranged differently. This variation in structure allows them to function differently.

T-CELL LYMPHOCYTE

After it develops from a bone marrow stem cell, the **T-cell lymphocyte** (T cell) travels to the **thymus** and is processed into a mature cell (see Figure 3-1). The thymus is a primary lymphoid organ located high in the chest. It is quite large in infants and shrinks as an individual matures.

The T cell can be distinguished from other lymphocyte types, such as B cells and natural killer cells, by the presence of a special receptor on its cell surface that is called the *T-cell receptor* (TCR). Other receptors are also present on the surface of the T cell. Different types of T cells have different functions in the immune response. The different types of T cells include the T-helper cell, the T-suppressor cell, the T-cytotoxic cell, and the T-memory cell.

The T-helper cell increases the functioning of the B-cell, enhancing the antibody response. It is easily identifiable by the CD4 cell receptor on its surface (Figure 3-4). The T-suppressor cell (or T-regulator cell) carries the CD8 marker as well as other markers on its surface and suppresses the functioning of the B cell.

The T-cytotoxic cell also carries the CD8 marker. It is active in surveillance against virally infected cells and neoplastic cells, directly attacking these cells.

T cells within cell-mediated immunity also start, regulate, and coordinate the overall immune response.

NATURAL KILLER CELL

The **natural killer cell** (NK cell) is a large lymphocyte that plays a part in the innate immune response of the body. NK cells have the ability to destroy foreign cells soon after their appearance because they recognize them as foreign without

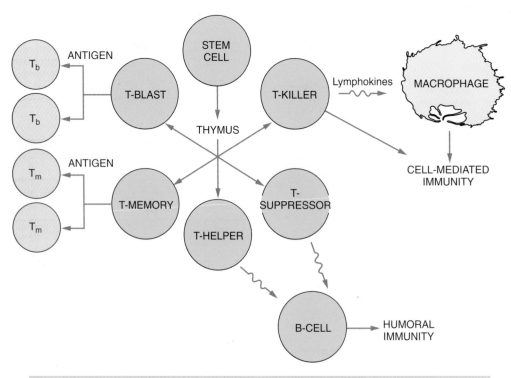

FIGURE 3-4 ■ Various types of T-cell lymphocytes and their involvement in the immune response.

first having to recognize them as specific antigens and go through any system checks. They are usually located only within the microcirculation and not in the outlying tissue. This cell type seems to be active against viruses and cancer cells. However, in several immunodeficiency diseases, including human immunodeficiency virus (HIV)-related acquired immunodeficiency syndrome (AIDS), NK cell function is abnormal.

MACROPHAGE

Not only is the white blood cell **macrophage** present in the connective tissue during inflammation, it is also involved in the evolving immune response to an antigen as an accessory cell (see Figure 3-1). The macrophage is active in phagocytosis of foreign substances and also assists both the B-cell and T-cell during the immune response.

Along with phagocytosis, the macrophage acts to process and present antigen material on its surface to the T-helper cell. This stimulates both types of lymphocytes to travel from the lymphoid tissue or surrounding blood vessels to the injury site. Thus the macrophage functions as an antigen-presenting cell, acting as a messenger between both the inflammatory response and immune response.

The macrophage carries receptors for lymphokines produced by the lymphocytes, which allow it to be activated into a single-minded pursuit of specific foreign material such as microorganisms or neoplastic cells (Table 3-2). When activated, the macrophage can function in many other different ways, always amplifying the immune response. Unlike lymphocytes, the macrophage does not retain memory of an encountered antigen and needs to be reactivated during each encounter.

DENDRITIC CELL

The **dendritic cell** (DC) is a white blood cell whose main function is to process antigenic material and present it on its surface to other cells of the immune system. Thus the dendritic cell functions as an antigen-presenting cell, acting as a messenger between innate immunity and acquired immunity. It is similar in function to a macrophage.

The dendritic cell is present in tissue that is in contact with the external environment, such as the skin and mucosa. It can also be found in an immature state in the blood. At certain developmental stages, it grows branched projections or dendrites. Once activated, it migrates to the lymph nodes or other lymphoid tissue, where it interacts with T cells and B cells to initiate and shape the acquired immune response. In mucosal tissue, including the oral mucosa, there is a specialized dendritic cell type called a **Langerhans cell.**

CYTOKINES

Cytokines are proteins that are made by cells and are able to affect the behavior of other cells; thus they are considered immunomodulating agents. Immunomodulating agents, or **immunomodulators,** alter the immune response by augmenting or reducing the functions of the response. Cytokines are produced by the cells of the immune system and play a prominent role in the activation of the immune response. They are one way that lymphocytes communicate with each other and with other immune system cells. B cells and T cells produce their own cytokines, called **lymphokines,** in varying levels (see Figure 3-4).

Different cytokines have differing functions within the immune response (see Table 3-2). They can activate macrophages and enhance the ability of macrophages to destroy foreign cells. These types of cytokines may also be involved in various other functions concerning leukocytes, fibroblasts, and endothelial cells. They are also responsible for the systemic effects of inflammation such as loss of appetite and increased heart rate. Monocytes/macrophages produce their own cytokines, called **monokines.** Dendritic cells, such as the Langerhans cells, also produce and react to cytokines.

One of the first cytokines to be discovered within the body was interferon. Produced by T cells and macrophages (as well as by cells outside the immune system), interferons are a group of proteins with antiviral properties. Chemokines are a group of cytokines that are named for their ability to induce chemotaxis in nearby responsive cells. They may be involved in controlling infection as part of the immune response as well as being involved in several developmental processes during embryogenesis.

MAJOR DIVISIONS OF THE IMMUNE RESPONSE

There are two major divisions of the immune response: (1) humoral immunity and (2) cell-mediated immunity (Figure 3-5). These two divisions differ in their reaction to an antigen. However, these divisions are interrelated, and present understanding of the immune response recognizes that these divisions do not function as distinctly separate mechanisms.

TABLE 3-2

Cytokines

CYTOKINE	FUNCTION
Interferons	Various functions involving leukocytes, fibroblasts, and endothelial cells
Interleukins	Stimulate leukocyte proliferation and other functions
Lymphotoxin	Destroys fibroblasts
Macrophage-activating factor	Activates macrophages to produce and secrete lysosomal enzymes
Macrophage chemotactic factor	Stimulates macrophage emigration
Migration inhibitory factor	Inhibits macrophage activity
Tumor necrosis factor	Various functions involving leukocytes and fibroblasts

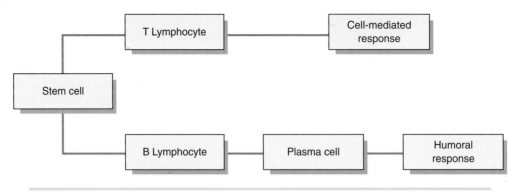

FIGURE 3-5 ■ The two major divisions of the immune response: humoral immunity and cell-mediated immunity.

Humoral immunity, or *antibody-mediated immunity,* involves the production of antibodies, with the B-cell lymphocytes as the primary cells. Humoral immunity is responsible for protection against many pathogenic microorganisms such as bacteria and viruses.

The other division of the immune system is **cell-mediated immunity,** or *cellular immunity;* it involves lymphocytes, usually T cells, working alone or assisted by macrophages. The cell-mediated division regulates both major divisions of the immune system.

MEMORY AND IMMUNITY

Memory is a characteristic function of the acquired immune response. This contrasts with the inflammatory response, which is not capable of memory. Certain lymphocytes retain the memory of an antigen after an initial encounter. For this reason, the immune response to that antigen is much more rapid and stronger the next time it is encountered. Immunity is this increased responsiveness that results from the retained memory of an already encountered antigen.

TYPES OF IMMUNITY

Two types of immunity can occur: (1) passive and (2) active. **Passive immunity** refers to the use of antibodies produced by another person to protect an individual against infectious disease. This type of immunity can occur naturally or it can be acquired. *Natural passive immunity* occurs when antibodies from a mother pass through the placenta to the developing fetus. These antibodies protect a newborn infant from disease while the infant's own immune system matures.

Passive immunity can also be acquired by injecting a person with antibodies against a microorganism to which the person has not previously been exposed. This is done to confer immediate protection against the disease caused by that microorganism. These antibodies are collected from individuals who have already had the disease and have naturally produced antibodies to the pathogenic microorganism. *Acquired passive immunity* is short-lived but can act immediately. It is used because the unprepared immune system of an individual takes longer to produce antibodies,

and in the meantime the disease may develop. Acquired passive immunity may be provided to dental personnel who do not have immunity to hepatitis B after needlestick or other occupational exposure incidents, using hepatitis B immunoglobulin.

Active immunity uses antibodies produced by one's own body to protect against infectious disease, and it can occur naturally or be acquired. It occurs naturally when a pathogenic microorganism causes disease. Protection against further attack by that microorganism is conferred to the individual if the body recovers from the disease. A less risky way of achieving active immunity is by an acquired or artificial means. This production of acquired active immunity is called **immunization.** A person is injected with or ingests either altered pathogenic microorganisms or products of those microorganisms. The altered microorganism or products of the microorganisms cannot produce infection but is able to act as an antigen. This is called a *vaccine,* and the process is called *vaccination.* When the pathogenic microorganism is encountered after vaccination, the immune system produces a stronger, faster response and prevents development of the disease.

Immunization lowers the risk of a microorganism causing disease because it safely prepares the immune system to fight future attacks by the disease-causing microorganism. In some cases more than one exposure to the antigen is needed to ensure adequate immunity; a repeated exposure by way of a vaccination is called a *booster.* Immunization by vaccination is used to protect children and adults against many diseases. Dental personnel should be vaccinated against the hepatitis B virus because of their high risk of occupational exposure to that virus.

Killed-type vaccines consist of heat- or chemical-treated microorganisms or toxins; these treatments make killed-type vaccines safe but in some cases they may be less effective than live-**attenuated** vaccines. Live-attenuated vaccines consist of genetically altered microorganisms that have lost virulence but still undergo limited replication. Molecular vaccines are composed of critical antigenic determinants, derived as recombinant (from cloned bacteria or yeast) or synthetic peptides; adjuvants may be used to stimulate immune responses.

IMMUNOPATHOLOGY

The immune response helps defend the body against disease-producing antigens, but it can also malfunction and cause tissue damage resulting in the production of lesions. **Immunopathology** is the study of diseases caused by the malfunctioning of the immune system. These immunopathologic conditions include (1) hypersensitivity, (2) autoimmune disease, and (3) immunodeficiency. Examples of each of these immunopathological conditions, in which damage is directly caused by the immune response, are discussed next. Some of these conditions fall into the category of a **syndrome,** which is a group of signs and symptoms that occur together to define the disease state. Many different syndromes are described in various chapters in this text.

HYPERSENSITIVITY

Hypersensitivity or **allergy** comprises the same basic types of reactions that occur when the immune response is fighting microorganisms and protecting the body against disease. However, these hypersensitivity or allergenic reactions are exaggerated immune responses causing an immunopathologic condition, along with tissue destruction. Four main types of hypersensitivity reactions occur; they are classified by the nature of the immune response that causes the disease (Table 3-3).

TYPE I HYPERSENSITIVITY

Type I hypersensitivity or *anaphylactic type hypersensitivity* is a reaction that occurs immediately—within minutes—after exposure to a previously encountered antigen, or **allergen** in this case, such as pollen, latex, or penicillin. With type I hypersensitivity plasma cells produce IgE as a response to the allergen. The newly produced IgE binds to mast cells located in tissue, causing them to release their granules containing histamine, a potent biochemical mediator of inflammation. This results in edema caused by increased dilation and permeability of blood vessels and in constriction of smooth muscle in the bronchioles of the lungs.

This type of hypersensitivity includes hay fever, urticaria (hives), and more serious conditions, including asthma and anaphylaxis. **Anaphylaxis** is a type of hypersensitivity that can be life-threatening because the individual may not be able to breathe as a result of the oropharyngeal tissue swelling and constriction of the bronchioles, which requires immediate treatment with epinephrine.

Drugs that suppress inflammation, such as antihistamines and corticosteroids, may be helpful in reducing symptoms of some forms of type I hypersensitivity.

TYPE II HYPERSENSITIVITY

With type II hypersensitivity or *cytotoxic type hypersensitivity*, antibody combines with an antigen that is bound to the surface of tissue cells, usually a circulating red blood cell. Activated complement components as well as both IgG and IgM antibodies in blood participate in this type of hypersensitivity reaction. The result is the destruction of the tissue that has the antigen on the surface of its cells. A type II reaction occurs in incompatible blood transfusions and in rhesus (Rh) incompatibility. In the latter case, the mother's antibodies cross the placenta and destroy the newborn's red blood cells, resulting in possibly fatal hemolytic anemia.

TYPE III HYPERSENSITIVITY

Type III hypersensitivity or *immune complex type hypersensitivity* is marked by the formation of immune complexes between microorganisms and antibody in the circulating blood. The complexes leave the blood and are deposited in various types of tissue or even in a localized area in an organ. In either case the deposition results in the initiation of an acute inflammatory response. Neutrophils are attracted to the tissue in which the complexes have been deposited. As a result of phagocytosis and death of the neutrophils, lysosomal enzymes are released, causing tissue destruction.

TYPE IV HYPERSENSITIVITY

Type IV hypersensitivity or *cell-mediated type hypersensitivity* involves a cell-mediated immune response rather than a humoral response that produces antibodies. T-cell lymphocytes that have been introduced to an antigen previously either directly cause damage to the tissue cells or recruit other cells that cause the damage. This type of hypersensitivity reaction is also called **delayed hypersensitivity** and is used when diagnosing tuberculosis. A visible skin reaction occurs if the individual tested has previously been exposed to the microorganism that causes tuberculosis.

This type of hypersensitivity is also responsible for the rejection of tissue grafts and transplanted organs as well as an allergy to nickel in dental restorations. New strategies for prevention of rejection, such as synthetic production of therapeutic antibodies against specific T-cell receptors, may produce fewer long-term side effects than the chemotherapies now routinely used.

HYPERSENSITIVITY TO DRUGS

Drugs can act as allergens and cause a hypersensitivity reaction. Many factors influence the risk of a hypersensitivity or allergic reaction to a drug. The route of administration influences how the reaction will be manifested and its severity. Topical administration of drugs (via the skin or mucous

---

TABLE 3-3

Hypersensitivity Reactions

TYPE OF REACTION	EXAMPLE(S)
Type I or anaphylactic type	Hay fever, asthma, anaphylaxis
Type II or cytotoxic type	Autoimmune hemolytic anemia
Type III or immune complex type	Autoimmune diseases such as systemic lupus erythematosus
Type IV or cell-mediated type	Granulomatous diseases such as tuberculosis as well as graft and organ transplant rejection

membranes) may cause a greater number of reactions than the oral (swallowed) or parenteral (administered by injection) route of administration; however, the reaction that occurs after parenteral administration may be more widespread and severe because the allergen can be carried quickly to many parts of the body by the circulating blood.

Patients with multiple allergies are more likely to have allergic reactions to drugs, and patients with autoimmune diseases such as systemic lupus erythematosus commonly have adverse reactions to medication. Children, with their newer levels of immunity, are less likely than adults to have an allergic reaction to a drug.

Drugs can be involved in any of the previously described hypersensitivity reactions. Type I hypersensitivity to a drug can include anaphylaxis, urticaria (hives), and angioedema (localized swelling). A systemic anaphylactic reaction is more likely to occur with an injected drug but can also occur with a drug administered orally, and can be fatal. For example, the drug penicillin may cause a systemic anaphylactic reaction in approximately 1 in 10,000 patients and causes about 300 deaths per year in the United States.

The classic example of type III hypersensitivity is **serum sickness,** which involves a drug allergy. This name was given to a reaction that occurred frequently when patients were given large amounts of horse antitoxin serum to provide passive immunity in the treatment of diphtheria and tetanus. This is no longer the method by which passive immunity to these diseases is provided. The drug penicillin is the single most common cause of serum sickness. Other drugs such as barbiturates can also cause this reaction. The signs and symptoms of serum sickness include rash or urticaria, fever, painful swelling of the joints (arthritis), renal disturbance or failure, edema around the eyes, and cardiac inflammation. Drugs can also be involved in a type IV hypersensitivity reaction. This T-cell–mediated allergic reaction can occur in response to topically applied substances and can produce contact dermatitis (skin inflammation) and contact **mucositis,** which is an inflammation of the mucosal tissues.

AUTOIMMUNE DISEASES

The immune system learns to differentiate between one's own cells or tissue and foreign substances early in embryologic development. This recognition and the nonresponsiveness of the immune system to one's own cells or tissue usually produce a type of *immunologic tolerance.*

In an **autoimmune disease** the recognition mechanism breaks down, and certain body cells are no longer tolerated. The immune system now treats body cells as antigens, creating an immunopathologic condition. An autoimmune disease may involve a single cell type or a single organ or may be even more extensive, involving multiple organs. Certain types of tissue and even entire organs may be damaged. Genetic factors may play a role in the predisposition of an individual to autoimmune disease, and viral infection may also be involved. Some autoimmune diseases are also called **connective tissue diseases.** Several

autoimmune diseases have oral manifestations and are described later in this chapter.

IMMUNODEFICIENCY

Immunodeficiency is a type of immunopathologic condition that involves a deficiency in number, function, or interrelationships of the involved white blood cells of the immune system and their products. This condition may be congenital (present at birth) or acquired (developed after birth). Immunodeficiency may be inherited genetically, or it can be caused by numerous other environmental factors.

When a person's immune system is not functioning adequately, infections and neoplasms may develop. In addition, research has shown that stress and depression may be associated with decreased levels of immune function. AIDS is an example of an immunodeficiency that has numerous oral manifestations.

ORAL IMMUNOLOGIC LESIONS AND DISEASES

APHTHOUS ULCERS, RECURRENT APHTHOUS ULCERS

Recurrent aphthous ulcers, also known as canker sores or *aphthous stomatitis,* are a painful type of oral ulcers for which the cause remains unclear. Aphthous ulcers are one of the most common oral lesions, occurring in about 20% of the general population. They frequently occur in episodes. The first episode of these ulcers usually occurs in adolescence, and they are somewhat more common in females than in males. The clinical appearance and location are important in establishing the diagnosis.

Trauma is the most commonly reported precipitating factor in the development of aphthous ulcers. They are often reported to occur after trauma to the oral mucosa during dental procedures (e.g., in the area of film or sensor placement or at the injection site for local anesthetics) or with the manipulation of oral tissue during dental hygiene treatment. Some patients associate the initiation of aphthous ulcers with eating certain foods such as citrus fruits. However, it is possible that patients perceive these foods as causative because of the sensitivity of the ulcers to foods with a high acid content, or the foods themselves may have caused trauma to the oral mucosa. The recurrence of aphthous ulcers has been associated with menstruation, whereas pregnancy has been found to produce a decrease in the episodes. These ulcers also occur in association with certain systemic diseases as well as with tobacco cessation. Emotional stress has also been suggested as a contributing factor.

Substantial evidence indicates that aphthous ulcers have an immunologic pathogenesis. Patients in whom aphthous ulcers develop have slightly elevated levels of antibodies to oral mucous membranes. Microscopically, an infiltrate of lymphocytes is present in the lesion, suggesting that cell-mediated immunity may be important in development of the ulcers. The infiltrate contains mainly T-helper cells in the prodromal stage and T-cytotoxic cells in the ulcerative phase; T-helper cells return in the healing stage. The T-cytotoxic cells are probably responsible for the ulceration. However, the specific antigen to which they are responding has not yet been identified. Research has not identified a link between microbes and aphthous ulcers. However, the potential role of microbes in the pathogenesis of aphthous ulcers is an area that is still being explored.

TYPES OF APHTHOUS ULCERS

There are three forms of recurrent aphthous ulceration: (1) minor, (2) major, and (3) herpetiform, with the three forms differing in the size and duration of the ulcers.

Minor aphthous ulcers are the most commonly occurring type. They appear as discrete, "punched-out," round-to-oval ulcers that can be as large as 1 cm in diameter and exhibit a yellowish-white fibrin surface (pseudomembrane) surrounded by a halo of erythema (Figure 3-6). Minor aphthous ulcers are more common in the anterior than the posterior part of the mouth. The ulcers often have a prodromal period of 1 to 2 days, which is characterized by a burning sensation or soreness in the area in which the ulcer will eventually form. Although they are small, these ulcers can be exquisitely painful, and single or multiple lesions may be present. They heal spontaneously in 7 to 10 days.

Major aphthous ulcers (also known as *Sutton disease*, and *periadenitis mucosa necrotica recurrens*) are larger than 1 cm in diameter and are deeper and last longer than minor aphthous ulcers (Figure 3-7). In addition, they can be more painful, often occur in the posterior part of the mouth, and are less common compared with minor aphthous ulcers. They can take several weeks to heal and frequently result in scarring. Ulcers that resemble major aphthous ulcers have been reported to occur in patients with HIV infection.

Herpetiform aphthous ulcers are the smallest at 1 to 2 mm and the least common type (Figure 3-8). They are mistakenly called *herpetiform* because they resemble ulcers caused by the herpes simplex virus, but like the other types of aphthous ulcers they do not have a known cause. They are painful and may develop anywhere in the oral cavity.

DIAGNOSIS

The diagnosis of the type of aphthous ulcers is made on the basis of their distinctive clinical appearance, the location of the lesions, and a complete patient history (Table 3-4). It is important to note that laboratory results are not specific for any form of aphthous ulcer.

The location of the ulcers is important in differentiating between recurrent aphthous ulcers and recurrent intraoral ulceration caused by the herpes simplex virus. The differentiation between aphthous ulcers and herpes simplex ulcers is described in Chapter 4 (see Table 4-2). Aphthous ulcers appear on nonkeratinized oral mucosa that is nonattached, that is, not fixed to bone, such as the buccal and labial mucosa, vestibular tissue, and the floor of the mouth as well as the lateral and ventral surfaces of the tongue. In contrast, ulcers resulting from the herpes simplex virus, when they occur intraorally, appear on keratinized mucosa such as the oral mucosa of the palate and gingival tissue (i.e., the mucosa fixed to bone). Because major aphthous ulcers may clinically resemble squamous cell carcinoma or deep fungal infections a biopsy may be necessary to rule out these conditions. However, as with minor aphthous ulcers, biopsy and microscopic features are nonspecific and not diagnostic for major aphthous ulcers.

Herpetiform aphthous ulcers may also be difficult to distinguish clinically from primary herpetic gingivostomatitis. However, no systemic signs or symptoms exist as in primary herpes simplex infection. Herpetiform aphthous ulcers have been reported to respond to topical application of liquid tetracycline, which may be helpful in confirming the diagnosis of herpetiform aphthous ulcers.

When a patient develops multiple aphthous ulcers, it is important to consider that they might be associated

FIGURE 3-6 ■ Minor aphthous ulcers. **A,** On the floor of the mouth. **B,** On the buccal mucosa, on the papilla of the Stenson duct.

FIGURE 3-7 ■ Major aphthous ulcers. **A,** On the labial mucosa. **B,** On the soft palate. **C,** On the buccal mucosa.

FIGURE 3-8 ■ Herpetiform aphthous ulcers on the palate. These are the smallest of the aphthous ulcers.

with a systemic disease. Other signs and symptoms that may suggest systemic disease should be considered when reviewing the patient's medical history. These include the presence of chronic gastrointestinal symptoms such as diarrhea and discomfort (Crohn disease, gluten-sensitive enteropathy/celiac disease, inflammatory bowel syndrome, intestinal lymphoma, ulcerative colitis), arthritis and skin lesions (Behçet syndrome), and childhood periodic fevers (cyclic neutropenia and PFAFA [periodic fever, aphthous stomatitis, pharyngitis, and adenitis] syndrome).

TREATMENT AND PROGNOSIS

The local application of topical corticosteroids and topical nonsteroidal antiinflammatory agents is helpful in the management of aphthous ulcers, and topical anesthetics such as lidocaine and benzocaine can help to decrease the pain. Topical corticosteroids and nonsteroidal antiinflammatory agents are most effective when applied very early in the development of the ulcer, during the prodromal or preulcerative period; systemic steroids may be necessary for managing patients with major aphthous ulcers.

TABLE 3-4

Clinical Features of the Three Types of Recurrent Aphthous Ulcers

	TYPE OF RECURRENT APHTHOUS ULCER		
FEATURE	MINOR	MAJOR	HERPETIFORM
Size	Small, 3 to 5 mm	Large, 5 to 10 mm	Smallest, 1 to 2 mm
Location on nonkeratinized mucosa	More anterior	More posterior	Anywhere
Number	1 to 5	1 to 10	1 to 100
Appearance	Shallow	Deep	Shallow
Scarring	No	Yes	No
Pain	Yes	Yes	Yes

FIGURE 3-9 ■ **A** and **B,** Two examples of urticaria (hives).

FIGURE 3-10 ■ Angioedema. (Courtesy Dr. Edward V. Zegarelli.)

Nicotine replacement therapy has been suggested to be helpful when aphthous ulcers occur in association with tobacco cessation.

URTICARIA AND ANGIOEDEMA

Urticaria and angioedema have a similar causal background in that they are skin and oral mucosal hypersensitivity reactions. The lesions are caused by localized areas of increased vascular permeability in the superficial connective tissue beneath the epithelium.

Urticaria, also called *hives,* appears as multiple areas of well-demarcated edema and erythema of the skin, usually accompanied by itching **(pruritus)** (Figure 3-9). **Angioedema** appears as a diffuse edema (swelling) of tissue caused by permeability of deeper blood vessels (Figure 3-10). The skin covering the swelling appears normal, and angioedema is usually not accompanied by itching. Urticaria and angioedema both may occur in acute self-limited episodes. On occasion, chronic or recurrent forms may occur each time the patient comes in contact with the allergen.

In many cases of urticaria and angioedema the cause cannot be identified. Infection, trauma, emotional stress, and certain systemic diseases have been reported to cause these lesions, and ingested allergens are frequent causes of urticaria.

Several mechanisms are capable of causing the increased vascular permeability that results in both urticaria and angioedema, including the release of the chemical mediator histamine from mast cells stimulated by IgE antibodies (type I hypersensitivity) and the activation of IgG or IgM antibodies along with trauma, causing vascular permeability. Acetylsalicylic acid (aspirin) and nonsteroidal antiinflammatory drugs, such as ibuprofen, can produce a nonspecific effect that can cause vascular permeability. A rare hereditary form of angioedema exists in which uncontrolled activation of the complement cascade occurs, resulting in prolonged vascular permeability.

DIAGNOSIS

The diagnoses for both urticaria and angioedema are based on the clinical appearance of the lesions and the patient's history. Avoidance of the causative agent, if identified, is important in managing patients with recurring urticaria and angioedema.

TREATMENT AND PROGNOSIS

Antihistaminic drugs (e.g., diphenhydramine [Benadryl]) are the standard drugs used to treat urticaria and angioedema. Immediate treatment is important. Angioedema involving the larynx and pharynx can cause asphyxiation and therefore may be fatal. Immediate treatment with epinephrine is necessary in these cases.

CONTACT MUCOSITIS AND DERMATITIS

Contact mucositis as well as **contact dermatitis** are lesions that result from the direct contact of an allergen with the oral mucosa and skin, respectively. The development of these conditions involves a T cell within a cell-mediated immune response and is an example of type IV hypersensitivity. The exact underlying immunologic basis is not always clear.

In contact mucositis the mucosa becomes erythematous and edematous, often accompanied by burning and pruritus (Figure 3-11, *A*). The mucositis occurs where the offending agent has contacted the mucosa, giving it a smooth, shiny appearance that is firm to palpation. Small vesicles and ulcers may appear in the affected areas. In contact dermatitis the initial lesion may be erythematous, with swelling and vesicles. Later the area becomes crusted, scaly, and white.

Preservatives in local anesthetics, and components of topical medication are common causes of allergic reactions. Acrylics, metal-based alloys, epoxy resins, and the flavoring agents in chewing gum and dentifrices all have been reported to cause contact mucositis.

Contact dermatitis, particularly affecting the hands, may occur in response to the materials used in dentistry. The routine use of gloves in dental care has decreased the incidence of this type of dermatitis; however, latex gloves and glove powder have also been responsible for contact dermatitis in some individuals (Figure 3-11, *B*).

DIAGNOSIS

When the cause of the contact mucositis or dermatitis is suspected, skin testing for sensitivity to the particular substance can help confirm the agent that has caused the lesion.

TREATMENT AND PROGNOSIS

Topical and systemic corticosteroids may be used in the management of these lesions in some patients.

FIXED DRUG ERUPTIONS

Fixed drug eruptions are lesions that appear in the same site each time a drug is introduced. The lesions generally appear suddenly after a latent period of several days and

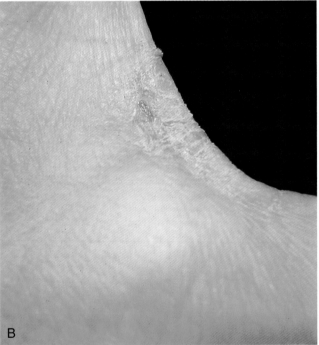

FIGURE 3-11 ▪ **A,** Contact mucositis on the labial mucosa, from acrylic. **B,** Contact dermatitis on the skin between the thumb and index finger, from latex gloves. (**A,** Courtesy Dr. Edward V. Zegarelli.)

subside when the drug is discontinued. They appear again when the drug is reintroduced, usually with greater intensity. Clinically there may be single or multiple slightly raised, reddish patches or clusters of macules on the skin or rarely the mucous membranes in the oral cavity. Pain and pruritus may be associated with these lesions.

The fixed drug eruption is a type III hypersensitivity reaction in which immune complexes are deposited along the endothelial wall of blood vessels. The ensuing inflammatory reaction causes vasculitis and subsequent damage to the vessel wall, giving rise to erythema and edema of the superficial layers of the skin or mucosa. If possible, the drug causing the reaction should be identified, and its use discontinued.

ERYTHEMA MULTIFORME

Erythema multiforme (EM) is an acute, self-limited disease that affects the skin and mucous membranes. The cause is not clear, but some evidence exists that it is a hypersensitivity reaction; however, the type has not been determined.

Erythema multiforme most commonly occurs in young adults and affects men more commonly than women. The characteristic skin lesion is called a *target,* or *bull's-eye* lesion, which consists of concentric rings of erythema alternating with normal skin color, with the darkest color at the center of the lesion. The term *erythema multiforme* refers to the variety of skin lesions that can occur, which range from target lesion macules to plaques to bullae (Figure 3-12). Erythema multiforme can affect the oral mucosa either alone or in association with skin lesions. Skin lesions can occur without the presence of any oral lesions. The oral lesions are usually ulcers (Figure 3-13, *A* and *B*). However, erythematous areas may also occur. The ulcers frequently form on the lateral borders of the tongue. Crusted and bleeding lips are frequently seen in erythema multiforme, and gingival involvement is rare.

This condition usually has an explosive onset of lesions on the oral mucosa, lips, and skin. Systemic symptoms are mild or lacking. It may be chronic on occasion, or there may be recurrent acute episodes because it seems to be related to persistent antigenic stimulus.

In the past a condition known as Stevens-Johnson syndrome was considered a very severe form of erythema multiforme. More recently, Stevens-Johnson syndrome has been separated from the erythema multiforme spectrum and classified as a variant of toxic epidermal necrolysis (TEN) (Figure 3-13, *C*), a rare and usually severe adverse reaction to certain drugs. Stevens-Johnson syndrome presents with mucosal lesions that are more extensive and painful than erythema multiforme. Lesions involving the genital mucosa and the mucosa of the eyes may also be involved. In Stevens-Johnson the lips are generally more extensively encrusted and bloody than in erythema multiforme.

Although the cause of erythema multiforme is not clear, in some cases triggering factors can be identified. Herpes simplex virus (HSV) infection, tuberculosis, and histoplasmosis have been associated with episodes of erythema multiforme, as have malignant neoplasms and drugs such as barbiturates and sulfonamides.

DIAGNOSIS

The diagnosis of erythema multiforme is made on the basis of the clinical features and the exclusion of other diseases; the microscopic appearance is nonspecific. Biopsy and microscopic examinations are helpful in some cases for excluding other diseases with similar clinical features but more distinctive microscopic features.

TREATMENT AND PROGNOSIS

If a cause can be identified, first remove the cause if possible. Topical corticosteroids may be helpful in mild cases of erythema multiforme, but systemic corticosteroid treatment is usually needed. Systemic antiviral medication is used in some cases to attempt to decrease recurrent episodes that are suspected of being stimulated by an HSV infection.

FIGURE 3-12 ■ Skin lesions of erythema multiforme. **A,** Target lesion *(arrow).* **B,** Bullae. (**A,** Courtesy Dr. Edward V. Zegarelli.)

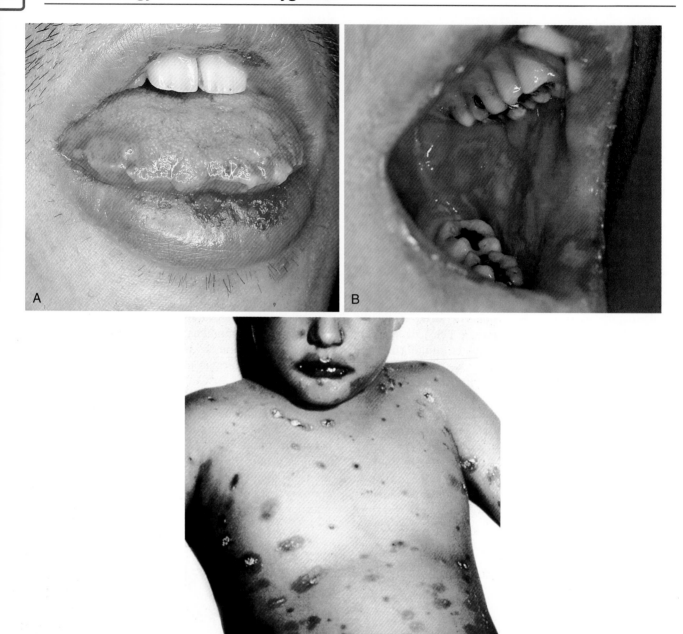

FIGURE 3-13 ■ Oral lesions of erythema multiforme. **A,** Crusted lip lesions with edema, ulceration, and erythema. **B,** Erythematous and ulcerated lesions of the lips and buccal mucosa. **C,** Stevens-Johnson syndrome. (**C,** Courtesy Dr. Sidney Eisig.)

LICHEN PLANUS

Lichen planus is a benign, chronic disease affecting the skin and oral mucosa. In some patients this disease may affect both the skin and the oral mucosa; in others either oral mucosa or skin alone may be affected.

The classic appearance of lichen planus affecting the oral mucosa is an arrangement of interconnecting white lines and circles (sometimes referred to as a lacelike pattern) (Figure 3-14). The slender white lines are called *Wickham striae*. The fundamental lesion is a small, papular, pinhead-sized, domed or hemispheric, glistening white nodule on the mucosa. The clinical appearance depends on the arrangement of these minute papules and striae. The most common location is the buccal mucosa. However, lichen planus also occurs on the tongue, lips, floor of the mouth, and gingiva. Lesions of lichen planus are frequently distributed symmetrically in the oral cavity.

The prevalence of lichen planus in the general population of the United States has been reported to be about 1%, with individuals ranging in age from 13 to 78 years. The disease is most common in middle age and has a slight female predilection. Most cases are asymptomatic, discovered on routine oral examination. There are also skin lesions.

FIGURE 3-14 ■ **A** and **B,** Two examples of the oral lesions of lichen planus. **C,** The plaquelike lesions on the tongue of a patient with lichen planus. (**A,** Courtesy Dr. Edward V. Zegarelli.)

Many factors have been implicated in lichen planus; however, the cause remains unknown. Erosive lesions tend to worsen with emotional stress. Many drugs and chemicals have been shown to produce lichenoid lesions (lesions that resemble lichen planus), but these have a different microscopic appearance from true lichen planus.

TYPES OF LICHEN PLANUS

Several forms of lichen planus have been described. The most common form is **reticular lichen planus.** In this form oral lesions are composed of Wickham striae along with slightly raised white plaquelike areas that do not rub off. The raised lines of Wickham striae are composed of 2- to 4-mm papules that, strung together, form the raised lines of Wickham striae. Plaquelike lesions are sometimes seen on the tongue of patients with lichen planus (Figure 3-14, *C*).

Erosive lichen planus and **bullous lichen planus** are those forms in which the epithelium separates from the connective tissue, resulting in erosions, bullae, or ulcers. These forms are less common (Figure 3-15). The striated lesions commonly occur on the buccal mucosa and may also occur on other mucosal tissue and the lips. Lichen planus can also present with gingival lesions that are clinically described as **desquamative gingivitis** (Figure 3-16).

With the skin lesions of lichen planus, itching or pruritus may be present. Scaly purplish lesions can occur anywhere on the skin, but the most common sites are the lumbar region, the flexor surfaces of the wrist and elbow, and the

FIGURE 3-15 ■ Erosive lichen planus on the buccal mucosa.

anterior surface of the ankles (Figure 3-17). Some patients with lichen planus have only skin lesions, some have only oral lesions, and others have both skin and oral lesions.

DIAGNOSIS

The diagnosis of lichen planus is made on the basis of both the distinctive clinical features and the microscopic

FIGURE 3-16 ■ Desquamative gingivitis seen in lichen planus. (Courtesy Dr. Edward V. Zegarelli.)

FIGURE 3-17 ■ Skin lesions of lichen planus presenting as scaly purplish lesions.

FIGURE 3-18 ■ Microscopic appearance of lichen planus. Degeneration of the basal cell layer of the epithelium (B) and the bandlike infiltrate of lymphocytes (L).

appearance of the tissue obtained through scalpel biopsy (Figure 3-18). The epithelium is generally parakeratotic and may be either hyperplastic or atrophic. The characteristic microscopic features include degeneration of the basal cell layer of the epithelium in small-to-extensive areas, sawtooth-shaped rete ridges, and a broad band of lymphocytes in the connective tissue immediately subjacent to the degenerated basal cell layer epithelium.

In erosive areas the separation of the epithelium from the connective tissue occurs at the interface of the epithelium and connective tissue. Epithelial atypia and dysplasia may also occur in lesions that appear clinically as lichen planus, and it has been suggested that these lesions may be premalignant.

TREATMENT AND PROGNOSIS

Lichen planus is a chronic disease. Treatment is indicated only when lesions are symptomatic. Erosive lesions usually respond quickly when topical corticosteroid medication is applied. Improvement of gingival lesions with meticulous oral hygiene has been reported. If a drug can be identified as the causative agent of lichenoid-appearing lesions, discontinuation of the drug should cause the lesions to disappear. However, at times it is not possible to discontinue the drug.

Research has been reported that suggests that patients with lichen planus, especially the erosive form, may be at increased risk for the development of squamous cell carcinoma. Therefore regular oral soft tissue examination and biopsy of any lesions not consistent with lichen planus are recommended.

REACTIVE ARTHRITIS (REITER SYNDROME)

Reactive arthritis, or Reiter syndrome, is a chronic disease that classically comprises the triad of three features: (1) arthritis, (2) urethritis, and (3) conjunctivitis.

All the components of the syndrome may not be present with a case of reactive arthritis but polyarthritis is generally the most prominent component of this syndrome. The cause of this syndrome is not clear; no infectious organisms can be identified. An antigenic marker called HLA-B27 is present in most patients with reactive arthritis, suggesting a strong genetic influence. An abnormal immune response to a microbial antigen is considered the most likely mechanism of occurrence. Reactive arthritis is far more prevalent in men than in women.

Reactive arthritis characteristically develops 1 to 4 weeks after sexually transmitted or gastrointestinal infection and is usually benign and self-limited. The arthritis of this condition usually involves the joints of the lower extremities such as the knees and ankles and may be asymmetric and migratory, chronic or recurrent.

Radiographically, a periosteal proliferation can be detected on the heels, ankles, metatarsals, phalanges, knees, and elbows. Fever, malaise, and weight loss may be associated with the arthritis; the urethritis usually precedes the other lesions. The conjunctivitis is usually mild, but some individuals experience iritis or inflammation of the iris.

Skin and mucous membrane lesions are seen in many patients with reactive arthritis. Oral lesions occur almost anywhere in the oral cavity (Figure 3-19). Aphthous-like ulcers, erythematous lesions, and areas of depapillation of the dorsal surface of the tongue that mimic geographic

FIGURE 3-19 ■ Reactive arthritis. **A,** Ulcerative lesions on the palate. **B,** Lesion on the tongue.

tongue have been described in patients with reactive arthritis.

DIAGNOSIS

The diagnosis of reactive arthritis is made on the basis of the clinical signs and symptoms along with identification of the HLA-B27 antigenic marker.

TREATMENT AND PROGNOSIS

Reactive arthritis lasts from weeks to months. During that time, the patient may experience spontaneous remission, but recurrent attacks are common. Aspirin or other nonsteroidal antiinflammatory drugs are generally used for treatment as well as antibiotics for possible coexistent infection. Physical therapy may help to reduce the arthritis.

LANGERHANS CELL HISTIOCYTOSIS (LANGERHANS CELL DISEASE)

Langerhans cell histiocytosis (LCH), formerly called *histiocytosis X,* is a group of rare disorders characterized by the presence of both Langerhans cells and eosinophils. Langerhans cells are not histiocytes or macrophages, and therefore these diseases are also called **Langerhans cell disease.** There are three main forms of LCH: (1) acute disseminated form (Letterer-Siwe disease), (2) chronic disseminated or multifocal form (Hand-Schüller-Christian disease), and (3) solitary eosinophilic granuloma. Langerhans cells were originally called *histiocytes* and were responsible for the past name of these diseases. In all three disorders the proliferating cell is the Langerhans cell (Figure 3-20).

The Langerhans cell is an immunologically competent cell of the mononuclear phagocyte series and participates

FIGURE 3-20 ■ Langerhans cell histiocytosis (Langerhans cell disease) microscopic appearance (high magnification) with a combination of Langerhans cells and eosinophils.

in cell-mediated immunity. The cause and pathogenesis of Langerhans cell histiocytosis remain unclear; a reactive process, a primary immunodeficiency disease, and a neoplastic process have all been suggested. The presence of eosinophils is thought to result from the production of an eosinophilic chemotactic factor produced by the Langerhans cell.

Letterer-Siwe disease is the acute disseminated form that usually affects children younger than 3 years of age. The course of the disease is usually so rapid that significant oral involvement does not often occur. The disease resembles a lymphoma in that it generally has a rapidly fatal course that may, in some cases, respond to chemotherapy.

FIGURE 3-21 ■ Langerhans cell histiocytosis (Langerhans cell disease): chronic disseminated form also known as Hand-Schüller-Christian disease. **A,** Skull radiograph. **B,** Ulcerated lesion of the mandible. (Courtesy Dr. Sidney Eisig.)

FIGURE 3-22 ■ Langerhans cell histiocytosis (Langerhans cell disease) in the solitary or chronic localized form of an eosinophilic granuloma, showing a well-circumscribed radiolucency. (Courtesy Drs. Paul Freedman and Stanley Kerpel.)

Hand-Schüller-Christian disease is the chronic disseminated or multifocal form. It occurs in children, usually younger than 5 years of age. A classic triad is seen in about 25% of patients. All changes are caused by localized collections of Langerhans cells. The triad includes single to multiple, well-defined or "punched-out" radiolucent areas of the skull (especially in the jawbones) that are caused by collections of macrophages in the sella turcica area, affecting the pituitary gland (Figure 3-21, *A*). In addition, unilateral or bilateral exophthalmos and diabetes insipidus may be present.

Oral manifestations of the chronic disseminated form of the disease include erythema of the oral mucosa with or without ulcerative lesions, and halitosis. Other oral manifestations include gingivitis, an unpleasant taste in the mouth, mobile and sensitive teeth, early exfoliation of teeth, and nonhealing extraction sites. A characteristic loss of supporting alveolar bone occurs, mimicking advanced periodontal disease (Figure 3-21, *B*).

The **eosinophilic granuloma of bone** is the solitary or chronic localized form. It affects mainly older children and young adults, with males affected twice as commonly as females. The skull and its mandible are typically involved with eosinophilic granuloma. The radiographic appearance varies, and the lesion may resemble periodontal disease or periapical inflammatory disease; or it may appear as a

well-circumscribed radiolucency with or without a sclerotic border (Figure 3-22). Cases of multifocal eosinophilic granuloma have also been reported.

TREATMENT AND PROGNOSIS

Eosinophilic granuloma is treated by conservative surgical excision; recurrence is rare. Low-dose radiation therapy may also be used for treatment of severe and persistent cases.

AUTOIMMUNE DISEASES WITH ORAL MANIFESTATIONS

Several autoimmune diseases affect the oral cavity (Table 3-5). In this type of disease tissue damage occurs because the immune system treats the person's own cells and tissue types as antigens. It is important to note that an individual with one autoimmune disease has an increased risk of developing another, so dental personnel must keep a patient's medical history current and ask for a medical consultation if warranted.

SJÖGREN SYNDROME

Sjögren syndrome is an autoimmune disease that affects the salivary and lacrimal glands, resulting in a decrease in

TABLE 3-5

Autoimmune Diseases with Oral Manifestations

DISEASE	ORAL MANIFESTATION
Sjögren syndrome	Xerostomia and parotid gland enlargement
Systemic lupus erythematosus	White erosive oral lesions
Pemphigus vulgaris	Mucosal ulceration with bullae
Benign mucous membrane pemphigoid	Mucosal ulceration and desquamative gingivitis
Behçet syndrome	Aphthous-like ulcers
Pernicious anemia*	Mucosal atrophy and ulceration with loss of both filiform and fungiform lingual papillae

*Described in Chapter 9.

FIGURE 3-23 ■ Sjögren syndrome with severe xerostomia and a lack of papillae on the dorsal tongue.

saliva and tears. This combination of dry mouth and dry eyes with Sjögren syndrome is also called **sicca syndrome** (*sicca,* dry). Decreased salivary flow, or **hyposalivation,** results in dry mouth, or **xerostomia;** decreased lacrimal flow results in dry eyes **(xerophthalmia)** with resultant damage to the eyes **(keratoconjunctivitis sicca).** The specific cause of Sjögren syndrome is not known. Both cellular and humoral immunity are involved in the pathogenesis.

In some patients only the mouth and eyes are involved. In others the autoimmune process can be more extensive. Salivary and lacrimal gland involvement without the presence of another autoimmune disease, is considered **primary Sjögren syndrome.** When another autoimmune disease accompanies salivary and lacrimal gland involvement, the combination is considered **secondary Sjögren syndrome.** About 50% of individuals with Sjögren syndrome have another autoimmune disease.

The oral manifestation of Sjögren syndrome is xerostomia (dry mouth), which occurs as a result of hyposalivation (decreased salivary flow) and causes the mucosa to become erythematous. Patients have oral discomfort and lack of saliva causes the mouth to feel sticky. Lips are cracked and dry, and a generalized loss of both filiform and fungiform papillae occurs on the dorsal surface of the tongue (Figure 3-23). Patients with xerostomia are at high risk for the development of caries, periodontal disease, and oral candidiasis.

Both major and minor salivary glands are affected. Parotid salivary gland enlargement, usually bilateral and symmetric, occurs in about 50% of the patients (Figure 3-24). The characteristic microscopic appearance of these enlarged parotid glands consists of replacement of the glands by lymphocytes, and changes in the epithelium of the ducts that appear as islands of epithelium (epimyoepithelial islands). Biopsy of the minor salivary glands is sometimes performed to assist in the diagnosis of Sjögren syndrome. The minor glands show aggregates of lymphocytes surrounding the salivary gland ducts (Figure 3-25).

In addition to the oral findings, patients with decreased lacrimal flow experience xerophthalmia causing burning

FIGURE 3-24 ■ Bilateral parotid gland enlargement seen in Sjögren syndrome. (Courtesy Dr. Louis Mandel.)

FIGURE 3-25 ■ Microscopic appearance (high magnification) of a minor salivary gland in Sjögren syndrome, showing aggregates of lymphocytes surrounding the salivary gland ducts. (Courtesy Dr. Harry Lumerman.)

and itching of the eyes and photophobia (abnormal visual intolerance of light). Severe ocular involvement may lead to keratoconjunctivitis sicca with ulceration and opacification of the cornea.

In some patients with Sjögren syndrome the **Raynaud phenomenon,** a disorder affecting the fingers and toes, may also occur. Both cold and emotional stress tend to trigger the reaction, which is characterized by an initial pallor of the skin that results from vasoconstriction and reduced blood flow. The initial pallor is followed by cyanosis, which occurs because of the decreased blood flow. When the skin is rewarmed, the blood vessels dilate, and the hyperemia results in a reddening of the skin. Finally, in minutes to hours the color returns to normal. The Raynaud phenomenon can occur alone or in association with autoimmune diseases other than Sjögren syndrome. Patients with Sjögren syndrome may also have myalgia (muscle pain or tenderness), arthralgia (joint pain), and chronic fatigue.

Laboratory abnormalities are important in the diagnosis of Sjögren syndrome. A positive result for **rheumatoid factor,** a serum antibody to IgG (i.e., an antibody to an antibody), is found in 90% of patients with Sjögren syndrome. Rheumatoid factor is also found in patients with other autoimmune diseases such as rheumatoid arthritis. **Autoantibodies,** called *anti–Sjögren syndrome A* and *anti–Sjögren syndrome B*, are also found in patients with Sjögren syndrome. Other laboratory abnormalities include mild anemia, a decreased white blood cell count, an elevated erythrocyte sedimentation rate, and a diffuse elevation of serum immunoglobulins.

DIAGNOSIS

The diagnosis of Sjögren syndrome is made when at least two of its three components are present: (1) xerostomia, (2) keratoconjunctivitis sicca, and (3) rheumatoid arthritis or another autoimmune disease. Xerostomia can result from conditions other than autoimmune disease, such as with many prescribed medications. Measurement of stimulated and unstimulated salivary flow and biopsy of minor salivary glands can be helpful in the diagnosis of Sjögren syndrome (see Figure 3-25). In addition, a characteristic pattern is seen in a parotid gland sialogram, with its pattern reflecting a lack of functioning glandular elements (Figure 3-26).

Keratoconjunctivitis is confirmed by eye examination. Lacrimal flow is measured using filter paper, but special examination techniques are necessary to demonstrate the corneal erosions.

TREATMENT AND PROGNOSIS

Sjögren syndrome is usually treated symptomatically. Nonsteroidal antiinflammatory agents are used for the arthritis; in severe cases corticosteroids and other immunosuppressive drugs may be necessary. Saliva substitutes are helpful, and for some patients the use of a humidifier at night makes the xerostomia more tolerable. Pilocarpine has been used to attempt to increase salivary flow in some patients. Sugarless gum or lozenges may be used to stimulate saliva production. However, the greater the destruction of salivary gland tissue,

FIGURE 3-26 ■ Sialogram of the parotid gland in Sjögren syndrome. (Courtesy Dr. Louis Mandel.)

the less saliva will be stimulated. An "artificial tears" formula containing methylcellulose helps to protect the eye from the drying effects of the disease. Glasses provide shielding and are helpful to minimize the drying effects of wind.

Maintaining good oral hygiene and using fluoride toothpaste and rinses can minimize the effects of xerostomia, as does the use of xylitol and remineralizing compounds. The interval between recall appointments should be sufficiently short to ensure early detection and treatment of root caries. The toothbrush and other oral hygiene aids may need modification if arthritis affects the movement of hands and arms.

For most patients the course of the disease is chronic and benign. However, patients are at risk for the development of other, more serious autoimmune diseases, such as lupus erythematosus, and for lymphoma and Waldenström macroglobulinemia, a disorder characterized by a high concentration of IgM in serum. Therefore, patients with Sjögren syndrome should be closely monitored by a physician.

SYSTEMIC LUPUS ERYTHEMATOSUS

Systemic lupus erythematosus (SLE) is an acute and chronic inflammatory autoimmune disease of unknown cause.

Systemic lupus erythematosus affects women eight times more frequently than men, predominantly during the childbearing years. It occurs three times more frequently in black women than in white women. SLE is a syndrome rather than a specific disease entity and includes a wide spectrum of disease activity and signs and symptoms that range from lesions confined to the skin, such as discoid lupus erythematosus, to a widespread, debilitating, life-threatening disease with multiple organ involvement. SLE is usually chronic and progressive, with periods of remission and exacerbation.

Both cellular and humoral immunity are impaired in SLE. It has been suggested that cellular immunity is mainly affected, resulting in deregulation of humoral immunity. Antigen-antibody complexes are deposited in various organs and stimulate an inflammatory response, which may be responsible for the tissue damage that occurs in SLE. Autoantibodies to the patient's DNA (anti-nuclear antibodies) are present in serum. These circulating antibodies are responsible for the positive anti-nuclear antibody and lupus erythematosus laboratory test results. Production of these antibodies is enhanced by estrogen. Antibodies to lymphocytes are present in some patients. Evidence exists for a genetic component in the pathogenesis of SLE as well as for changes in levels of circulating neutrophils (neutropenia).

Skin lesions are among the most common signs of the disease (Figure 3-27). The most common skin lesion is an erythematous rash involving areas of the body exposed to sunlight; the classic "butterfly" rash occurs over the bridge of the nose, and there may be erythematous lesions on the fingertips. The lesions can heal with scarring in the center as they continue to spread at the periphery. They tend to worsen when exposed to sunlight. Atrophy and hypopigmentation or hyperpigmentation can follow these lesions. Other skin lesions such as bullae, purpura, a discoid rash, vitiligo, or subcutaneous nodules can also occur.

Arthritis and arthralgia are common manifestations of SLE. Any joint can be involved, and symptoms resemble rheumatoid arthritis but without severe deformities. The Raynaud phenomenon occurs in 15% of patients. Myalgia and myositis (inflammation of muscle) also occur. A retinal vasculitis causes degeneration of the nerve fiber layer of the retina and can cause loss of vision. Psychoses and depression are signs of central nervous system involvement, and seizures can be present. Involvement of the pleura may cause shortness of breath and chest pain. Pericarditis, cardiac arrhythmias, and endocarditis may be seen late in the disease. Kidney involvement is common. Thrombocytopenia may also occur in patients with SLE.

Oral lesions accompany skin lesions in about 25% of patients with discoid lupus erythematosus, which is the mildest form of this autoimmune disease. Oral lesions appear as erythematous plaques or erosions. White striae radiating from the center of the lesion are usually present. The lesions may resemble lichen planus but are less symmetric in their distribution. The involvement of the oral mucosa in this disease is usually mild (Figure 3-28). Petechiae and gingival bleeding may be present in patients with severe thrombocytopenia. Sjögren syndrome may be present in some patients with SLE.

DIAGNOSIS

The diagnosis of systemic lupus erythematosus is usually based on the classic multiorgan involvement and the presence of anti-nuclear antibodies in serum. **LE cells,** mature neutrophils that have phagocytized spherical inclusions derived from other neutrophils, may be identified in circulating blood. However, the diagnosis of SLE is difficult if the onset is slow and insidious.

The microscopic appearance of oral lesions resembles that of lichen planus because it also involves destruction of the basal cells. However, the inflammatory infiltrate is distributed around blood vessels in the connective tissue rather than in a subepithelial band. In addition, direct immunofluorescence and immunohistochemical testing of skin and mucosal lesions shows granular and linear deposits of immunoglobulins along the basement membrane area.

FIGURE 3-27 ■ **A** and **B,** Skin lesions of lupus erythematosus. (**B,** Courtesy Dr. Edward V. Zegarelli.)

FIGURE 3-28 ■ **A** and **B,** Oral lesions of lupus erythematosus.

TREATMENT AND PROGNOSIS

Once the diagnosis of systemic lupus erythematosus is made, the decision as to whether treatment is indicated depends on the degree of disease activity. This once-fatal disease is now managed with several drugs. Aspirin and nonsteroidal antiinflammatory agents are used for mild signs and symptoms. Hydroxychloroquine, an antimalarial agent, and corticosteroids combined with other immunosuppressive agents such as azathioprine and cyclophosphamide are also used.

If the course of the disease is mild and only a few organs are involved, the prognosis is excellent; however, the disease can also be fatal. Kidney involvement can be associated with severe hypertension and rapid onset of renal failure, which is a cause of death in patients with SLE. Other common causes of death include hemorrhage secondary to thrombocytopenia, nervous system involvement, and infection.

SLE is an extremely complex disease. A medical consultation may be needed before dental treatment to identify the extent of systemic involvement and to clarify which drugs should be used for treatment.

PEMPHIGUS VULGARIS

Pemphigus vulgaris is a severe, progressive autoimmune disease that affects both the skin and mucous membranes. Pemphigus vulgaris is characterized by intraepithelial vesicle formation that results from breakdown of the cellular adhesion between epithelial cells. This type of epithelial cell separation is called **acantholysis.** The patient with pemphigus vulgaris has circulating autoantibodies that are reactive against components of the epithelial cell attachment mechanism. The higher the titer of circulating antibodies, the greater the epithelial destruction. These autoantibodies are also found in surrounding epithelial cells. *Pemphigus vulgaris* is the type of pemphigus seen most frequently. Three other forms of pemphigus are *pemphigus vegetans, pemphigus foliaceus,* and *pemphigus erythematosus.* These are much rarer conditions overall, but all are characterized by epithelial acantholysis (breakdown of cellular adhesion within the prickle cell layer of the epithelium).

No gender predilection exists. A broad age range has been reported, including both children and elderly individuals, with most cases occurring between age 40 and 50. Genetic and ethnic factors have been reported;. It is a relatively rare condition. Pemphigus vulgaris is often present in Ashkenazi Jews.

In more than 50% of cases of pemphigus vulgaris the first signs of disease occur in the oral cavity; oral lesions can precede cutaneous lesions by many months. The appearance of oral lesions ranges from shallow ulcers to fragile vesicles or bullae. Because the bullae are so fragile, they rupture soon after they form; the detached epithelium remains as a gray membrane (Figure 3-29). The ulcers are painful and range in size from small to very large. Gentle finger pressure with movement on clinically normal mucosa can produce a cleavage in the epithelium and result in the formation of a bulla. This is called the **Nikolsky sign.**

Skin lesions in pemphigus vulgaris include erythema, vesicles, bullae, erosions, and ulcers. Microscopically, the tissue shows an intact basal layer of epithelium attached to the underlying connective tissue (Figure 3-30). The loss of attachment between the epithelial cells results in detached cells that appear rounded. These rounded, acantholytic cells are **Tzanck cells,** and are present in the area of separation. Tzanck cells may also be seen on cytologic smear, but the diagnosis must be confirmed by biopsy.

FIGURE 3-29 ■ **A-C,** Oral lesions in pemphigus vulgaris. (**B,** Courtesy Dr. Fariba Younai; **C,** courtesy Dr. Sidney Eisig.)

DIAGNOSIS

The diagnosis of pemphigus vulgaris is made by biopsy, and microscopic examinations. Direct or indirect immunofluorescence is also used in the diagnosis. Direct immunofluorescence is performed on biopsy tissue and identifies autoantibodies present in the tissue. The tissue is viewed through a special microscope, with fluorescence seen surrounding the cells in the prickle cell layer. The tissue must be placed in a different fixative solution than tissue submitted for routine microscopic examination, and is usually sent to a specialized laboratory. In indirect immunofluorescence the patient's serum is used to detect the presence of circulating autoantibodies. These circulating autoantibodies are present in 80% of patients with pemphigus vulgaris, and therefore this is a very useful diagnostic test for this disease.

TREATMENT AND PROGNOSIS

The treatment of pemphigus vulgaris generally involves high doses of corticosteroids, often in combination with

FIGURE 3-30 ■ Microscopic appearance of pemphigus vulgaris (low magnification), showing acantholysis of the epithelium and the intact basal layer attached to the connective tissue.

other immunosuppressive drugs such as azathioprine and methotrexate. The amount of autoantibodies present in the patient's serum correlates with the severity of lesions; therefore the concentration (titer) of autoantibodies is used to determine disease activity and response to the drug therapy.

Pemphigus vulgaris was at one time a life-threatening disease. The mortality rate is now about 8 to 10% within the first 5 years and is related to the complications of corticosteroid treatment rather than to the disease itself. As with other autoimmune diseases, patients with pemphigus vulgaris may develop another autoimmune disease.

MUCOUS MEMBRANE PEMPHIGOID

Mucous membrane pemphigoid, also known as **cicatricial pemphigoid** and **benign mucous membrane pemphigoid,** is a chronic autoimmune disease that affects the oral mucosa, conjunctiva, genital mucosa, and skin. Mucous membrane pemphigoid is not as severe a disease as pemphigus vulgaris. However, lesions may heal with scarring,. The name *cicatricial pemphigoid* refers to this healing with scarring. Autoantibodies and complement components have been identified at the basement membrane of the epithelium. Lesions occur as a result of cleavage of the epithelium from the underlying connective tissue in this area.

The most common site for oral mucous membrane pemphigoid lesions is the gingiva. The gingival lesions have been called *desquamative gingivitis* (Figure 3-31). The appearance ranges from erythema to ulceration and involves both the marginal and attached gingiva. However, desquamative gingivitis is a clinical and descriptive term, and similar lesions can be seen in lichen planus and pemphigus vulgaris. In this disease, as in pemphigus vulgaris, a Nikolsky sign can be produced on normal-appearing tissue by gentle friction. Bullae, erosions, and ulcers can also occur in other locations in the oral cavity. The bullae of mucous membrane pemphigoid are thick-walled, much less fragile, and persist longer than those of pemphigus vulgaris.

DIAGNOSIS

The diagnosis of mucous membrane pemphigoid is made by biopsy and microscopic examination. On microscopic examination the epithelium appears to separate from the connective tissue at the basement membrane, with no degeneration of the basal cells of the epithelium as in lichen planus or acantholysis as in pemphigus vulgaris (Figure 3-32). An inflammatory infiltrate, usually including prominent plasma cells and eosinophils, is seen in the connective tissue. In mucous membrane pemphigoid, direct immunofluorescence shows a linear pattern of fluorescence at the basement membrane. Indirect immunofluorescence, identifying autoantibodies in serum, is usually not helpful in the diagnosis of mucous membrane pemphigoid.

TREATMENT AND PROGNOSIS

Mucous membrane pemphigoid is a chronic disease that follows a benign course. Gingival involvement can occur alone, or more extensive lesions can be present elsewhere on the body such as the eyes. Topical corticosteroid application is helpful in the management of mild cases. In more severe cases high doses of systemic corticosteroids may be necessary. The disease may be difficult to control and slow to respond to therapy.

Patients may experience episodes of exacerbation followed by periods of remission. An ophthalmologic consultation to rule out the presence of ocular lesions should be done in all patients diagnosed with oral lesions of mucous membrane pemphigoid.

BULLOUS PEMPHIGOID

Some investigators have suggested that bullous and mucous membrane pemphigoid are variants of a single disease. However, differences exist between the two diseases that make this inference questionable.

Most patients with bullous pemphigoid are older than age 60, and no gender predilection exists. Oral lesions are less common in bullous pemphigoid than in mucous membrane pemphigoid, occurring in only about one-third of patients. When they occur, the gingival lesions are very similar to those of mucous membrane pemphigoid, and other mucosal lesions are more extensive and painful.

FIGURE 3-31 ■ Desquamative gingivitis in mucous membrane pemphigoid. (Courtesy Dr. Victor M. Sternberg.)

FIGURE 3-32 ■ Microscopic appearance of mucous membrane pemphigoid (low magnification), showing a separation of the epithelium from the connective tissue at the basement membrane area.

DIAGNOSIS

As in mucous membrane pemphigoid, the microscopic appearance of bullous pemphigoid shows a cleavage of the epithelium from the connective tissue at the basement membrane. Unlike mucous membrane pemphigoid, in bullous pemphigoid circulating autoantibodies are usually detectable; and unlike pemphigus vulgaris, the circulating autoantibodies do not correlate with disease activity.

TREATMENT AND PROGNOSIS

High doses of systemic corticosteroids and nonsteroidal antiinflammatory drugs are used in the management of bullous pemphigoid. The disease is chronic, with periods of remission, and is usually not life-threatening.

BEHÇET SYNDROME

Behçet syndrome is a chronic, recurrent autoimmune disease consisting mainly of oral ulcers, genital ulcers, and ocular inflammation and skin lesions.

With Behçet syndrome, no gender predilection exists and the mean age of onset is 30 years. There is an increased prevalence of this syndrome in individuals from the Mediterranean region and Asia, but it is rare in the United States. Evidence for an immunologic pathogenesis includes the identification of antibodies to human mucosa in patients with Behçet syndrome and the association between Behçet syndrome HLA-B5 and HLA-B51. Most symptoms of the disorder are caused by inflammation of the blood vessels.

The oral ulcers that occur in Behçet syndrome are very similar in appearance to aphthous ulcers (Figure 3-33). They are painful and recurrent and range in size from 1 mm to 2 cm. The genital ulcers are usually small, and the ocular lesions usually begin with photophobia and can develop into conjunctivitis and uveitis. The skin lesions show a papular pattern of pustules and are most common on the trunk, genitals, and limbs.

DIAGNOSIS

The diagnosis of Behçet syndrome requires that two of the three principal manifestations be present: (1) oral ulcers, (2) genital ulcers, and (3) ocular inflammation. A pustular lesion that develops after a needle puncture, such as with local anesthesia administration in the oral cavity, is highly suggestive of Behçet syndrome.

TREATMENT AND PROGNOSIS

Systemic and topical corticosteroids as well as immuno-suppressive drugs are used in the management of Behçet syndrome. Chlorambucil is used for the ocular lesions; occasionally other immunosuppressive drugs are needed. Behçet disease is a lifelong disorder with a series of remissions and exacerbations.

SELECTED REFERENCES

Books

Cawson RA: *Essentials of oral pathology and oral medicine,* ed 8, Philadelphia, 2008, Churchill Livingstone.

Bath-Balogh M, Fehrenbach MJ: *Illustrated dental embryology, histology, and anatomy,* ed 3, St. Louis, 2011, Saunders.

Fehrenbach MJ, Herring SW: *Illustrated anatomy of the head and neck,* ed 4, St. Louis, 2012, Saunders.

Fehrenbach MJ, Weiner J: *Saunders review of dental hygiene,* ed 2, St. Louis, 2009, Saunders.

Kumar V, Cotran RS, Robbins SL: *Robbins basic pathology,* ed 9, Philadelphia, 2013, Saunders.

McCance K, Huether S: *Pathophysiology,* ed 6, St. Louis, 2010, Mosby.

Neville BW, Damm DD, Allen CM, et al: *Oral and maxillofacial pathology,* ed 3, St. Louis, 2009, Saunders.

Parham P: *The immune system,* ed 3, New York, 2009, Garland Science.

Journal Articles
Immunity

Chaplin DD: Part 1. Overview of the human immune response, *J Allergy Clin Immunol* 117(2 Suppl Mini-Primer):S430, 2006.

Eisenstein M: Vaccines: a moving target, *Nature* 474:S16, 2011.

Grivennikov SI, Greten FR, Karin M: Immunity, inflammation, and cancer, *Cell* 140:883, 2010.

Yamanaka N: Moving towards a new era in the research of tonsils and mucosal barriers, *Adv Otorhinolaryngol* 72:6, 2011.

Immunologic Oral Lesions

Al-Johani KA, Fedele S, Porter SR: Erythema multiforme and related disorders, *Oral Surg Oral Med Oral Pathol Oral Radiol Endod* 103:642, 2007.

Bosch X: Systemic lupus erythematosus and the neutrophil, *N Engl J Med* 365:758, 2011.

Chavan M, Jain H, Diwan N, et al: Recurrent aphthous stomatitis: a review, *J Oral Pathol Med* 418:577, 2012.

Epstein JB, Wan LS, Gorsky M, et al: Oral lichen planus: progress in understanding its malignant potential and the implications for clinical management, *Oral Surg Oral Med Oral Pathol Oral Radiol Endod* 96:32, 2003.

Konidena A, Pavani BV: Hepatitis C virus infection in patients with oral lichen planus, *Niger J Clin Pract* 14:228, 2011.

Mockenhaupt M: The current understanding of Stevens-Johnson syndrome and toxic epidermal necrolysis, *Expert Rev Clin Immunol* 7:803, 2011.

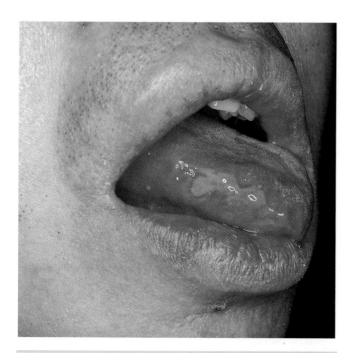

FIGURE 3-33 ▪ Aphthous-like ulcer on the tongue in Behçet syndrome.

Iwai S, Sueki H, Watanabe H, et al: Distinguishing between erythema multiforme major and Stevens-Johnson syndrome/toxic epidermal necrolysis immunopathologically, *J Dermatol* 39:1, 2012.

Tasher D, Somekh E, Dalal I: PFAPA syndrome: new clinical aspects disclosed, *Arch Dis Child* 91:981, 2006.

Wolf R, Lipozencic J: Shape and configuration of skin lesions: targetoid lesions, *Clin Dermatol* 29:504, 2011.

Websites

Centers for Disease Control and Prevention. Frequently asked questions about multiple vaccinations and the immune system. Available at http://www.cdc.gov/vaccinesafety/Vaccines/multiplevaccines.html

Grivennikov SI, Greten FR, Karin M: Immunity, inflammation, and cancer, *Cell* 140:883, 2010. Available at http://www.ncbi.nlm.nih.gov/pubmed/20303878

Medscape: Aphthous stomatitis. Available at http://emedicine.medscape.com/article/1075570-overview

Midgley A, McLaren Z, Moots RJ, et al: The role of neutrophil apoptosis in juvenile-onset systemic lupus erythematosus, *Arthritis Rheum* 60:2390, 2009. Available at http://onlinelibrary.wiley.com/doi/10.1002/art.24634/full

National Institute of Arthritis and Musculoskeletal and Skin Diseases: Understanding autoinflammatory diseases. Available at http://www.niams.nih.gov/Health_Info/Autoinflammatory/default.asp

Review Questions

1. The immune system usually defends the body against foreign substances that are called
  A. Plasma cells
  B. Antibodies
  C. Antigens
  D. Lymphocytes

2. Memory is an important function of the immune system because it
  A. Retains the memory of the antibody
  B. Allows faster future immune responses
  C. Allows faster inflammatory responses
  D. Weakens future immune responses

3. Immunization with a vaccine works by
  A. Increasing the risk of an antigen-causing disease
  B. Using antibodies produced by another person
  C. Passing antibodies from the mother to the fetus
  D. Producing active acquired immunity

4. Which of the following is an important fact about the B-cell lymphocyte?
  A. It is derived from a precursor stem cell.
  B. It matures and resides in the thymus.
  C. It is produced from plasma cells.
  D. It is active in foreign substance surveillance.

5. A macrophage is a cell of the immune system that
  A. Retains a memory of an encountered antigen
  B. Produces antibodies
  C. Undergoes B-cell phagocytosis initially during inflammation
  D. Can be activated by lymphokines

6. Which statement is *correct* when applied to natural killer cells?
  A. They do not circulate within the body.
  B. They secrete antibodies.
  C. They are part of the body's innate immunity.
  D. They are a type of T-cell lymphocyte.

7. In which type of immunopathology are the cells of the body no longer tolerated and treated by the immune system as antigens?
  A. Hypersensitivity
  B. Immunodeficiency
  C. Hyperplasia
  D. Autoimmune disease

8. During the anaphylactic type of hypersensitivity reaction, the plasma cells
  A. Produce antibody called IgE
  B. React with lymphocytes
  C. Combine with antigen
  D. Form immune complexes with antigen

9. Which type of hypersensitivity reaction involves activated complement?
  A. Type I
  B. Cytotoxic
  C. Type III
  D. Anaphylactic

10. What type of lymphocyte matures in the thymus, produces lymphokines, and can increase or suppress humoral immunity?
  A. T-cell lymphocyte
  B. Plasma cell
  C. Natural killer cell
  D. Macrophage

11. In the immune system, antibodies are proteins that are
  A. Also called immunoglobulins
  B. Also called cytokines
  C. Directly produced by lymphocytes
  D. Directly produced from mast cells

12. Which of the following types of immunologic disease involve a decreased number or activity of lymphoid cells?
  A. Autoimmune
  B. Hypersensitivity
  C. Immunodeficiency
  D. Reactive hyperplasia

Review Questions—cont'd

13. Humoral immunity involves the production of
    A. Antigens
    B. Antibodies
    C. Autoimmune cells
    D. Toxins

14. The laboratory measurement of a specific antibody level in the blood is called
    A. Phagocytosis
    B. Immunization
    C. Titer
    D. Pavementing

15. Which type of immunity may be provided immediately to dental personnel after needlestick accidents?
    A. Natural passive immunity
    B. Acquired passive immunity
    C. Natural active immunity
    D. Acquired active immunity

16. Which of the following situations would result in the *least* risk of drug allergy?
    A. Application of topical medication
    B. Presence of infection
    C. Presence of multiple allergies
    D. Use with children

17. Which of the following is involved in the regulation of *both* humoral and cell-mediated immunity?
    A. Humoral immunity
    B. Cell-mediated immunity
    C. Innate immunity
    D. Bone marrow cells

18. Which of the following is involved in the communication between lymphocytes within the immune system?
    A. Histamine
    B. Complement
    C. Bradykinin
    D. Cytokines

19. All of the following are examples of hypersensitivity reactions *except*
    A. Systemic lupus erythematosus
    B. Urticaria
    C. Angioedema
    D. Contact dermatitis and mucositis

20. Reactive arthritis is known for being
    A. An infectious disease
    B. An immunodeficiency disease
    C. An immunologic disorder
    D. More common in women than in men

21. Which one of the following types of hypersensitivity reactions is referred to as delayed hypersensitivity?
    A. Type I
    B. Type II
    C. Type III
    D. Type IV

22. A target lesion on the skin is associated with which of the following diseases?
    A. Behçet syndrome
    B. Systemic lupus erythematosus
    C. Lichen planus
    D. Erythema multiforme

23. Tzanck cells are seen in which of the following conditions?
    A. Pemphigus vulgaris
    B. Erythema multiforme
    C. Systemic lupus erythematosus
    D. Behçet syndrome

24. The oral lesions in Reiter syndrome may resemble
    A. Pemphigus vulgaris
    B. Lichen planus
    C. Angioedema
    D. Geographic tongue

25. Aphthous ulcers are seen in each all of the following systemic diseases *except*
    A. Behçet syndrome
    B. Langerhans cell histiocytosis
    C. Ulcerative colitis
    D. Cyclic neutropenia

26. The two cell types that microscopically characterize Langerhans cell histiocytosis are
    A. Lymphocytes and plasma cells
    B. Fibroblasts and lymphocytes
    C. Eosinophils and mononuclear cells
    D. Neutrophils and lymphocytes

27. Which one of the following is the form of Langerhans cell histiocytosis that is characterized by a triad of symptoms?
    A. Letterer-Siwe disease
    B. Hand-Schüller-Christian disease
    C. Eosinophilic granuloma
    D. Behçet syndrome

28. The most benign type of Langerhans cell histiocytosis is
    A. Hand-Schüller-Christian disease
    B. Eosinophilic granuloma
    C. Letterer-Siwe disease
    D. Chronic disseminated reticulosis

Continued

LESION	CAUSE	AGE/RACE/GENDER	LOCATION
Sjögren syndrome	Autoimmune disease Decreased lacrimal flow Decreased salivary flow	*	Eyes Oral cavity
Systemic lupus erythematosus	Autoimmune disease	Affects women more than men (8:1), blacks more than whites (3:1)	Multiple sites Skin Mucous membranes Joints Eyes Central nervous system Kidneys, heart, and other organs
Pemphigus vulgaris	Autoimmune disease	Affects children and adults Most common in fourth to fifth decade More common in Ashkenazi Jews	Mucous membranes Skin
Mucous membrane pemphigoid (cicatricial pemphigoid, benign mucous membrane pemphigoid)	Autoimmune disease	Adults	Mucous membranes Most common: gingiva May affect eyes
Bullous pemphigoid	Autoimmune disease	80% affected are over 60 yr old	Mucous membranes Skin
Behçet syndrome	Autoimmune disease	Mean age of onset, 30 yr	Mucous membranes Oral Genital Ocular

*No significant information.
†See reference materials.

CLINICAL FEATURES	RADIOGRAPHIC FEATURES	MICROSCOPIC FEATURES	TREATMENT	DIAGNOSTIC PROCESS
Primary Sjögren syndrome: dry eyes (xerophthalmia), dry mouth (xerostomia) Secondary Sjögren syndrome: dry eyes (xerophthalmia), dry mouth (xerostomia) Along with another autoimmune disease	Sialogram shows characteristic features (see text)	Salivary gland changes: lymphocytic infiltration and epimyoepithelial islands	Xerostomia: saliva substitutes Saliva stimulation: pilocarpine	Clinical Radiographic Microscopic Laboratory
Oral lesions Erythematous plaques or erosions White striations radiating from center of lesion	N/A	Destruction of the basal layer of the epithelium with inflammatory infiltrate around blood vessels Immunohistochemical testing Granular and linear deposits of immunoglobulins along basement membrane zone	Antiinflammatory and immunosuppressive agents	Laboratory Microscopic Clinical
Progressive involvement of mucous membranes and skin Oral lesions Painful, erythema, vesicles, bullae, erosions Positive Nikolsky sign	N/A	Intact basal layer attached to the underlying connective tissue Acantholysis of the prickle cell layer Tzanck cells	Corticosteroids and other immunosuppressive agents	Laboratory Microscopic
Oral lesions Desquamative gingivitis Bullae, erosions, ulcers Lesions heal with scarring	N/A	Epithelium detaches from the connective tissue at the basement membrane	Topical/systemic corticosteroids	Microscopic
Oral lesions as in cicatricial pemphigoid but less common	N/A	Epithelium detaches from the connective tissue at the basement membrane	Systemic corticosteroids and other antiinflammatory agents	Microscopic
Oral lesions: aphthous-like ulcers	N/A	†	Corticosteroids and other immunosuppressive agents	Clinical

Chapter 4

Infectious Diseases

Joan Andersen Phelan

OBJECTIVES

After studying this chapter, the student will be able to:

1. State the difference between an inflammatory and an immune response to infection.
2. Describe the factors that allow opportunistic infection to develop.
3. List two examples of opportunistic infections that can occur in the oral cavity.
4. For each of the following infectious diseases, name the organism causing it, list the route or routes of transmission of the organism and the oral manifestations of the disease, and describe how the diagnosis is made: impetigo, tuberculosis, actinomycosis, syphilis (primary, secondary, tertiary), verruca vulgaris, condyloma acuminatum, and primary herpetic gingivostomatitis.
5. Describe the relationship between streptococcal tonsillitis, pharyngitis, scarlet fever, and rheumatic fever.
6. List and describe four forms of oral candidiasis.
7. Describe the clinical features of herpes labialis.
8. Describe the clinical features of recurrent intraoral herpes simplex infection and compare them with the clinical features of minor aphthous ulcers.
9. Describe the clinical characteristics of herpes zoster when it affects the skin of the face and oral mucosa.
10. List two oral infectious diseases for which a cytologic smear may assist in confirming the diagnosis.
11. List four diseases associated with the Epstein-Barr virus.
12. List two diseases caused by coxsackieviruses that have oral manifestations.
13. Describe the spectrum of human immunodeficiency virus (HIV) disease, including initial infection and the development of acquired immunodeficiency syndrome (AIDS).
14. List and describe the clinical appearance of five oral manifestations of HIV infection.

VOCABULARY

Granuloma (gran″u-lo′mə) A tumor-like mass of inflammatory tissue consisting of a central collection of macrophages, often including multinucleated giant cells, surrounded by lymphocytes.

Granulomatous disease (gran″u-lom′ə-təs dĭ-zēz′) A disease characterized by the formation of granulomas.

Herpetic whitlow (hər-pe′tik hwit′lo) An infection caused by herpes simplex virus infection that involves the distal phalanx of a finger.

Incubation period (in″ku-ba′shən pe′re-od) The period between the infection of an individual by a pathogen and the manifestation of the disease it causes.

VOCABULARY—cont'd

Malaise (mah-lāz′) A vague, indefinite feeling of discomfort, debilitation, or lack of health.

Opportunistic infection (op″ər-too-nis′tik in-fek′shən) A disease caused by a microorganism that does not ordinarily cause disease but becomes pathogenic under certain circumstances.

Paresthesia (par″əs-the′zhə) An abnormal sensation such as burning, prickling, or tingling.

Pathogenic microorganism (path-o-jen′ik mi″kro-or′gən-iz-əm) A microorganism that causes disease.

Pruritus (proo-ri′təs) Itching.

Subclinical infection (səb-klin′ĭ-kəl in-fek′shən) An infectious disease not detectable by the usual clinical signs.

Humans are surrounded and inhabited by an enormous number of microorganisms. The ability of these organisms to cause disease depends on both the microorganism and the state of the body's defenses. The organism must be capable of causing disease, and the individual must be susceptible to the disease. Microorganisms are traditionally divided into those that produce disease (pathogenic microorganisms) and those that do not (nonpathogenic microorganisms). To cause disease the organism must gain access to the body, accommodate to growth in the human environment, and avoid multiple host defenses. These defense mechanisms include intact skin and mucosal surfaces, antimicrobial secretory and excretory products on the skin and mucosa, the competition among the components of the normal microflora, the inflammatory response, and the immune response.

Numerous infectious diseases can affect the tissues of the oral cavity. Bacterial, fungal, and viral infections are the most common; but even protozoan and helminthic infections, although extremely rare, have been reported.

The oral cavity can be the primary site of involvement of an infectious disease, or a systemic infection can have oral manifestations. These infections are transmitted from one individual to another by several different routes. Organisms can be transferred through the air on dust particles or water droplets. Some organisms require intimate and direct contact to be transferred. Some can be transferred on hands and objects, and others such as hepatitis B must be transferred from one person to another in blood or other body fluids. Microorganisms that initially invade the oral tissues can cause a local infection, systemic infection, or both. Microorganisms circulating in the bloodstream can cause lesions in the oral cavity, and microorganisms causing infection in the lungs can be transferred to oral tissues when they are present in sputum. The oral cavity contains numerous microorganisms that make up the normal oral microflora. Changes such as a decrease in salivary flow, antibiotic administration, and immune system alterations affect the oral microflora so that organisms that are usually nonpathogenic are able to cause disease. This type of infection is called an **opportunistic infection.**

Microorganisms penetrating epithelial surfaces act as foreign material and stimulate the inflammatory and immune responses. The inflammatory response is nonspecific, resulting in edema and the accumulation of a large number of white blood cells at the site. The responses of the immune system, both humoral and cell mediated, are highly specific; microorganisms are antigens, and specific antibodies are formed in response to specific antigens.

Humoral immunity (immunity that is mediated by antibodies) is an effective defense against some microorganisms, and cell-mediated immunity (immunity in which T lymphocytes are responsible for the response) is the primary defense against others, such as intracellular bacteria (tuberculosis), viruses, and fungi. Microbial infections are responsible for many more diseases than those included in this chapter. The diseases discussed here are common, cause specific oral lesions, and help to illustrate principles of infectious disease. Dental caries and periodontal disease clearly are infectious diseases that are important to dental hygienists. However, they are not included in this text because they are usually studied in courses other than oral pathology. The dental hygienist frequently encounters oral infectious diseases and must be able to recognize their clinical features and significance.

BACTERIAL INFECTIONS

IMPETIGO

Impetigo is a bacterial skin infection caused primarily by *Staphylococcus aureus* and occasionally by *Streptococcus pyogenes*. Impetigo most commonly involves the skin of the face or extremities and is usually seen in young children. The organisms are present on skin. Nonintact skin is necessary for infection; areas of trauma such as cuts and abrasions and areas of dermatitis are likely sites of this infection. The lesions of impetigo are infectious. Direct contact is required for transmission. Impetigo presents as either vesicles that rupture, resulting in thick, amber-colored crusts, or as longer lasting bullae. Lesions may itch **(pruritus),** and regional lymphadenopathy may be present. Systemic manifestations such as fever and **malaise** generally do not occur with this infection. When impetigo affects the perioral skin, the lesions may resemble recurrent herpes simplex infection (herpes simplex infection is discussed later in this chapter). However, recurrent herpes simplex infection is much less common than impetigo in small children. The diagnosis of impetigo is made on the basis of the clinical presentation or by identification of the bacteria from cultures of the lesions. Topical or systemic antibiotics are used for treatment.

TONSILLITIS AND PHARYNGITIS

Tonsillitis and **pharyngitis** are inflammatory conditions of the tonsils and pharyngeal mucosa. Many different organisms cause them, including streptococci, adenoviruses, influenza viruses, and Epstein-Barr virus. The clinical features include sore throat, fever, tonsillar hyperplasia, and erythema of the oropharyngeal mucosa and tonsils.

Streptococcal tonsillitis and pharyngitis are common bacterial infections that are spread by contact with infectious nasal or oral secretions. The appearance of streptococcal tonsillitis and pharyngitis (i.e., "strep throat") closely resembles tonsillitis and pharyngitis caused by other infections such as viral infections. Specific laboratory tests, including a rapid antigen detection test, are available for diagnostic confirmation of streptococcal infection. Antibiotics are used to treat streptococcal infection.

Tonsillitis and pharyngitis caused by group A β-hemolytic streptococci are significant because of their relationship to scarlet fever and rheumatic fever. **Scarlet fever** usually occurs in children. In addition to fever, patients with scarlet fever develop a generalized red skin rash that is caused by a toxin released by the bacteria. In addition to streptococcal tonsillitis and pharyngitis, oral manifestations of scarlet fever include petechiae on the soft palate and an appearance of the tongue that has been called **strawberry tongue.** The fungiform papillae are red and prominent, with the dorsal surface of the tongue exhibiting either a white coating or erythema. Throat culture is helpful in confirming the diagnosis of streptococcal pharyngitis in a patient with scarlet fever.

Rheumatic fever is a childhood disease that follows a group A β-hemolytic streptococcal infection, usually tonsillitis and pharyngitis. Rheumatic fever is characterized by an inflammatory reaction involving the heart, joints, and central nervous system. Rheumatic fever may result in permanent damage to heart valves.

TUBERCULOSIS

Tuberculosis is an infectious chronic **granulomatous disease** usually caused by the organism *Mycobacterium tuberculosis.* The chief form of the disease is a primary infection of the lung. Inhaled droplets containing bacteria lodge in the alveoli of the lungs. After undergoing phagocytosis by macrophages, the organisms are resistant to destruction and multiply in the macrophages. They then disseminate in the bloodstream. After a few weeks dissemination ceases. The signs and symptoms of this lung infection include fever, chills, fatigue and malaise, weight loss, and persistent cough. The bacteria can be carried to widespread areas of the body and cause involvement of organs such as the kidneys and liver. This is called **miliary tuberculosis.** Involvement of the submandibular and cervical lymph nodes (usually as a result of ingesting the organism in nonpasteurized milk)

FIGURE 4-1 ▪ This ulcer on the tongue tested positive for tuberculosis organisms.

causes enlargement of those nodes and is called **scrofula** or **tuberculous lymphadenitis.** The lung infection can occur at any age. Most commonly, foci of infection in the lungs become completely walled off and heal by fibrosis and calcification. A reactivation of the primary lesion can occur years after the initial infection. This reactivation is usually the result of a compromised immune response.

Oral lesions associated with tuberculosis occur but are rare. They most likely appear when organisms are carried from the lungs in sputum and transmitted to the oral mucosa (Figure 4-1). The tongue and palate are the most common sites for oral lesions of tuberculosis, but they may occur anywhere in the oral cavity, even in bone as in osteomyelitis. Oral lesions appear as painful, nonhealing, slowly enlarging ulcers that can be either superficial or deep.

DIAGNOSIS

Oral lesions of tuberculosis are identified by biopsy and microscopic examination of the tissue. The characteristic histopathologic lesions of tuberculosis are **granulomas.** The granulomas are composed of areas of necrosis surrounded by macrophages, multinucleated giant cells, and lymphocytes. Similar lesions occur in deep fungal infections and foreign-body reactions. Staining the tissue to be examined microscopically with a special stain may reveal the organisms. Tissue culture to diagnose tuberculosis requires a specialized laboratory.

A skin test is used to determine whether an individual has been exposed and infected with *M. tuberculosis.* An antigen called **purified protein derivative** is injected into the skin. If the individual's immune system has previously encountered the antigen, a positive inflammatory skin reaction occurs (a type IV delayed-hypersensitivity reaction). This skin reaction indicates previous infection with the bacteria but not necessarily active disease. When a skin test result is positive, chest radiographs are taken to determine whether active tuberculosis disease is present. Once the skin test result is positive, it will always test positive.

Effective drug treatment for tuberculosis became available in the 1940s. In the United States most tuberculosis treatment centers had closed by the mid-1970s. State health departments reported a dramatic increase in new cases in the mid-1980s, particularly in densely populated urban areas. This increase was suggested to be related to human immunodeficiency virus infection and to noncompliance of patients with therapy. Recent public health efforts have focused on ensuring compliance with antituberculosis drug treatment; as a result the number of new cases reported has decreased.

Tuberculosis is an infectious disease that can be transmitted occupationally to dental health care personnel. Routine use of universal precautions, including eye protection, mask, or facial shield, is important in preventing the transmission of airborne droplet infections such as tuberculosis. However, for patients with active tuberculosis, routine dental treatment is deferred. When emergency dental treatment is needed, the use of a special mask is recommended to ensure prevention of transmission of the tuberculosis organism.

TREATMENT AND PROGNOSIS

Oral lesions resolve with treatment of the patient's primary (usually pulmonary) disease. Combinations of several different medications, including isoniazid and rifampin, are used to treat tuberculosis. Treatment continues for many months and may continue for as long as 2 years. Patients usually become noninfectious shortly after treatment begins. Consultation with the patient's physician should confirm that treatment is ongoing and that the patient is no longer infectious.

ACTINOMYCOSIS

Actinomycosis is an infection caused by a filamentous bacterium called *Actinomyces israelii*. These organisms were at one time thought to be fungi; therefore the name ends in the suffix "mycosis," which usually indicates a fungal infection.

The most characteristic form of the disease is the formation of abscesses that tend to drain by the formation of sinus tracts (Figure 4-2). The colonies or organisms appear in the pus as tiny, bright yellow grains and are called *sulfur granules* because of their yellow color. The organisms can also be identified by microscopic examination. These organisms are common inhabitants of the oral cavity. It is not clear why they only occasionally cause disease. Predisposing factors have not been identified. The infection is often preceded by tooth extraction or an abrasion of the mucosa.

In general, the clinician makes a diagnosis of actinomycosis by identifying the colonies in the tissue from the lesion. Actinomycosis is treated with long-term, high doses of antibiotics.

FIGURE 4-2 ■ Actinomycosis. The skin lesion is over the mandible, and the incision and drainage site is seen below the lesion. "Sulfur granules" were noted in the exudate draining from the site, and the condition was treated with long-term antibiotic therapy.

TABLE 4-1

Stages of Syphilis

STAGE	ORAL LESION
Primary	Chancre
Secondary	Mucous patch
Latent	None
Tertiary	Gumma

SYPHILIS

Syphilis is a disease caused by the spirochete *Treponema pallidum*. The organism is transmitted from one person to another by direct contact. The spirochete, a corkscrew-like bacterium, can penetrate mucous membranes but requires a break in the continuity of the skin surface to invade through the skin. The organisms die quickly when exposed to air and changes in temperature. Syphilis is usually transmitted through sexual contact with a partner who has active lesions. It can also be transmitted by transfusion of infected blood or by transplacental inoculation of a fetus from an infected mother.

The disease occurs in three stages: (1) primary, (2) secondary, and (3) tertiary (Table 4-1). The lesion of the primary stage, called the **chancre,** is highly infectious and forms at the site at which the spirochete enters the body (Figure 4-3). Regional lymphadenopathy accompanies the chancre. The lesion heals spontaneously after several weeks without treatment, and the disease enters a latent period.

FIGURE 4-3 ■ **A,** Chancre on tongue seen in primary syphilis. **B,** Chancre on lip. (**A,** Courtesy Dr. Norman Trieger; **B,** courtesy Dr. Edward V. Zegarelli.)

The secondary stage occurs about 6 weeks after the primary lesion appears. In the secondary stage diffuse eruptions of the skin and mucous membranes occur. The skin lesions have many forms. The oral lesions are called **mucous patches** and appear as multiple, painless, grayish-white plaques covering ulcerated mucosa. The lesions of secondary syphilis are the most infectious. They undergo spontaneous remission but can recur for months or years. After remission the disease may remain latent for many years.

The tertiary lesions occur years after the initial infection if the infection has not been treated. They chiefly involve the cardiovascular system and the central nervous system. The localized tertiary lesion is called a **gumma** and is noninfectious. A gumma can occur in the oral cavity; the most common sites are the tongue and palate. The lesion appears as a firm mass that eventually becomes an ulcer. The gumma is a destructive lesion and can lead to perforation of the palatal bone.

CONGENITAL SYPHILIS

Syphilis can be transmitted from an infected mother to the fetus because the organism can cross the placenta and enter the fetal circulation. **Congenital syphilis** often causes serious and irreversible damage to the child, including facial and dental abnormalities. The developmental disorders that result from fetal and neonatal syphilis are described in Chapter 5.

DIAGNOSIS AND TREATMENT

The diagnosis of syphilitic lesions occurring on skin can be made by a special microscopic technique called a **dark-field examination** to identify the spirochetes. However, other spirochetes are present in the oral cavity; therefore this examination is not reliable for oral lesions. Two of the serologic (blood) tests that are commonly used to confirm the diagnosis of syphilis include (1) the Venereal Disease

Research Laboratory (VDRL) test, and (2) the fluorescent treponemal antibody absorption (FTA-ABS) test. These tests may produce negative results in primary syphilis because sufficient antibodies may not have formed for the test result to be positive. If syphilis continues to be suspected, retesting is done.

Syphilis is generally treated with penicillin. The VDRL test is used again to evaluate the success of treatment. The antibody titer decreases if treatment has been successful. The FTA test remains positive after treatment.

NECROTIZING ULCERATIVE GINGIVITIS

Necrotizing ulcerative gingivitis (NUG) was formerly called **acute necrotizing ulcerative gingivitis** (ANUG). This condition is more chronic than acute and therefore, is most appropriately called NUG. It is a painful erythematous gingivitis with necrosis of the interdental papillae (Figure 4-4). NUG is usually caused by a combination of a fusiform bacillus and a spirochete *(Borrelia vincentii)* and is associated with decreased resistance to infection.

The gingiva is painful and erythematous, with necrosis of the interdental papillae generally accompanied by a foul odor and metallic taste. The necrosis results in cratering of the interdental papillae area. Sloughing of the necrotic tissue presents as a pseudomembrane over the tissues. Systemic manifestations of infection such as fever and cervical lymphadenopathy may be present. Clinical features distinguish NUG from acute marginal gingivitis and the gingival component of acute primary herpes simplex infection (see Figure 4-20, *B*).

PERICORONITIS

Pericoronitis is an inflammation of the mucosa around the crown of a partially erupted, impacted tooth (Figure 4-5). The soft tissue around the mandibular third molar is the most common location for pericoronitis. The inflammation is usually the result of infection by bacteria that are part of the normal oral microflora, which proliferate in the pocket between the soft tissue and the crown of the tooth. Compromised host defenses, ranging from minor illnesses to immunodeficiency, are associated with an increased risk of pericoronitis. Trauma from an opposing molar and impaction of food under the soft tissue flap (operculum) covering the distal portion of the third molar may also precipitate pericoronitis.

DIAGNOSIS

The diagnosis of pericoronitis is made on the basis of the clinical presentation. The tissue around the crown of a partially erupted tooth is swollen, erythematous, and painful.

FIGURE 4-4 ■ Necrotizing ulcerative gingivitis.

FIGURE 4-5 ■ Pericoronitis. (Courtesy Dr. Kenneth Fleisher.)

TREATMENT AND PROGNOSIS

Treatment of pericoronitis includes mechanical debridement and irrigation of the pocket and systemic antibiotics. Extraction of the impacted molar is usually necessary to prevent recurrence.

ACUTE OSTEOMYELITIS

Acute osteomyelitis involves acute inflammation of the bone and bone marrow (Figure 4-6, *A*). Acute osteomyelitis of the jaws is most commonly a result of the extension of a periapical abscess. It may follow fracture of the bone or surgery, and may also result from bacteremia.

DIAGNOSIS

The diagnosis of the specific organism causing acute osteomyelitis is based on culture results, and treatment is based on antibiotic sensitivity testing. Microscopic examination shows nonviable bone, necrotic debris, acute inflammation, and bacterial colonies in the marrow spaces. No change is seen on the radiograph unless the disease has been present for more than 1 week.

A

B

FIGURE 4-6 ■ **A,** Low-power microscopy of acute osteomyelitis, showing nonviable bone. Bacterial colonies and inflammatory cells are seen between trabeculae of bone. **B,** Diffuse, irregular radiographic changes seen in chronic osteomyelitis.

TREATMENT AND PROGNOSIS

The treatment of acute osteomyelitis involves drainage of the purulent exudate from the area and the use of appropriate antibiotics.

CHRONIC OSTEOMYELITIS

Chronic osteomyelitis is a long-standing inflammation of bone. It may occur in inadequately treated acute osteomyelitis, long-term inflammation of bone with no recognized acute phase, Paget disease, sickle cell disease, or bone irradiation that results in decreased vascularity. The involved bone is painful and swollen, and radiographic examination reveals a diffuse and irregular radiolucency that can eventually become radiopaque as bone forms within the chronically inflamed tissue (Figure 4-6 *B*). When radiopacity develops, the condition is called **chronic sclerosing osteomyelitis.** Recently, cases of osteonecrosis of the mandible and maxilla have been reported in patients taking bisphosphonate medication. This may appear clinically similar to chronic osteomyelitis. Bisphosphonate-associated osteonecrosis is described in Chapter 9.

DIAGNOSIS

The diagnosis of chronic osteomyelitis is based on biopsy results and the microscopic examination, which shows chronic inflammation of bone and marrow. Bacterial culture may be helpful, but the bacteria may be difficult to identify.

TREATMENT

Treatment of chronic osteomyelitis involves debridement and administration of systemic antibiotics. In some patients the use of hyperbaric oxygen may be needed to successfully treat this condition.

FUNGAL INFECTIONS

CANDIDIASIS

Candidiasis, also called **candidosis, moniliasis,** and **thrush,** occurs as a result of an overgrowth of the yeastlike fungus *Candida albicans*. It is the most common oral fungal infection. This fungus is part of the normal oral microflora in many individuals, particularly those individuals with diabetes mellitus and those who wear dentures. Overgrowth of *Candida albicans* is associated with many different conditions (Box 4-1).

Newborn infants are particularly susceptible to an overgrowth of this fungus because they do not have either an established oral microflora or a fully developed immune system. Pregnant women often have *Candida* vaginitis because they are somewhat immunosuppressed in order to maintain the fetus. The organism is transmitted to the infant while it passes through the birth canal. Antibiotics can alter the bacteria of the oral microflora, which can allow the overgrowth of *Candida albicans*. Systemic and topical corticosteroids,

diabetes, and cell-mediated immune system deficiency are other factors that allow the overgrowth of this fungus. Candidiasis is one of the most common oral lesions that occur in association with immunodeficiency. Candidiasis generally affects the superficial layers of the epithelium; therefore, when it is present, the proliferating organisms are easily identified in a sample obtained by scraping the surface (mucosal smear) of the lesion.

TYPES OF ORAL CANDIDIASIS

Several forms of oral candidiasis exist; recognition of their clinical features is important so that candidiasis is appropriately included in the differential diagnosis of a variety of clinical presentations. The types of oral candidiasis are as follows:

- Pseudomembranous
- Erythematous
- Denture stomatitis (chronic atrophic candidiasis)
- Chronic hyperplastic (*Candida* leukoplakia)
- Angular cheilitis

Box 4-1

Conditions Associated with Overgrowth of *Candida albicans*

- Antibiotic therapy
- Cancer chemotherapy
- Corticosteroid therapy
- Dentures
- Diabetes mellitus
- Human immunodeficiency virus infection
- Hypoparathyroidism
- Infancy (newborn)
- Malignancies involving bone marrow
- Primary T-lymphocyte deficiency
- Xerostomia

FIGURE 4-7 ■ Pseudomembranous candidiasis.

FIGURE 4-8 ■ Erythematous candidiasis. **A,** Recent-onset and erythematous lesions elsewhere in the oral cavity differentiate this from median rhomboid glossitis. **B,** Response to antifungal treatment confirmed the diagnosis of oral candidiasis in this patient.

Pseudomembranous Candidiasis

A white curdlike material is present on the mucosal surface in **pseudomembranous candidiasis** (Figure 4-7). The underlying mucosa is erythematous. On occasion, a burning sensation is felt, and the patient may complain of a metallic taste.

Erythematous Candidiasis

An erythematous, often painful, mucosa is the presenting complaint in **erythematous candidiasis** (Figure 4-8). This type of candidiasis may be localized to one area of the oral mucosa or be more generalized. Irregular, patchy

FIGURE 4-9 ■ Chronic atrophic candidiasis (denture stomatitis). **A,** Full denture. **B,** Partial denture.

depapillation of the tongue is often seen in this type of candidiasis.

Denture Stomatitis

Denture stomatitis is the most common type of candidiasis affecting the oral mucosa. It is also called **chronic atrophic candidiasis** (Figure 4-9). This type of candidiasis also presents as erythematous mucosa, but the erythematous change is limited to the mucosa covered by a full or partial denture. The lesions may vary from petechiae-like to more generalized and granular. It is most common on the palate and maxillary alveolar ridge. Denture stomatitis is asymptomatic and is usually discovered by the dentist or dental hygienist during a routine oral examination.

Chronic Hyperplastic Candidiasis

Chronic hyperplastic candidiasis (Figure 4-10) appears as a white lesion that does not wipe off the mucosa. **Candidal leukoplakia** and **hypertrophic candidiasis** are other names for this type of oral candidiasis. An important diagnostic feature of this type of candidiasis is its response to antifungal medication: when leukoplakia is caused by candidiasis, it disappears when treated with antifungal medication (therapeutic diagnosis). If the lesion does not respond to antifungal therapy, biopsy should be considered to establish the diagnosis of the lesion.

FIGURE 4-10 ■ Chronic hyperplastic candidiasis. The white appearance of the tongue did not wipe off, and it disappeared with antifungal treatment.

FIGURE 4-12 ■ Median rhomboid glossitis.

FIGURE 4-11 ■ Angular cheilitis.

Angular Cheilitis

Candida organisms are often the cause of **angular cheilitis** (Figure 4-11), especially if saliva collects at the corners of the mouth. It appears as erythema or fissuring at the labial commissures. Angular cheilitis may be caused by other factors such as nutritional deficiency or a combination of candidiasis and bacterial infection; however, it most commonly results from *Candida* infection. Angular cheilitis frequently accompanies intraoral candidiasis.

Chronic Mucocutaneous Candidiasis

A severe form of candidiasis that usually occurs in patients who are severely immunocompromised is called **chronic mucocutaneous candidiasis.** The patient has skin lesions as well as chronic oral and genital mucosal candidiasis. Oral involvement may appear as pseudomembranous, erythematous, or hyperplastic candidiasis; and angular cheilitis is common. The skin lesions usually involve the nails and skinfolds.

Median Rhomboid Glossitis (Central Papillary Atrophy)

Several studies have reported an association between **median rhomboid glossitis** (Figure 4-12) also called *central papillary atrophy* and candidiasis. It appears as an erythematous, often rhombus-shaped, flat-to-raised area on the midline of the posterior dorsal tongue. *Candida* organisms have been identified in some lesions, and some lesions disappear with antifungal treatment. However, the response to antifungal treatment is not consistent; therefore, although this lesion has been associated with candidiasis, the cause is not yet clear.

DIAGNOSIS AND TREATMENT

Because *Candida* is part of the oral microflora in many individuals, a culture is not useful for diagnosis. A positive culture result indicates that the organisms are present but not that they are causing infection. Clinical features and the use of the mucosal smear/cytologic preparation (Figure 4-13) are usually more helpful. The surface of the lesion is scraped vigorously with a tongue blade, wooden spatula, or specially designed brush; and the scrapings are spread on a glass slide and fixed with alcohol. The slide is then sent to an oral pathology laboratory for staining and examination. In addition to the smear, the response of the lesion to antifungal treatment is important in confirming the diagnosis of candidiasis. Lesions caused by *Candida* should resolve with antifungal treatment. Both topical and systemic

FIGURE 4-13 ■ Photomicrograph of a smear showing epithelial cells and *Candida* organisms.

FIGURE 4-14 ■ Oral lesions of histoplasmosis in this patient clinically resemble squamous cell carcinoma. (Courtesy Dr. A. Ross Kerr.)

medications are used for candidiasis. However, in some patients, particularly those who are immunocompromised, candidiasis is persistent and recurrent.

Although the final diagnosis and management of a patient with oral candidiasis is the responsibility of the dentist, dental hygienists are often the first to recognize the oral changes characteristic of this condition. Recurrent oral candidiasis may be an early sign of a severe underlying medical problem.

DEEP FUNGAL INFECTIONS

Oral lesions occur in some deep fungal infections (e.g., *histoplasmosis, coccidioidomycosis, blastomycosis,* and *cryptococcosis*). They are all characterized by primary involvement of the lungs. Oral lesions are caused by implantation of the organism carried by sputum from the lungs to the oral mucosa.

Infections caused by these organisms are more common in certain areas of the United States than in others. Histoplasmosis is widespread in the midwestern United States, and coccidioidomycosis is more prevalent in parts of the western United States, particularly the San Joaquin Valley of California. Blastomycosis is common in the Ohio and Mississippi River basin areas. Therefore oral lesions caused by these organisms are most likely seen in areas of the country in which the infection is most common.

Cryptococcosis is transmitted through inhalation of organisms contained in dust from bird droppings, particularly from pigeons. In addition to the regional distribution of these infections, reactivation, including the development of oral lesions, can also occur in patients who are immunocompromised.

DIAGNOSIS

The initial signs and symptoms of these deep fungal infections are usually related to the primary lung infection. Oral lesions are preceded by pulmonary involvement. These oral lesions are chronic, nonhealing ulcers that can resemble squamous cell carcinoma (Figure 4-14). Diagnosis is made by biopsy and microscopic examination. Special staining

of the tissue reveals the organisms, which can be identified by their microscopic appearance. The tissue can also be cultured; this is useful in establishing the diagnosis.

TREATMENT

Systemic antifungal medications such as amphotericin B or ketoconazole or itraconazole are used to treat these infections. However, latent infections may remain even after treatment and may reappear if the individual's immune system becomes deficient.

MUCORMYCOSIS

Mucormycosis, also called **phycomycosis,** is a rare fungal infection. The organisms are a common inhabitant of soil and are usually nonpathogenic. However, infection with this organism occurs in diabetic and severely debilitated patients. The disease often involves the nasal cavity, maxillary sinus, and hard palate and can present as a proliferating or destructive mass in the maxilla. The diagnosis is made by biopsy and identification of the organisms in the tissue.

VIRAL INFECTIONS

HUMAN PAPILLOMAVIRUS INFECTION

Human papillomavirus (HPV) selectively infects skin and oral mucosa. Infection occurs by direct contact. More than 150 different types of HPV have been identified; some of these types have been found to cause neoplasia and therefore are called *high-risk types.* Others that cause benign lesions or are not associated with lesions are called *low-risk types.* At least 40 different types of HPV have been identified in oral mucosa. A recent study that examined both high-risk and low-risk types of HPV in the oral cavity found the overall prevalence of HPV in the oral cavity to be 6.9%. This included both high-risk and low-risk types. HPV has been clearly associated with carcinoma of the vaginal cervix (cervical cancer). High-risk types have been identified and associated with squamous cell carcinomas that form in the oropharyngeal region (see Chapter 7). Evidence of their role in the pathogenesis of these cancers is emerging, but is not yet completely clear.

For HPV to infect skin and oral mucosa, it must infect the basal cells of the epithelium. This usually requires a break in the surface of these tissues. HPV matures in the spinous layer and then the virus is released on the surface of the tissue. Proliferation of the basal cells of the infected epithelium is a characteristic of benign lesions that are caused by HPV infection.

Like other viruses, HPV incorporates itself into the nuclear material of infected cells. HPV-infected cells, called *koilocytes,* are characterized microscopically by an irregular nucleus surrounded by clear cytoplasm (Figure 4-15).

Three benign lesions caused by HPV infection are seen in the oral cavity. These include the verruca vulgaris, condyloma acuminatum, and focal epithelial hyperplasia. These are described in this chapter. The benign squamous papilloma, described in Chapter 7, is also most likely caused by HPV infection. The relationship between HPV and oral cancer is further described in Chapter 7.

VERRUCA VULGARIS

The **verruca vulgaris,** or common wart, is a papillary oral lesion caused by several different human papillomaviruses. It is a common skin lesion. Oral lesions are less common than skin lesions, but they do occur. The virus is inoculated by direct contact and may be transmitted from skin to oral mucosa. The lips are one of the most common intraoral sites for this lesion. Autoinoculation occurs through finger sucking or fingernail biting in patients with verrucae on the hands or fingers (Figure 4-16). The verruca vulgaris is usually a white, papillary, exophytic lesion (Figure 4-17)

FIGURE 4-17 ■ Verruca vulgaris on the lateral aspect of the tongue in an adult.

FIGURE 4-15 ■ Koilocytes in oral epithelium indicate human papilloma virus infection.

FIGURE 4-16 ■ **A** and **B,** Verruca vulgaris on the tongue of a child with a similar lesion on the thumb. (Courtesy Dr. Edward V. Zegarelli.)

FIGURE 4-18 ■ Condyloma acuminatum. The presence of condyloma acuminatum in a child is strongly suggestive of sexual abuse. (Courtesy Dr. Sidney Eisig.)

FIGURE 4-19 ■ Multifocal epithelial hyperplasia. (Courtesy Dr. Stanley Kerpel.)

that closely resembles and is related to the benign tumor of squamous epithelium called the **papilloma** (see Chapter 7).

Microscopically, the verruca vulgaris consists of finger-like projections of markedly keratotic, stratified squamous epithelium that exhibits a prominent granular cell layer; numerous cells with clear cytoplasm, called *koilocytes*, are present in the upper spinous layer of the epithelium. These cells contain viral particles that are visible by electron microscopic examination. Each of the projections contains a central core of fibrous connective tissue containing many blood vessels. The vacuolated cells in the epithelium contain the viral particles.

Diagnosis

Biopsy and microscopic examination reveal the light microscopic features of this lesion. Immunologic staining is also useful in identifying these viruses.

Treatment and Prognosis

Conservative surgical excision is the treatment of choice for verruca vulgaris. These lesions may recur. In addition, patients with skin lesions should be instructed to refrain from finger sucking or fingernail biting to prevent reinoculation and development of new lesions.

CONDYLOMA ACUMINATUM

The **condyloma acuminatum** is a benign papillary lesion caused by other human papillomaviruses. The virus is generally transmitted by sexual contact and is most commonly found in the anogenital region. It is transmitted to the oral cavity through oral-genital contact or self-inoculation.

Oral condylomas appear as papillary, bulbous masses and can occur anywhere in the oral mucosa (Figure 4-18). Multiple lesions may be present. They have been reported to occur on the tongue, buccal mucosa, palate, gingiva, and alveolar ridge. The oral condyloma tends to be more diffuse

than the papilloma or verruca vulgaris and is generally not as well keratinized as the verruca vulgaris. The condyloma is pink, whereas the verruca vulgaris is usually white.

Microscopically, the condyloma acuminatum is composed of fingerlike (papillary) projections of epithelium covering cores of connective tissue. The epithelium is thickened, and cells with clear cytoplasm are seen throughout the epithelium. These clear cells contain viral particles that can be identified through immunologic staining.

When the condyloma acuminatum occurs in the oral cavity, it is generally treated by conservative surgical excision. However, recurrence is common, and multiple lesions make management difficult. Patients should be instructed to avoid oral-genital contact with an infected partner to prevent reinoculation.

MULTIFOCAL EPITHELIAL HYPERPLASIA

Multifocal epithelial hyperplasia, also called *Heck disease,* is characterized by the presence of multiple whitish to pale pink nodules distributed throughout the oral mucosa (Figure 4-19). The disease is most common in children and was first described in Native Americans, but it has since been described in many different areas of the world. This disease is caused by another human papillomavirus. The lesions are generally asymptomatic and do not require treatment. They resolve spontaneously weeks to months after onset. Microscopically, the lesions show thickened epithelium with broad, connected rete ridges. Cells in the epithelium that have clear cytoplasm, consistent with koilocytes, may also be seen in the lesions of multifocal epithelial hyperplasia.

HERPES SIMPLEX INFECTION

Two major forms of the herpes simplex virus exist: type 1 and type 2. Oral infections are generally caused by type 1, and genital infections are most commonly caused by type 2.

Oral infection with the herpes simplex virus occurs in an initial (primary) form and a recurrent (secondary) form. The herpes simplex virus is one of a group of viruses called human herpesviruses (HHVs). Other herpesviruses include varicella-zoster virus (VZV), Epstein-Barr virus (EBV), cytomegalovirus (CMV), and Kaposi sarcoma–associated herpesvirus (KSHV; human herpesvirus 8). Herpes simplex viruses have the ability to persist in an individual in a clinically quiescent or latent state. For many individuals, the primary infection undergoes remission without the virus being completely eliminated.

PRIMARY HERPETIC GINGIVOSTOMATITIS

The oral disease caused by initial infection with the herpes simplex virus is called **primary herpetic gingivostomatitis** (Figure 4-20). Painful, erythematous, and swollen gingivae and multiple tiny vesicles on the perioral skin, vermilion border of the lips, and oral mucosa characterize the disease. These vesicles progress to form ulcers. Systemic symptoms such as fever, malaise, and cervical lymphadenopathy generally occur first, followed by gingival involvement and the appearance of mucosal vesicles and ulcers. The disease most commonly occurs in children between the ages of 6 months and 6 years. However, it may occur at any age if an individual who has not been previously exposed to the virus comes into contact with it or if a sufficient level of antibodies has not developed to confer protection against reinfection. Because many more individuals have antibodies to herpes simplex than have a history of the disease, the majority are thought to be **subclinical infections.** The disease is usually self-limited. The lesions heal spontaneously in 1 to 2 weeks.

RECURRENT HERPES SIMPLEX INFECTION

In many individuals, after the primary infection, the herpes simplex virus tends to persist in a latent state, usually in the nerve tissue of the trigeminal ganglion, and causes localized recurrent infections. It has been estimated that one third to one half of the population of the United States experience **recurrent herpes simplex infection.** The most common type of recurrent oral herpes simplex infection occurs on the vermilion border of the lips and is called **herpes labialis** (Figure 4-21), which is also called a **cold sore** or **fever blister.** Recurrent infections are often produced by certain stimuli such as sunlight, menstruation, fatigue, fever, and emotional stress. These stimuli are thought to trigger viral replication and immunologic changes that result in clinical lesions.

Recurrent herpes simplex infection can also occur intraorally (Figure 4-22). The appearance and location of these lesions are important to distinguish them from aphthous ulcers (Table 4-2). Recurrent intraoral herpes simplex occurs on keratinized mucosa that is fixed to bone, most commonly the hard palate and gingiva. The lesions appear as painful clusters of tiny vesicles or ulcers that can coalesce to form a single ulcer with an irregular border. Usually patients experience prodromal symptoms such as pain, burning, or tingling in the area in which the vesicles develop.

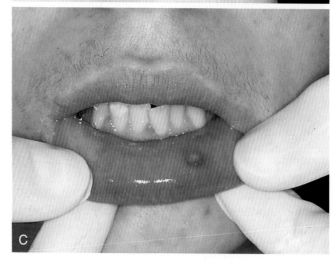

FIGURE 4-20 ■ **A,** Primary herpetic gingivostomatitis in a child. **B** and **C,** Primary herpetic gingivostomatitis in an adolescent. (**A,** Courtesy Dr. Edward V. Zegarelli.)

The lesions heal without scarring in 1 to 2 weeks. Episodes of recurrence vary from once a month in some individuals to once a year in others.

Herpes simplex virus is transmitted by direct contact with an infected individual, and the lesions of the primary infection occur at the site of inoculation. The herpes simplex

FIGURE 4-21 ■ Herpes labialis. **A,** Twelve hours after onset. **B,** Forty-eight hours after onset.

FIGURE 4-22 ■ **A** and **B,** Recurrent intraoral herpes simplex.

virus can be isolated from both primary and recurrent lesions. The amount of virus present is highest in the vesicle stage. In some individuals the virus is present in the oral cavity, even when no lesions are present. Herpes simplex virus can cause a painful infection of the fingers called a **herpetic whitlow.** Before the routine use of gloves during dental treatment, this was an occupational hazard for dentists and dental hygienists (Figure 4-23). Herpetic whitlow can be either a primary or a recurrent infection. Herpes simplex virus can also cause eye infection (Figure 4-24). Routine barrier infection control procedures (mask, eye protection, and gloves) are important in preventing the transmission of the herpes simplex virus to dental health care providers.

Diagnosis

The diagnosis of herpes simplex infection, both primary and recurrent, is generally based on the clinical characteristics of the disease (see Table 4-2). In immunocompromised patients the characteristic clinical features may be lacking. A viral culture can be performed to confirm the diagnosis. This procedure requires a special culture medium and at least 2 days before results are available.

Herpes simplex virus causes changes in epithelial cells that can be seen microscopically. These virally altered cells can be seen in tissue obtained by biopsy or on a smear taken by scraping the basal cells of the lesion and spreading them on a glass slide, fixing them with alcohol, and submitting

TABLE 4-2

Comparison of the Clinical Features of Recurrent Minor Aphthous Ulcers and Recurrent Herpes Ulceration

FEATURE	MINOR APHTHOUS ULCERS	HERPES SIMPLEX ULCERATION
Location	Nonkeratinized mucosa	Keratinized mucosa
Number	One to several	Multiple (crops)
Vesicle precedes ulcer	No	Yes
Pain	Yes	Yes
Size	<1 cm	1-2 mm
Borders	Round to oval	Clusters of ulcers coalesce to form a large irregular ulcer
Recurrent	Yes	Yes

FIGURE 4-23 ■ **A,** Herpetic whitlow in a dental hygienist (initial lesion). **B,** Recurrent lesion occurred many, many years later. (Courtesy Susan Rod Graham.)

them to an oral pathology laboratory for staining and examination (Figure 4-25). The virally altered epithelial cells that are seen on a cytologic preparation (smear) from patients with herpes simplex infection are called **Tzanck cells.** These are different from the Tzanck cells that are seen in pemphigus vulgaris (see Chapter 3) but have the same name. Smears of herpes simplex ulceration have been reported to be positive for virally altered cells only about 50% of the time.

Treatment

Antiviral drugs such as acyclovir are available for the treatment of herpes simplex infection and are used for treating genital herpes simplex infection. Antiviral drugs have not been shown to be consistently effective in treating the

FIGURE 4-24 ■ Herpetic eye infection. (Courtesy Dr. Sidney Eisig.)

FIGURE 4-25 ■ Cytologic smear preparation showing a virally altered cell (Tzanck cell) resulting from herpes simplex infection. (Courtesy Dr. Harry Lumerman.)

intraoral lesions of herpes simplex infection except in immunocompromised patients. The use of sunscreens may prevent the development of herpes labialis. Systemic antiviral medication has been approved by the U.S. Food and Drug Administration for treating and preventing herpes labialis. Topical application of antiviral drugs may prevent or decrease the duration of herpes labialis when they are administered very early in the development of the lesion (prodrome), before epithelial damage has occurred.

VARICELLA-ZOSTER VIRUS

The **varicella-zoster virus** (VZV) causes both chickenpox (varicella) and shingles (herpes zoster). Respiratory aerosols and contact with secretions from skin lesions transmit the virus. Both chickenpox and herpes zoster are contagious.

CHICKENPOX

Chickenpox is a highly contagious disease that causes vesicular and pustular eruptions of the skin and mucous membranes, along with systemic symptoms such as headache, fever, and malaise (Figure 4-26). The **incubation period** is about 2 weeks. Chickenpox usually occurs in children; although oral lesions occur, they generally do not cause severe discomfort. Usually an individual has only a single episode of chickenpox; but second, milder forms have also been described. Recovery generally occurs in 2 to 3 weeks.

HERPES ZOSTER

Although chickenpox has been described in adults, the virus usually causes a different form of disease in this population. The form that usually occurs in adults is called **herpes zoster** or **shingles**. It is characterized by a unilateral, painful eruption of vesicles along the distribution of a sensory nerve (Figure 4-27). Whether or not the varicella-zoster virus is harbored in the sensory ganglia (during the interval between chickenpox and herpes zoster) in a manner similar to that of the herpes simplex virus is not clear. However, herpes zoster often occurs in association with immunodeficiency or certain malignancies such as Hodgkin disease and leukemia. A vaccine is available to prevent varicella-zoster infections. The vaccine is given to children to prevent chickenpox and to older adults to prevent the recurrence of the infection as herpes zoster.

The depression of cell-mediated immunity appears to be important in the development of herpes zoster. Any of the three branches of the trigeminal nerve may be affected: (1) the ophthalmic branch, (2) the maxillary branch, or (3) the mandibular branch (Figure 4-28). Oral lesions occur when the maxillary and/or mandibular branches are affected (Figure 4-29). Skin lesions on the forehead and around the eye occur when the ophthalmic branch is involved. The oral lesions, like the skin lesions, are characterized by their unilateral distribution. Prodromal symptoms of pain, burning, or both, called **paresthesia**, often precede the development of vesicles. Oral lesions are painful

FIGURE 4-26 ■ Chickenpox. **A,** Skin lesions. **B,** Gingival lesion. (Courtesy Dr. Roger S. Kitzis.)

FIGURE 4-27 ■ Herpes zoster. **A,** Unilateral distribution of vesicles along the distribution of a sensory nerve. **B,** Many vesicles coalesce to form large lesions.

Ophthalmic branch

Maxillary branch

Mandibular branch

FIGURE 4-28 ■ Diagram of the branches of the trigeminal nerve.

FIGURE 4-29 ■ Herpes zoster. **A,** Unilateral facial lesions occurring along the distribution of the maxillary branch of the trigeminal nerve. **B,** Intraoral lesions in the same patient illustrate the unilateral distribution of herpes zoster.

and begin as vesicles that progress to ulcers. The disease usually lasts for several weeks, and in some patients, neuralgia, which takes months to resolve, may follow the resolution of the lesions.

Diagnosis

The diagnosis of varicella (chicken pox) and herpes zoster is generally made on the basis of the clinical features. Biopsy or a cytologic mucosal smear of the lesion may show the same type of virally altered epithelial cells that are seen in herpes simplex infection (Tzanck cells). Laboratory identification of varicella zoster virus is also helpful.

Treatment

Varicella generally requires only supportive treatment. Antiviral drugs are used for immunocompromised patients and for patients with herpes zoster. In some patients corticosteroids have been used in an attempt to prevent the pain of postherpetic neuralgia.

EPSTEIN-BARR VIRUS INFECTION

The **Epstein-Barr virus** (EBV) has been implicated in several diseases that occur in the oral region, including infectious mononucleosis, nasopharyngeal carcinoma, Burkitt lymphoma, and hairy leukoplakia. Nasopharyngeal carcinoma and Burkitt lymphoma are rare malignant

neoplasms. Infectious mononucleosis and hairy leukoplakia are discussed here.

INFECTIOUS MONONUCLEOSIS

Infectious mononucleosis is an infectious disease caused by the Epstein-Barr virus. It is characterized by sore throat, fever, generalized lymphadenopathy, enlarged spleen, malaise, and fatigue. Palatal petechiae occur in infectious mononucleosis, usually appearing early in the course of the disease. The mechanism for the development of these petechiae is unclear. The diagnosis is confirmed by the identification in the blood of mononucleosis cells, which are atypical activated T lymphocytes. Severe complications such as hepatitis occur in some patients. In developed countries infectious mononucleosis occurs principally in late adolescence, among young adults in the upper socioeconomic classes. The virus is transmitted by close contact. Contact with saliva during kissing is a frequent route of transmission of Epstein-Barr virus. In most patients infectious mononucleosis is a benign, self-limited disease

FIGURE 4-30 ■ Hairy leukoplakia seen here in an HIV-infected patient is an oral epithelial lesion caused by the Epstein-Barr virus.

FIGURE 4-31 ■ Herpangina.

that resolves within 4 to 6 weeks. In some patients fatigue lasts much longer. Multiple recurrences occur in some patients.

HAIRY LEUKOPLAKIA

Hairy leukoplakia is characterized by an irregular, corrugated white lesion most commonly occurring on the lateral border of the tongue (Figure 4-30). Epstein-Barr virus has been identified in the epithelial cells of hairy leukoplakia and is considered to be the cause of the lesion. Hairy leukoplakia was first identified in patients infected with human immunodeficiency virus (HIV) and occurs most commonly in these patients; it has also been reported in immunocompromised patients not infected with HIV (i.e., organ transplant patients). Hairy leukoplakia is discussed later in this chapter as an oral manifestation of HIV infection.

COXSACKIEVIRUS INFECTIONS

The **coxsackieviruses,** named for the town in New York state where the virus was first discovered, cause several different infectious diseases. Three of these have distinctive oral lesions and are discussed here. Fecal-oral contamination, saliva, and respiratory droplets can all be the means of transmission.

HERPANGINA

Herpangina characteristically includes vesicles on the soft palate (Figure 4-31), along with fever, malaise, sore throat, and difficulty swallowing (dysphagia). An erythematous pharyngitis is also present. The disease is usually mild to moderate and resolves in less than 1 week without treatment.

HAND-FOOT-AND-MOUTH DISEASE

Hand-foot-and-mouth disease usually occurs in epidemics in children younger than 5 years of age. Oral lesions are generally painful vesicles and ulcers that can occur anywhere in the mouth. Multiple macules or papules occur on the skin, typically on the feet, toes, hands, and fingers. Lesions resolve spontaneously within 2 weeks.

Diagnosis

Although the oral lesions may resemble herpes simplex infection, the distribution of the skin lesions and the mild systemic symptoms usually help to differentiate the two conditions. Viral culture and measurement of circulating antibodies to the type of coxsackievirus that causes hand-foot-and-mouth disease may help to confirm the diagnosis but generally are not necessary.

Treatment

The disease is generally mild and of short duration. Treatment usually is not required.

ACUTE LYMPHONODULAR PHARYNGITIS

Acute lymphonodular pharyngitis is another coxsackievirus infection that is characterized by fever, sore throat, and mild headache. Hyperplastic lymphoid tissue of the soft palate or tonsillar pillars appears as yellowish or dark pink nodules. The disease generally lasts several days to 2 weeks and does not usually require treatment.

OTHER VIRAL INFECTIONS THAT MAY HAVE ORAL MANIFESTATIONS

MEASLES

Measles is a highly contagious disease causing systemic symptoms and a skin rash that results from a type of virus called a **paramyxovirus.** The disease most commonly occurs in childhood. Early in the disease, **Koplik spots,** which are small erythematous macules with white necrotic centers, may occur in the oral cavity.

MUMPS

Mumps, or **epidemic parotitis,** is a viral infection of the salivary glands that is also caused by a paramyxovirus. The disease most commonly occurs in children and is characterized by painful swelling of the salivary glands, most commonly bilateral swelling of the parotid glands.

HUMAN IMMUNODEFICIENCY VIRUS AND ACQUIRED IMMUNODEFICIENCY SYNDROME

The virus associated with **acquired immunodeficiency syndrome (AIDS)** was identified in 1983; in 1986 it was designated as **human immunodeficiency virus (HIV).** HIV is transmitted by sexual contact with infected persons, by contact with infected blood and blood products, and to infants of infected mothers. HIV infects cells of the immune system. The most important of the cells of the immune system that the virus infects is the CD4⁺ T-helper lympho-cyte. This lymphocyte is important both in cell-mediated immunity and in regulating the immune response. As the disease progresses, this lymphocyte becomes depleted. Other cells that may be infected with HIV include macrophages, Langerhans cells, dendritic cells, and cells of the nervous system.

THE SPECTRUM OF HUMAN IMMUNODEFICIENCY VIRUS

Many individuals experience an acute disease that occurs shortly after infection with HIV, whereas other individuals remain asymptomatic. The acute disease resolves, and infected individuals may have no signs or symptoms of disease for some time. In most patients infected with HIV, a progressive immunodeficiency eventually develops. As the immune system begins to fail, the number of CD4⁺ lymphocytes decreases; nonspecific problems such as fa-tigue and opportunistic infections such as oral candidiasis may develop. As the immune system becomes profoundly deficient, life-threatening opportunistic infections and cancers occur. The most severe result of infection with HIV is AIDS.

DIAGNOSING AIDS

The diagnosis of AIDS is well defined. The definition of AIDS has been established by the Centers for Disease Control and Prevention (CDC) and is given in Box 4-2. Since it was iden-tified in the early 1980s, this definition has been changed several times as knowledge of the disease has grown. The most recent definition of AIDS in adults and adolescents includes HIV infection with severe CD4⁺ lymphocyte deple-tion (less than 200 CD4⁺ lymphocytes per microliter [μl] of blood). The normal CD4⁺ lymphocyte count is between about 550 and 1000 lymphocytes/μl blood. The revised definition continues to include a number of opportunistic diseases such as *Pneumocystis carinii* pneumonia, esopha-geal candidiasis, and Kaposi sarcoma. Also included is HIV-related wasting syndrome. In addition to including the CD4⁺ lymphocyte count, the revised definition includes pul-monary tuberculosis, recurrent pneumonia, and invasive cervical cancer.

Box 4-2

Definition of Acquired Immunodeficiency Syndrome

Acquired immunodeficiency syndrome (AIDS) is an illness characterized by one or more of the following diseases or conditions:

With Laboratory Evidence of Human Immunodeficiency Virus Infection

1. Fewer than 200 CD4⁺ T lymphocytes/μl or a CD4⁺ T-lymphocyte percentage of total lymphocytes less than 14%
2. Any of the diseases listed below or those that follow here:
   a. Multiple bacterial infections of certain types affecting a child less than 13 yr of age
   b. Coccidioidomycosis, disseminated
   c. Human immunodeficiency virus (HIV) encephalopathy (HIV dementia)
   d. Histoplasmosis, disseminated
   e. Isosporiasis with diarrhea persisting longer than 1 mo
   f. Lymphoma of the brain at any age
   g. Kaposi sarcoma
   h. Certain types of lymphoma
   i. Mycobacterial disease other than tuberculosis, disseminated
   j. Extrapulmonary tuberculosis
   k. *Salmonella* septicemia, recurrent
   l. HIV-related wasting syndrome
   m. Pulmonary tuberculosis
   n. Recurrent pneumonia
   o. Invasive cervical cancer

Human Immunodeficiency Virus Laboratory Tests Not Performed or Results Inconclusive and the Patient Has No Other Cause of Immunodeficiency

1. Candidiasis of the esophagus, trachea, bronchi, or lungs
2. Cryptococcosis, extrapulmonary
3. Cryptosporidiosis with diarrhea persisting longer than 1 mo
4. Cytomegalovirus disease of an organ other than liver, spleen, or lymph nodes in a patient older than 1 mo of age
5. Herpes simplex virus infection causing a mucocutaneous ulcer that persists longer than 1 mo or bronchitis, pneumonitis, or esophagitis for any duration affecting a patient older than 1 mo of age
6. Kaposi sarcoma affecting a patient less than 60 yr of age
7. Lymphoma of the brain affecting a patient less than 60 yr of age
8. Lymphoid interstitial pneumonia, pulmonary hyperplasia, or both, affecting a child less than 13 yr of age
9. *Mycobacterium avium* or *Mycobacterium kansasii* disease, disseminated
10. *Pneumocystis carinii* pneumonia
11. Progressive multifocal leukoencephalopathy
12. Toxoplasmosis of the brain affecting a patient older than 1 mo of age

Adapted from Centers for Disease Control and Prevention: 1993 revised classification system for HIV infection and expanded surveillance case definition for AIDS among adolescents and adults, *MMWR Recomm Rep* 41(RR-17):1, 1992.

HUMAN IMMUNODEFICIENCY VIRUS TESTING

Tests that identify antibody to HIV are the tests generally used to determine whether a person has been infected with HIV. More recently, a rapid HIV test has been approved. This test identifies antibody to HIV either in oral fluid or in blood. The oral test uses a collector specially designed to obtain a sample of transudate through the oral mucosa. Oral fluid testing has been approved as a test that can be done by people at home. A positive oral test is confirmed by a blood test using a more specific test called a **Western blot test.** A negative test does not require confirmation. Routine HIV testing of blood generally uses a blood test called an **enzyme-linked immunosorbent assay (ELISA).** When this test is positive twice, it is followed by the more specific **Western blot test.** To be considered seropositive for HIV, a person must have two positive ELISA results followed by a positive Western blot test result. Other tests such as the polymerase chain reaction (PCR) identify virus rather than antibody. HIV testing is now becoming a component of the laboratory tests that accompany routine physical examinations. In the United States different states have different laws concerning HIV testing. Informed consent by the patient and pretest counseling may be required before HIV testing can be done. HIV testing is an important means of controlling HIV infection by allowing infected individuals to be treated and as a result, their viral load and potential infectivity are decreased.

CLINICAL MANIFESTATIONS

The initial infection with HIV may be completely asymptomatic. However, early in HIV infection the amount of circulating virus is very high, and the risk of transmission to others may be very high. In some individuals lymphadenopathy may develop; in still others an acute illness resembling infectious mononucleosis and lasting 8 to 14 days can occur. When this acute illness develops, the patient may have sore throat, general malaise, myalgia and arthralgia, lymphadenopathy, and fever. Patients with acute infection can also have oral candidiasis, skin rash, nausea, and diarrhea. After this acute illness, some individuals have persistent lymphadenopathy, but many become completely asymptomatic.

The virus infects cells of the immune system; as a result this system stops protecting the individual against certain infections and tumors. In time, as the immune system becomes deficient, a variety of signs and symptoms can develop, signaling changes in the immune system. Several of these signs and symptoms occurring together are sometimes called *AIDS-related complex.* They include oral candidiasis, fatigue, weight loss, and lymphadenopathy. HIV can also infect cells of the nervous system, resulting in dementia in some patients.

Antibodies to HIV generally begin to be detectable in blood about 6 weeks after the initial infection. However, in some individuals antibodies may not be detectable for 6 months and occasionally for up to 1 year or more.

The spectrum of HIV infection includes the full range of problems that result from infection with this virus, from asymptomatic infection to AIDS (Figure 4-32). AIDS represents terminal HIV infection in this spectrum. It is not yet known how many of the persons who become infected with HIV go on to experience immunodeficiency, opportunistic diseases, or dementia. Some patients who are HIV-seropositive appear to remain immunocompetent for many years. Cofactors that can contribute to the development of the immunodeficiency are being studied. The results of natural history studies have shown that without treatment most HIV infected individuals will develop AIDS.

MEDICAL MANAGEMENT

Tests such as polymerase chain reaction (PCR) are used to measure the amount of HIV circulating in serum. This is called the *viral load.* Measurement of viral load along with the $CD4^+$ lymphocyte count is used to assess HIV infection. Patients with HIV infection are managed with combinations of different types of antiretroviral (anti-HIV) drugs and drugs that prevent and treat opportunistic diseases. The combination of drugs is called *highly active*

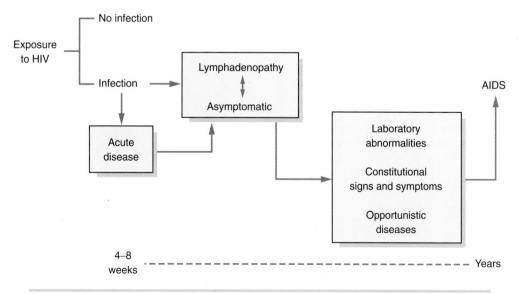

FIGURE 4-32 ▪ Spectrum of human immunodeficiency virus *(HIV)* disease. *AIDS,* acquired immunodeficiency syndrome.

antiretroviral therapy (HAART or ART). Measurement of viral load is used to evaluate the effectiveness of antiretroviral therapy. Management of HIV infection is continually changing in response to the results of ongoing clinical drug trials. With antiretroviral treatment, many individuals infected with HIV may live long and relatively healthy lives.

ORAL MANIFESTATIONS

Oral lesions are prominent features of AIDS and HIV infection (Box 4-3). Some of these lesions are known to be indicators of developing immunodeficiency and predictors of the development of AIDS in individuals who are HIV seropositive. The oral lesions that occur develop because of the deficiency in cell-mediated immunity and the deregulation of immunologic responses that occurs when the T-helper cells (CD4$^+$ lymphocytes) become depleted. Oral lesions include opportunistic infections, tumors, and autoimmune-like diseases. As a result of management of HIV infection with antiviral therapy, oral manifestations of HIV are much less common than earlier in the history of this disease.

ORAL CANDIDIASIS

Oral candidiasis occurs frequently in individuals with cell-mediated immunodeficiency and is one of the most common oral lesions seen in persons with HIV infection (Figure 4-33). It is also called *thrush*. All of the different types of oral candidiasis described earlier in this chapter, including mucocutaneous candidiasis, can occur. It is important to remember that candidiasis can be associated with a variety of conditions other than HIV infection, such as uncontrolled diabetes, other immunodeficiency diseases, antibiotic treatment, and xerostomia. Both topical and systemic antifungal treatment can be used to control oral candidiasis in the patient

with immunodeficiency caused by HIV infection. Recurrence is common.

In persons who are known to be infected with HIV, the development of oral candidiasis is worrisome because it generally signals the beginning of a progressively severe immunodeficiency. It may also be a sign of acute HIV infection. Persons with unexplained oral candidiasis should be referred to a physician for evaluation if the cause of the candidiasis cannot be determined. Studies have shown oral candidiasis to be a very early sign of developing immunodeficiency and predictive of the development of AIDS in a person who is infected with HIV. Oral lesions caused by other fungal infections such as histoplasmosis and coccidioidomycosis have also been reported in persons with HIV infection, but they are rare.

HERPES SIMPLEX INFECTION

Ulcers caused by the herpes simplex virus occur in persons with HIV infection (Figure 4-34). Herpes labialis and lesions

FIGURE 4-33 ■ Candidiasis in a patient with human immunodeficiency virus infection. Removable white plaques are present on the mucosa of the soft palate.

Box 4-3

Oral Lesions Associated with Human Immunodeficiency Virus Infection

- Candidiasis
- Herpes simplex infection
- Herpes zoster
- Hairy leukoplakia
- Human papillomavirus lesions
- Atypical gingivitis and periodontitis
- Other opportunistic infections reported:
  - *Mycobacterium avium, M. intracellulare*
  - Cytomegalovirus
  - *Cryptococcus neoformans*
  - *Klebsiella pneumoniae*
  - *Enterobacter cloacae*
  - *Histoplasma capsulatum*
- Kaposi sarcoma
- Non-Hodgkin lymphoma
- Aphthous ulcers
- Mucosal pigmentation
- Bacterial salivary gland enlargement and xerostomia
- Spontaneous gingival bleeding resulting from thrombocytopenia

FIGURE 4-34 ■ Herpes simplex ulceration of the hard palate in a patient with human immunodeficiency virus infection. *Arrows* point to the periphery of the ulcer.

consistent with intraoral recurrent herpes simplex infection can also develop in persons with HIV infection. The clinical characteristics of these lesions are the same as those occurring in immunocompetent individuals. However, when the immune system, particularly cell-mediated immunity, becomes deficient, HIV-infected individuals are at risk for the development of ulcers caused by the herpes simplex virus that do not have the same clinical characteristics as those seen in immunocompetent persons. These appear as persistent, superficial, painful ulcers that can be located anywhere in the oral cavity. Small, characteristic herpes simplex–like ulcers can be seen surrounding larger ulcers, but their presence cannot be depended on for diagnosis. The diagnosis of these ulcers is made by several methods, including viral culture, cytologic smear, biopsy, and response to the antiviral medication acyclovir.

Ulceration of the oral mucosa from herpes simplex infection that has been present for more than 1 month is an oral lesion that meets the criteria for the diagnosis of AIDS. This can occur only when a person has profound immunodeficiency. Oral ulcers caused by cytomegalovirus may also occur in HIV-infected individuals who are severely immunodeficient. These ulcers are much rarer than those caused by herpes simplex virus.

HERPES ZOSTER

Herpes zoster is caused by the varicella-zoster virus and is described earlier in this chapter. When herpes zoster occurs in a person with HIV infection, it generally follows the usual pattern (see Figures 4-27 to 4-29). Although the infection can disseminate, most cases are self-limited. In the facial and oral area the lesions appear as distinctly unilateral ones following the distribution of one or more branches of the trigeminal nerve. The development of herpes zoster in a person infected with HIV is a sign of developing immunodeficiency.

HAIRY LEUKOPLAKIA

Hairy leukoplakia is caused by Epstein-Barr virus and is discussed earlier in this chapter. It was first described in individuals with HIV infection; although it has been reported in HIV-negative individuals, most cases are an oral manifestation of HIV infection. It almost always occurs on the lateral borders of the tongue and may extend onto the dorsal and ventral tongue (Figure 4-35; and see Figure 4-30). On the lateral tongue it appears as an irregular white lesion that has a corrugated surface. The corrugations may not be present when the lesions extend onto the dorsal or ventral tongue. Microscopically, this lesion shows hyperkeratosis (often with hairlike projections), epithelial hyperplasia, vacuolated epithelial cells, and little or no inflammatory infiltrate in the underlying connective tissue.

Other white lesions such as those resulting from chronic tongue chewing and hyperplastic candidiasis can resemble hairy leukoplakia clinically. Biopsy of the lesions can reveal a microscopic appearance that is consistent with hairy leukoplakia. However, the most reliable method of diagnosis is identification of the Epstein-Barr virus in the lesion.

In general, hairy leukoplakia is not treated. Lesions may respond to antiviral medication such as acyclovir or zidovudine but recur when treatment is discontinued. Studies have shown hairy leukoplakia to be predictive of the development of AIDS in HIV-infected persons.

HUMAN PAPILLOMAVIRUS INFECTIONS

Lesions caused by human papillomaviruses are described earlier in this chapter. Papillary oral lesions resulting from several different papillomaviruses have been described in persons with HIV infection. They are either normal in color or have a slightly erythematous mucosa (Figure 4-36). These lesions may be persistent and may occur in multiple oral mucosal locations. Results of studies have suggested that the prevalence of these human papillomavirus lesions has not decreased with antiretroviral therapy as has the prevalence of most other HIV-associated oral lesions. Diagnosis of these lesions is made by biopsy and microscopic examination, with special tests to identify papillomavirus. HPV lesions in patients with HIV infection are difficult to control, and recurrence and proliferation are common.

FIGURE 4-35 ■ Hairy leukoplakia.

FIGURE 4-36 ■ Papillary lesion of the upper lip caused by human papillomavirus in a patient with human immunodeficiency virus infection.

FIGURE 4-37 ■ Kaposi sarcoma in a patient with acquired immunodeficiency syndrome. **A,** Skin. **B,** Gingiva. (Courtesy Dr. Fariba Younai.)

KAPOSI SARCOMA

Kaposi sarcoma is one of the opportunistic neoplasms that occur in patients with HIV infection. Human herpesvirus type 8 (HHV-8), or Kaposi sarcoma–associated herpesvirus (KSHV), has been associated with this neoplasm. Oral lesions appear as reddish-purple, flat or raised lesions and are seen anywhere in the oral cavity. The most common locations are the palate and gingiva (Figure 4-37). This lesion was common before antiretroviral therapy was available, but is now seen much less frequently.

The diagnosis is made by biopsy. However, the clinical appearance of the lesion can be used when it is characteristic and the diagnosis of Kaposi sarcoma has been made at another site. At present no effective treatment for Kaposi sarcoma exists. Surgical excision to decrease the size of the lesion is sometimes attempted, as are radiation treatment and chemotherapy. Kaposi sarcoma is one of the intraoral lesions that may fulfill the criteria for the diagnosis of AIDS.

LYMPHOMA

Non-Hodgkin lymphoma is another of the malignant tumors that occur in association with HIV infection. It occasionally occurs in the oral cavity. Epstein-Barr virus has been associated with this neoplasm. These tumors have appeared as nonulcerated, necrotic, or ulcerated masses and have been surfaced by either ulcerated or normal-colored erythematous mucosa (Figure 4-38).

The diagnosis is made by biopsy and microscopic examination. Treatment involves several different chemotherapeutic drugs. Oral lymphoma is another oral lesion that may meet the criteria for the diagnosis of AIDS.

FIGURE 4-38 ■ Intraoral lymphoma in a patient with acquired immunodeficiency syndrome.

GINGIVAL AND PERIODONTAL DISEASE

In patients with HIV infection unusual forms of gingival and periodontal disease can develop. These occur in HIV-infected individuals whose immune system has become deficient, and have been called **linear gingival erythema** and **necrotizing ulcerative periodontitis.** A condition resembling necrotizing ulcerative gingivitis (NUG) also occurs in individuals with HIV infection.

Linear gingival erythema has three characteristic features: (1) spontaneous bleeding, (2) punctate or

FIGURE 4-39 ■ Atypical periodontal disease in a patient with human immunodeficiency virus infection.

FIGURE 4-40 ■ Persistent, nonspecific (major aphthous-like) ulcers in a patient with human immunodeficiency virus infection. (Courtesy Dr. Sidney Eisig.)

petechiae-like lesions on the attached gingiva and alveolar mucosa, and (3) a bandlike erythema of the gingiva that does not respond to therapy. Linear gingival erythema is different from typical gingivitis in that gingivitis is generally not characterized by spontaneous bleeding, and the erythema of typical gingivitis responds within a few days to 1 week to scaling, root planing, and improvement of oral hygiene. Linear gingival erythema occurs independently of oral hygiene status.

Some patients experience gingivitis that resembles necrotizing ulcerative gingivitis, and it can be either generalized or localized to specific areas. Necrotizing ulcerative periodontitis resembles necrotizing ulcerative gingivitis in that patients experience pain, spontaneous gingival bleeding, interproximal necrosis, and interproximal cratering (Figure 4-39). Patients also experience intense erythema and, most characteristically, extremely rapid bone loss. **Necrotizing stomatitis** is characterized by extensive focal areas of bone loss along with the features of necrotizing ulcerative periodontitis.

The specific causes of these atypical gingival and periodontal diseases remain unclear. The microbiota associated with these diseases is being studied and has not been found to be distinctly different from that of inflammatory periodontal disease. These atypical gingival and periodontal conditions are not common in HIV-infected individuals and appear to occur in patients whose immune systems have become severely compromised.

Treatment of HIV gingivitis and periodontitis involves scaling, root planing, and soft tissue curettage. In addition, intrasulcular lavage with povidone-iodine, use of a chlorhexidine mouth rinse, and short-term systemic metronidazole administration have been helpful in the treatment of these conditions. Good oral hygiene, including the use of smaller toothbrushes and interproximal cleaning devices, has been a component of management.

Most HIV-infected patients do not have HIV-associated gingival and periodontal problems. However, recognition of early lesions is essential to prevent extensive bone loss, and frequent recall is helpful in early identification of gingival and periodontal disease. Lack of response to periodontal treatment is a clue to the recognition of HIV-associated gingivitis and periodontitis.

SPONTANEOUS GINGIVAL BLEEDING

A decrease in the number of platelets resulting from an autoimmune type of thrombocytopenic purpura is occasionally seen in patients with HIV infection. These patients can have bleeding gums or mucosal petechiae. Gingival bleeding not related to thrombocytopenia has also been described in linear gingival erythema and necrotizing ulcerative periodontitis. A platelet count should be considered before deep scaling procedures are performed.

APHTHOUS ULCERS

Characteristic minor aphthous ulcers occur in patients with HIV infection and AIDS. Studies have suggested that an increase in the incidence of these ulcers occurs in patients with HIV infection. The clinical appearance and behavior of minor aphthous ulcers in HIV-infected patients are the same as in other individuals (see Chapter 3). Minor aphthous ulcers are diagnosed on the basis of their clinical appearance.

Ulcers that resemble major aphthous ulcers also occur in patients with HIV infection (Figure 4-40). They appear as deep, persistent, painful ulcers and must be differentiated from infectious ulcers. Biopsy and microscopic examination of these ulcers do not show any evidence of an infectious

CHAPTER 4 *Synopsis—cont'd*

CONDITION/DISEASE	CAUSE	AGE/RACE/SEX	LOCATION
Deep Fungal Infections			
Histoplasmosis Coccidioidomycosis Blastomycosis Cryptococcosis	*Histoplasma capsulatum* *Coccidioides immitis* *Blastomyces dermatitidis* *Cryptococcus neoformans*	*	Primary: lung infection Secondary: oral mucosal involvement
Mucormycosis	†	*	Nasal cavity Maxillary sinus Hard palate
Viral Infections			
Verruca vulgaris	A human papillomavirus	Children and adults	Skin Lips: most common oral location
Condyloma acuminatum	A human papillomavirus	Usually adults	Oral mucosa: any location
Multifocal epithelial hyperplasia	A human papillomavirus	Occurs in children	Oral mucosa

Primary herpetic
    gingivostomatitis
	Herpes simplex virus
	Most oral infections are
	    type 1, some are type 2
		Generally in children
		Less common in
		    adolescents and adults
			Lips, Gingival and oral mucosa

Recurrent herpes
    simplex infection
	Herpes simplex virus	Usually seen in
		    adolescents and adults
			Herpes labialis: vermilion
			    of lips
			Recurrent intraoral form:
			    keratinized mucosa (hard
			    palate and gingiva)

Chickenpox	Varicella-zoster virus	Usually seen in children Less common in adolescents and adults	Skin Mucous membranes

N/A, Not applicable.
*No significant information.
†Not covered in this text.

CLINICAL FEATURES	RADIOGRAPHIC FEATURES	MICROSCOPIC FEATURES	TREATMENT	DIAGNOSTIC PROCESS
Chronic nonhealing ulcers	Irregular radiolucency if bone involvement	Causative organism identified in biopsy tissue	Appropriate antifungal agents	Microscopic
Proliferating mass with destruction of bone	Irregular radiolucency if bone involvement	Causative organism identified in biopsy tissue	Appropriate antifungal agent Management of underlying disease	Microscopic
White, papillary exophytic lesion resembling a papilloma	N/A	Finger-like projection of keratotic squamous epithelium with central cores of well-vascularized fibrous connective tissue Cells with clear cytoplasm in the upper spinous layer	Surgical excision Immunologic staining to identify presence of papillomavirus May recur	Microscopic
Pink, papillary lesion usually more diffuse than papilloma or verruca vulgaris There may be multiple lesions	N/A	Thickened epithelium with finger-like projections covering cores of connective tissue Cells with clear cytoplasm seen throughout the epithelium	Surgical excision Recurrence is common	Microscopic
Multiple whitish to pale pink nodules distributed throughout the oral mucosa	N/A	Thickened epithelium with broad, connected rete bridges Cells with clear cytoplasm seen in the epithelium	Self-limited disease	Clinical Microscopic
Multiple tiny vesicles that progress to form painful ulcers Painful, erythematous, swollen gingiva Fever, malaise, cervical lymphadenopathy	N/A	Virally altered epithelial cells in mucosal smear or biopsy tissue (Tzanck cells)	Self-limited disease	Clinical Microscopic
Focal crops of tiny vesicles that coalesce to form a single ulcer Prodromal symptoms	N/A	Virally altered epithelial cells in mucosal smear or biopsy tissue (Tzanck cells)	Self-limited disease	Clinical
Vesicular and pustular eruptions Oral lesions usually do not cause severe discomfort	N/A	Virally altered epithelial cells in mucosal smear or biopsy tissue (Tzanck cells)	Self-limited disease	Clinical

Continued

Chapter 5

Developmental Disorders

Olga A.C. Ibsen

OBJECTIVES

After studying this chapter, the student will be able to:

1. Define each of the words in the vocabulary list for this chapter.
2. Define inherited disorders.
3. Recognize developmental disorders of the dentition.
4. Describe the embryonic development of the face, oral cavity, and teeth.
5. Define each of the developmental anomalies discussed in this chapter.
6. Identify (clinically, radiographically, or both) the developmental anomalies discussed in this chapter.
7. Distinguish between intraosseous cysts and extraosseous cysts.
8. Describe the differences between odontogenic and nonodontogenic cysts.
9. Name four odontogenic cysts that are intraosseous.
10. Name two odontogenic cysts that are extraosseous.
11. Name four nonodontogenic cysts that are intraosseous.
12. Name four nonodontogenic cysts that are found in the soft tissues of the head, neck, and oral region.
13. List and define three anomalies that affect the number of teeth.
14. List and define two anomalies that affect the size of teeth.
15. List and define five anomalies that affect the shape of teeth.
16. Define and identify each of the following anomalies affecting tooth eruption: impacted teeth, embedded teeth, and ankylosed teeth.
17. Identify the diagnostic process that contributes most significantly to the final diagnosis of each developmental anomaly discussed in this chapter.

VOCABULARY

Ankyloglossia (ang″kə-lo-glos′e-ə) Extensive adhesion of the tongue to the floor of the mouth or the lingual aspect of the anterior portion of the mandible.

Ankylosed teeth (ang′kə-lōzd tēth) Teeth that are fused to the alveolar bone; a condition especially common with retained deciduous teeth.

Anodontia (an″o-don′shə) Congenital lack of teeth.

Anomaly (ə-nom′ə-le) Marked deviation from normal, especially as a result of congenital or hereditary defects.

Commissure (kom′i-sūr) The site of union of corresponding parts (e.g., the corners of the lips) (labial commissure, commissural lip pits).

Concrescence (kən-kres′əns) In dentistry, a condition in which two adjacent teeth become united by cementum.

VOCABULARY—cont'd

Congenital disorder (kən-jen′ĭ-təl dis-or′dər) A disorder that is present at and existing from the time of birth.

Cyst (sist) An abnormal sac or cavity lined by epithelium and surrounded by fibrous connective tissue.

Dens in dente (dens in den′te) "A tooth within a tooth"; a developmental anomaly that results when the enamel organ invaginates into the crown of a tooth before mineralization.

Dentinogenesis (den″tĭ-no-jen′ə-sis) The formation of dentin.

Differentiation (dif″ər-en″she-a′shən) The distinguishing of one tissue from another.

Dilaceration (di-las″ər-a′shən) An abnormal bend or curve, as in the root of a tooth.

Fusion (fu′zhən) The union of two adjacent tooth germs.

Gemination (jem″ĭ-na′shən) "Twinning"; when a single tooth germ attempts to divide, resulting in the incomplete formation of two teeth; the tooth usually has a single root and root canal.

Hypodontia (hi″po-don′shə) Partial anodontia; the lack of one or more teeth.

Impacted teeth (im-pak′təd tēth) Teeth that cannot erupt into the oral cavity because of a physical obstruction.

Macrodontia (mak″ro-don′shə) Abnormally large teeth.

Microdontia (mi″kro-don′shə) Abnormally small teeth.

Multilocular (mul″tĭ-lok′ū-lər) A radiographic appearance in which many circular radiolucencies exist; these can appear "soap bubble–like" or "honeycomb-like."

Nodule (nod′ūl) A small solid mass that can be detected through touch.

Oligodontia (ol″ĭ-go-don′she-ə) A subcategory of hypodontia in which six on more teeth are missing.

Predilection (prĕd-ĭ-lĕk′shən) A disposition in favor of something; preference.

Proliferation (pro-lif″ə-ra′shən) The multiplication of cells.

Stomodeum (sto″mo-de′əm) The embryonic invagination that becomes the oral cavity.

Supernumerary (soo″per-noo′mər-ar″e) In excess of the normal or regular number, as in teeth.

The development of the human body is an extremely complex process that begins when an egg is fertilized by a sperm. It continues with a series of cell divisions, multiplications, and **differentiation** into various tissues and structures. A failure or disturbance that occurs during these processes may result in a lack, excess, or deformity of a body part. These disorders are called **developmental disorders,** or **developmental anomalies.**

Inherited disorders are different from developmental disorders in that they are caused by an abnormality in the genetic makeup (genes and chromosomes) of an individual and transmitted from parent to offspring through the egg or sperm. Inherited disorders are discussed in Chapter 6.

A **congenital disorder** is one that is present at birth. It can be either inherited or developmental; however, the cause of most congenital abnormalities is unknown.

The complex process of **proliferation** and differentiation that takes place in the human body provides numerous possibilities for errors or defects in development. The head and neck region is a common location for such errors because of its intricate sequence and pattern of development. This chapter includes descriptions of developmental disorders of the face, oral cavity, and teeth with which the dental hygienist should be familiar.

Some of the developmental disturbances discussed in this chapter can be identified clinically, whereas others are identified by radiographic examination; still others require biopsy and microscopic examinations. A thorough clinical examination, including examination of extraoral and intraoral structures, is an essential component. Dental radiographs are an important part of the examination. Any developmental anomalies observed either clinically or radiographically are documented in the patient's record even if no treatment is indicated. The patient is informed of all dental anomalies, their possible implications, and the treatment necessary, if any. In some instances referral to a specialist is indicated. To better understand these developmental disorders, a brief review of the embryonic development of the face, oral cavity, and teeth is included in this chapter.

EMBRYONIC DEVELOPMENT OF THE FACE, ORAL CAVITY, AND TEETH

FACE

Development of the face is a process of selective growth or proliferation and differentiation (Figures 5-1 and 5-2). During the third week of embryonic life, an **invagination,** or infolding, of the ectoderm forms the primitive oral cavity, which is called the **stomodeum.** Just above the stomodeum is a process called the **frontal process,** and just below it is a structure called the first **branchial arch.** Additional branchial arches form below the first branchial arch. All of the face and most of the structures of the oral cavity develop from either the frontal process or the first branchial arch. The first branchial arch divides into two **maxillary processes** and the **mandibular process.** The maxillary processes give rise to the upper part of the cheeks, the lateral portions of the upper lip, and part of the palate. The mandibular arch forms the lower part of the cheeks, the mandible, and part of the tongue.

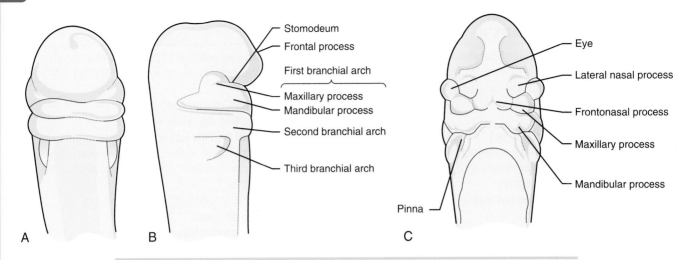

FIGURE 5-1 ■ In the third week of embryonic life an *invagination,* or infolding, of the ectoderm forms the primitive oral cavity, called the *stomodeum.* **A** and **B,** As facial development continues, the first branchial arch divides into two maxillary processes. **C,** The fourth week of development.

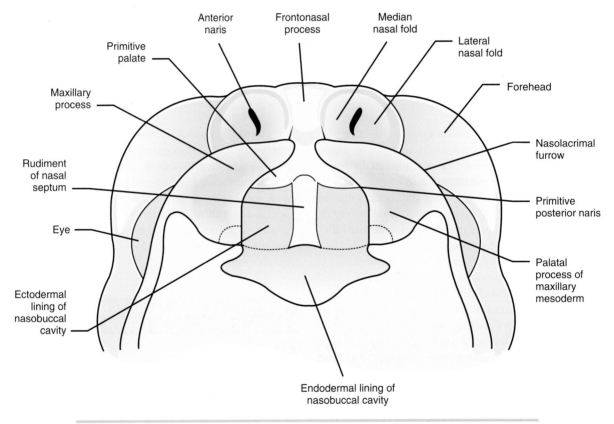

FIGURE 5-2 ■ The right and left palatine processes fuse to form the maxilla and premaxilla. A Y-shaped pattern results.

As development continues, two pits (called **olfactory pits**) mark the future openings of the nose that develop on the surface of the frontal process. They divide the frontal process into three parts: (1) the **median nasal process,** (2) the **right lateral nasal process,** and (3) the **left lateral nasal process.** The lateral nasal processes form the sides of the nose, whereas the median nasal process forms the center and tip of the nose. Later, the median nasal process grows downward between the maxillary processes to form a

pair of bulges called the **globular process.** This continues to grow downward, forming the portion of the upper lip called the **philtrum.** Most of these developments are completed by the end of the eighth week of embryonic life.

ORAL AND NASAL CAVITIES

The area of the palate called the **premaxilla** develops from the globular process. The lateral **palatine processes** (left and right) are formed from the maxillary processes. These lateral palatine processes then fuse with the premaxilla. The fusion creates a Y-shaped pattern (see Figure 5-2). The nasal septum arises from the median nasal process. The right and left maxillary processes fuse together with the nasal septum at the center of the palate.

The tongue develops from the first three branchial arches. The second and third branchial arches are located just below the first branchial arch (Figure 5-1, B). The body of the tongue forms from the first branchial arch, and the base of the tongue forms from the second and third branchial arches.

TEETH

Tooth development, or **odontogenesis,** in the human embryo begins at about the fifth week of embryonic life and involves both ectoderm and ectomesenchyme. The ectomesenchyme is derived from neural crest cells.

Odontogenesis begins with the formation of a band of ectoderm in each jaw called the **primary dental lamina.** Ten small knoblike proliferations of epithelial cells develop on the primary dental lamina in each jaw (Figure 5-3, A). Each of these proliferations extends into the underlying mesenchyme, becoming the early enamel organ for each of the primary teeth (Figure 5-3, B).

The tooth germ is composed of three parts: (1) the enamel organ, (2) the dental papilla, and (3) the dental sac, or *follicle* (Figure 5-3, C). The enamel organ develops from ectoderm, and the dental papilla and dental sac or follicle develop from mesoderm. Cell differentiation in the enamel organ progresses to produce ameloblasts, which form enamel. In the dental papilla odontoblasts are produced to form dentin. The permanent, or **succedaneous,** enamel organs form at the same time.

Formation of dental hard tissues occurs during the fifth month of gestation (Figure 5-4). **Dentinogenesis** is the formation of **dentin.** Dentin is the first mineralized tooth tissue to appear. When it begins to form, the mesenchymal tissue within the tooth germ is called the **dental papilla.** After dentin is produced, the dental papilla is called the *dental pulp.* **Enamel** is the product of the enamel organ. Enamel matrix begins to form shortly after dentin, and mineralization and maturation of enamel follow the formation of the matrix. **Amelogenesis** refers to the formation of enamel. The enamel is highly mineralized epithelial tissue and 90% of its volume is occupied by hydroxyapatite crystals.

The dental sac, or follicle, that surrounds the developing tooth germ provides cells that form cementum, the periodontal ligament, and alveolar bone. **Cementogenesis** (the formation of **cementum**) occurs after crown formation is complete. An epithelial structure called the **Hertwig epithelial root sheath** proliferates to shape the root of the tooth and induces the formation of the root dentin. Cells of the Hertwig epithelial root sheath must break up and pull away from the root surface before cementum can be produced. Very little cementum is produced until the tooth has erupted and is in occlusion and functioning. Root length is not completed until 1 to 4 years after the tooth erupts into the oral cavity.

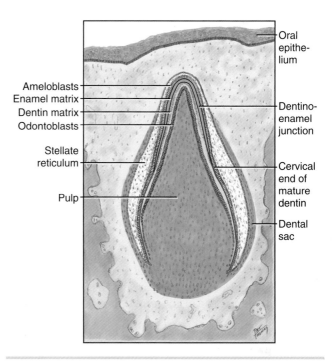

FIGURE 5-3 ■ Development of a tooth germ, showing initiation of dental lamina **(A),** proliferation of dental lamina **(B),** and differentiation of the components of the tooth germ **(C).** (From Bath-Balogh M, Fehrenbach MF: *Illustrated dental embryology, histology, and anatomy,* ed 3, St. Louis, 2012, Saunders.)

FIGURE 5-4 ■ Deposition of enamel and dentin. (From Bath-Balogh M, Fehrenbach MF: *Illustrated dental embryology, histology, and anatomy,* ed 3, St. Louis, 2012, Saunders.)

DEVELOPMENTAL SOFT TISSUE ABNORMALITIES

ANKYLOGLOSSIA

Ankyloglossia is a developmental anomaly of the tongue. It is an extensive adhesion of the tongue to the floor of the mouth, caused by a short lingual frenum. The condition is often referred to as "tongue-tied." Ankyloglossia is derived from the Greek words *ankylos*, meaning adhesion, and *glossa*, meaning tongue. This adhesion results from the complete or partial fusion of the lingual frenum to the floor of the mouth. It is four times more common in boys than girls. Total ankyloglossia is rare. Partial ankyloglossia appears clinically as a very short lingual frenum connecting the anteroventral portion of the tongue to the floor of the mouth (Figure 5-5). Patients with a short lingual frenum may exhibit no adverse effects, but some may have problems with speech. Gingival recession and bone loss can occur if the frenum is attached high on the lingual alveolar ridge. Surgical removal of a portion of the lingual frenum, known as **frenectomy**, is the usual treatment for ankyloglossia.

COMMISSURAL LIP PITS

Commissural lip pits are epithelium-lined blind tracts located at the corners of the mouth **(commissures)** (Figure 5-6). These tracts may be shallow, or they may be several millimeters deep. They are a relatively common developmental **anomaly.** The cause of commissural lip pits is not clear; both the incomplete fusion of the maxillary and mandibular processes and the defective development of the horizontal facial cleft have been suggested. They are more often seen in adult males. The commissural lip pit may be observed during examination.

Another lip pit that occasionally may be seen is the **congenital lip pit (paramedian lip pit).** It occurs near the midline of the vermilion border of the lower lip and may appear as either a unilateral or bilateral depression. They are inherited as an autosomal dominant trait. No treatment is indicated for lip pits.

LINGUAL THYROID

A **Lingual thyroid,** or **ectopic lingual thyroid nodule,** is a mass of thyroid tissue located on the tongue away from the normal anatomic location of the thyroid gland. It is an uncommon developmental anomaly that results from the failure of the primitive thyroid tissue to migrate from its developmental location in the area of the foramen cecum on the posterior portion of the tongue to its normal position in the neck.

Clinically, the lingual thyroid nodule appears as a smooth nodular mass at the base of the tongue posterior to the circumvallate papillae on or near the midline. It can be asymptomatic or can cause a feeling of fullness in the throat or difficulty in swallowing. Microscopically, the lingual thyroid is composed of immature or mature thyroid tissue.

FIGURE 5-5 ■ Ankyloglossia. The short lingual frenum is attached near the tip of the tongue. (Courtesy Dr. George Blozis.)

FIGURE 5-6 ■ Commissural lip pit. A deep depression is seen at the labial commissure.

On occasion, the size of the lingual thyroid necessitates its removal. However, this nodule may be the patient's only functioning thyroid tissue. Therefore it is necessary to establish the presence of functioning thyroid tissue elsewhere before any nodular lesion located in the posterior aspect of the tongue is removed. If a normally located thyroid gland is lacking or nonfunctional, the lingual thyroid is not removed.

DEVELOPMENTAL CYSTS

A **cyst** is an abnormal, pathologic sac or cavity lined by epithelium and surrounded by fibrous connective tissue. Cysts occur throughout the body, including the oral region.

TABLE 5-1

Classification of Developmental Cysts

ODONTOGENIC		NONODONTOGENIC	
INTRAOSSEOUS	**EXTRAOSSEOUS**	**INTRAOSSEOUS**	**EXTRAOSSEOUS**
• Dentigerous cyst	• Eruption cyst	• Nasopalatine duct cyst	• Nasolabial cyst
• Primordial cyst		• Median palatal cyst	• Branchial cleft cyst (cervical lymphoepithelial cyst and intraoral lymphoepithelial cyst)
• Odontogenic keratocyst (keratocystic odontogenic tumor)		• Globulomaxillary cyst	• Epidermal cyst
• Lateral periodontal cyst	• Gingival cyst	• Median mandibular cyst	• Thyroglossal tract cyst

The cysts discussed in this chapter are all related to the development of the face, jaws, and teeth. Some have a distinctive microscopic appearance, and a definitive diagnosis is based on microscopic examination of the tissue. Other cysts are lined by less distinctive epithelium. The diagnosis of these cysts is based on both the microscopic appearance of the tissue and the location of the cyst.

The most common cyst observed in the oral cavity is caused by pulpal inflammation and is called a **radicular cyst (periapical cyst).** This cyst is described in Chapter 2. It develops from a preexisting periapical granuloma found at the apex of a nonvital tooth. The radicular cyst is always associated with a nonvital tooth and diagnosis can be made only through microscopic examination because the radiographic appearance can be similar to other lesions. A **residual cyst** is a radicular cyst that remains after extraction of the offending tooth. Because cysts are commonly observed in the jaws and surrounding soft tissues, the dental hygienist should understand their diagnostic criteria, pathogenesis, and prognosis. The preliminary identification of a cystic lesion is within the scope of dental hygiene practice.

Developmental cysts are classified as **odontogenic** (related to tooth development) and **nonodontogenic** (not related to tooth development). Cysts are also classified according to location, cause, origin of the epithelial cells, and microscopic appearance (Table 5-1). Developmental cysts can vary in size from small, asymptomatic lesions to large lesions that can cause expansion of bone. Very large and long-standing lesions can resorb tooth structure or move teeth. Oral cysts that occur within bone are called **intraosseous cysts,** and cysts that occur in soft tissue are called **extraosseous cysts.**

Radiographically, cysts within bone generally appear as well-circumscribed radiolucencies. All cysts may appear **unilocular,** but some are more likely to appear as **multilocular** radiolucencies. When a cyst is found within soft tissue, there is no radiographic feature.

ODONTOGENIC CYSTS

DENTIGEROUS CYST

A **dentigerous cyst,** also called a **follicular cyst,** forms around the crown of an unerupted or developing tooth (Figure 5-7). It is the second most common odontogenic

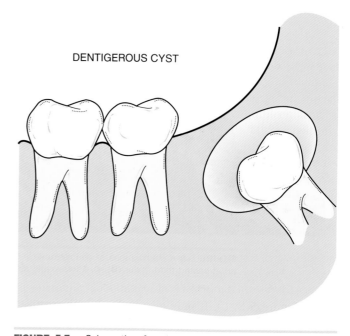

DENTIGEROUS CYST

FIGURE 5-7 ■ Schematic of a dentigerous cyst located around the crown of an unerupted or impacted tooth.

cyst after the radicular cyst. The epithelial lining originates from the reduced enamel epithelium after the crown has completely formed and calcified. Fluid accumulates between the crown and the reduced enamel epithelium. The reduced enamel epithelium results from remnants of the enamel organ. The most common location for the dentigerous cyst is around the crown of an unerupted or impacted mandibular third molar. However, a dentigerous cyst may form around the crowns of other unerupted or **impacted teeth** such as the maxillary cuspid or a supernumerary tooth. The cyst may develop in both males and females. However, there is a higher incidence in males and this cyst is most often seen in young adults in their twenties and thirties. The size of these cysts can range from small and asymptomatic to very large. When large, it is capable of displacing teeth or causing a fracture of the mandible.

Radiographically, the dentigerous cyst appears as a well-defined, unilocular radiolucency around the crown of an unerupted or impacted tooth (Figure 5-8, *A* and *B*). Microscopically, the lumen is most characteristically lined with cuboidal epithelium surrounded by a wall of connective

FIGURE 5-36 ■ Mottled enamel. The discoloration of the enamel in this patient occurred as a result of high fluoride intake.

FIGURE 5-37 ■ **A,** Hutchinson incisors. **B,** Mulberry molars. (Courtesy Dr. George Blozis.)

extent of the injury. The color of the enamel of these teeth may range from yellow to brown, or severe pitting and deformity may be involved. These enamel defects can frequently be identified radiographically before the eruption of the involved tooth. An anterior Turner tooth may be restored to provide an improved aesthetic appearance; a posterior Turner tooth may require a restoration to provide improved function.

Enamel Hypoplasia Resulting from Fluoride Ingestion

Enamel hypoplasia resulting from fluoride ingestion, or **dental fluorosis,** occurs as a result of the patient ingesting high concentrations of fluoride during tooth formation, usually in drinking water. Affected teeth exhibit a mottled discoloration of enamel (Figure 5-36). *Mottling* refers to irregular areas of discoloration. The more fluoride ingested, the more severe the mottling. The optimal range of fluoride in drinking water is 0.7 to 1.2 ppm. Ingestion of water with a fluoride concentration two to three times the recommended amount results in mild fluorosis that appears as white flecks and chalky opaque areas of enamel. Ingestion of water containing four times the recommended amount of fluoride causes brown or black staining and a pitted or overall corroded enamel appearance.

All permanent teeth are involved in this type of enamel hypoplasia. The teeth affected by fluorosis are generally decay resistant. To improve the aesthetic appearance of these teeth, bleaching, bonding, composites, porcelain veneers, or full-coverage crowns can be used.

Enamel Hypoplasia Resulting from Congenital Syphilis

Syphilis is a contagious sexually transmitted disease caused by the spirochete *Treponema pallidum.* It is described in detail in Chapter 4. **Congenital syphilis** is transmitted from an infected mother to her fetus via the placenta. Children with congenital syphilis have numerous developmental anomalies and may be blind, deaf, or paralyzed. In utero infection with *T. pallidum* results in enamel hypoplasia of the permanent incisors and first molars. This is so rare that a lengthy discussion is not warranted.

The affected incisors are shaped like screwdrivers: broad cervically and narrow incisally, with a notched incisal edge (Figure 5-37, *A*). They are called **Hutchinson incisors.** First molars appear as irregularly shaped crowns made up of multiple tiny globules of enamel instead of cusps (Figure 5-37, *B*). Because of their berrylike appearance, these molars are called **mulberry molars.** Not every case of congenital syphilis exhibits these dental findings, and similarly shaped teeth may be seen in individuals without congenital syphilis.

Treatment to improve the aesthetic appearance of these teeth includes full-coverage crowns.

Enamel Hypoplasia Resulting from Birth Injury, Premature Birth, or Idiopathic Factors

Enamel hypoplasia can occur as a result of trauma or change of environment at the time of birth or in premature infants. In addition, many cases of enamel hypoplasia do not have an identifiable cause despite careful and thorough history taking. The ameloblast is a sensitive cell that is easily damaged. For this reason even a mild illness or systemic problem can result in enamel hypoplasia. Such illnesses may be so insignificant that they are not known to the patient or remembered by the patient's parents.

FIGURE 5-38 ■ Regional odontodysplasia.

To improve the aesthetic appearance of these teeth, composites, porcelain veneers, or full-coverage crowns can be used.

ENAMEL HYPOCALCIFICATION

Enamel hypocalcification is a developmental anomaly that results in a disturbance of the maturation of the enamel matrix. It usually appears as a localized, chalky white spot on the middle third of smooth crowns. The underlying enamel may be soft and susceptible to caries. The cause of enamel hypocalcification is uncertain; however, trauma during the maturation of enamel matrix has been suggested. Bleaching, composites, porcelain veneers, or full-coverage crowns can be used to improve the aesthetic appearance of these teeth.

ENDOGENOUS STAINING OF TEETH

Endogenous or **intrinsic staining of teeth** occurs as a result of the deposition of substances circulating systemically during tooth development. For example, ingestion of tetracycline during tooth development causes a yellowish-green discoloration of dentin that is visible through the enamel. At the time of eruption the teeth fluoresce under ultraviolet light. Later the tetracycline is oxidized, the color changes from yellowish to brown, and the teeth no longer fluoresce. Other conditions such as rhesus (Rh) incompatibility (erythroblastosis fetalis), neonatal liver disease, and congenital porphyria (an inherited metabolic disease) also cause endogenous staining of teeth.

REGIONAL ODONTODYSPLASIA

Regional odontodysplasia, or **ghost teeth,** is an unusual developmental problem in which one or several teeth in the same quadrant are malformed and radiographically exhibit a marked reduction in radiodensity and a characteristic ghostlike appearance (Figure 5-38). Very thin enamel and dentin are present. On occasion, the enamel is not visible on the radiograph. The pulp chambers of these teeth are extremely large. Either the teeth do not erupt, or eruption is incomplete. If ghost teeth erupt into the oral cavity, they are typically nonfunctional and malformed.

FIGURE 5-39 ■ **A,** Horizontal impaction of the third molar. **B,** Mesioangular impaction of the third molar.

Regional odontodysplasia can affect either the deciduous or the permanent dentition. The maxilla, especially the anterior maxilla, is more often involved than the mandible. The cause of regional odontodysplasia is unknown. A vascular phenomenon has been suggested. Extraction usually is the treatment of choice for ghost teeth.

ABNORMALITIES OF TOOTH ERUPTION

IMPACTED AND EMBEDDED TEETH

Impacted teeth are teeth that cannot erupt because of a physical obstruction. **Embedded teeth** are those that do not erupt because of a lack of eruptive force. An impacted tooth is one of the most common developmental defects occurring in humans. Any tooth can be impacted. The most commonly impacted teeth are the maxillary and mandibular third molars, the maxillary cuspids, the maxillary and mandibular premolars, and supernumerary teeth. Impacted teeth are identified radiographically (Figure 5-39).

Third-molar impactions are classified according to the position of the tooth: mesioangular, distoangular, vertical, and horizontal. The most common position of an impacted third molar is mesioangular. The crown of the third molar points in a mesial direction and is in contact with the second molar, which is preventing its eruption. In a distoangular

FIGURE 5-40 ■ Ankylosis of deciduous molar. (Courtesy Dr. Margot Van Dis.)

impaction the crown of the third molar points in a distal direction toward the ramus, and the roots of the impacted tooth are adjacent to the distal root of the second molar. In a vertical impaction the crown of the third molar is in a normal position for eruption, but eruption is prevented by the distal aspect of the second molar or by the anterior border of the ramus. In a horizontal impaction the crown of the third molar is seen in a horizontal position relative to the inferior border of the mandible.

Teeth can be completely impacted in bone with no communication with the oral cavity, or they can be partially impacted. In a partial impaction the tooth lies partly in soft tissue and partly in bone. Partially impacted teeth often have communication with the oral cavity and are susceptible to infections, that is, pericoronitis. For unknown reasons some completely impacted teeth undergo resorption. This resorption usually begins in the crown portion of the tooth, and the tooth is slowly replaced by bone. Radiographically this resorption should not be confused with caries. Caries of an impacted tooth is impossible unless communication with the oral cavity occurs.

Impacted teeth are surgically removed to prevent odontogenic cyst and tumor formation or damage (resorption) to adjacent teeth or because the bone (in some cases) may be more susceptible to fracture. Partially impacted third molars are removed to prevent infections. Studies have shown that the optimal time to extract impacted third molars is between the ages of 12 and 24 years. With increased age a greater incidence of nerve paresthesia exists.

ANKYLOSED TEETH

Ankylosed teeth (or *submerged teeth*) are deciduous teeth in which bone has fused to cementum and dentin, preventing exfoliation of the deciduous tooth and eruption of the underlying permanent tooth (Figure 5-40). Deciduous molars are most often affected by ankylosis. The cause is unknown; trauma and infection of the periodontal ligament have been suggested.

Initially the tooth erupts into the oral cavity into normal occlusion. The ankylosed tooth is not exfoliated. When the permanent teeth erupt, those adjacent to the ankylosed tooth have taller occlusocervical heights. Compared with the adjacent teeth, the ankylosed tooth appears submerged and has a different, more solid sound when percussed.

The presence of an ankylosed tooth is usually suspected on the basis of the clinical appearance and is confirmed radiographically. The periodontal ligament space is lacking or indistinct because of the union of bone and cementum, and the tooth usually exhibits root resorption. Ankylosis may be seen in permanent teeth that have been avulsed and reimplanted.

Extraction of ankylosed deciduous teeth is necessary to allow eruption of the underlying permanent tooth. Extraction of ankylosed permanent teeth is often necessary to prevent malocclusion, caries, and periodontal disease.

SELECTED REFERENCES

Books

Alley KE, Melfi RC: *Permar's oral embryology and microscopic anatomy*, ed 10, Baltimore, 2000, Lippincott, Williams & Wilkins.

Darby M: *Mosby's comprehensive review of dental hygiene*, ed 7, St. Louis, 2012, Mosby.

Langlais RP, Miller CS: *Color atlas of common oral diseases*, ed 3, Baltimore, 2003, Lippincott, Williams & Wilkins.

Miller BF: *Miller-Keane encyclopedia and dictionary of medicine, nursing, and allied health*, revised reprint, ed 7, Philadelphia, 2005, Saunders.

Neville BW, Damm DD, Allen CM, et al: *Oral and maxillofacial pathology*, ed 3, St. Louis, 2009, Saunders.

Regezi JA, Sciubba JJ, Pogrel MA: *Atlas of oral and maxillofacial pathology*, Philadelphia, 2000, Saunders.

Regezi JA, Sciubba JJ, Jordan RCK: *Oral pathology: clinical-pathologic correlations*, ed 6, St. Louis, 2012, Saunders.

Scheid RC: *Woelfel's dental anatomy: its relevance to dentistry*, ed 7, Baltimore, 2007, Lippincott, Williams & Wilkins.

Journal Articles

Alexander WN, Lilly GE, Irby WB: Odontodysplasia, *Oral Surg* 22:814, 1966.

Alfors E, Larson A, Sjögren S: The odontogenic keratocyst: a benign cystic tumor? *J Oral Maxillofac Surg* 42:10, 1984.

Al-Talabani NG, Smith CJ: Experimental dentigerous cysts and enamel hypoplasia: their possible significance in explaining the pathogenesis of dentigerous cysts, *J Oral Pathol* 9:82, 1980.

Baker BR: Pits of the lip commissures in Caucasoid males, *Oral Surg* 21:56, 1966.

Barker GR: A radiolucency of the ascending ramus of the mandible associated with invested parotid salivary gland material and analogous with a Stafne bone cavity, *Br J Oral Maxillofac Surg* 26:81, 1988.

Baum BJ, Cohen MM: Patterns of size reduction in hypodontia, *J Dent Res* 50:779, 1971.

Bhargava D, Deshpande A: Keratocystic odontogenic tumor (KCOD)—a cyst to a tumor, *Oral Maxillofac Surg* 16:163, 2012.

Bodin I, Julin P, Thomsson M: Hyperdontia III: supernumerary anterior teeth, *Dentomaxillofac Radiol* 10:35, 1981a.

Bodin I, Julin P, Thomsson M: Hyperdontia IV: supernumerary premolars, *Dentomaxillofac Radiol* 19:99, 1981b.

Brannon RB: The odontogenic keratocyst—a clinicopathologic study of 312 cases. I. Clinical features, *Oral Surg* 42:54, 1976.

Brannon RB: The odontogenic keratocyst—a clinicopathologic study of 312 cases. II. Histologic features, *Oral Surg* 43:233, 1977.

Buchner A, Hansen LS: Lymphoepithelial cysts of the oral cavity: a clinicopathologic study of 38 cases, *Oral Surg* 50:441, 1980.

Burton DJ, Saffos RO, Scheffer RB: Multiple bilateral dens in dente as a factor in the etiology of multiple periapical lesions, *Oral Surg* 49:496, 1980.

Carter L, Carney Y, Perez-Pudlewski D: Lateral periodontal cyst: multifactorial analysis of a previously unreported series, *Oral Surg Oral Med Oral Pathol Oral Radiol Endod* 81:210, 1996.

Cavanha AO: Enamel pearls, *Oral Surg* 19:373, 1965.

Chi AC, Neville BW, Klinger BJ: A multilocular radiolucency, *J Am Dent Assoc* 138:1102, 2007.

Christ TF: The globulomaxillary cyst—an embryologic misconception, *Oral Surg Oral Med Oral Pathol* 30:515, 1970.

Conklin WW: Bilateral dens invaginatus in the mandibular incisor region, *Oral Surg* 45:905, 1978.

Dachi SF, Howell FV: A survey of 3874 routine full-mouth radiographs. II. A study of impacted teeth, *Oral Surg* 14:1165, 1961.

Darling AI, Levers BGH: Submerged human deciduous molars and ankylosis, *Arch Oral Biol* 18:1021, 1973.

Dean HT, Arnold FA: Endemic dental fluorosis or mottled teeth, *J Am Dent Assoc* 30:1278, 1943.

Dehlers FAC, Lee KW, Lee EC: Dens evaginatus (evaginated odontoma), *Dent Pract* 17:239, 1967.

Delany GM, Goldblatt LI: Fused teeth: a multidisciplinary approach to treatment, *J Am Dent Assoc* 103:732, 1981.

DiFiore PM, Hartwell GR: Median mandibular lateral periodontal cysts, *Oral Surg Oral Med Oral Pathol* 63:545, 1987.

Eisenbud LE, Attie J, Garlick J, et al: Aneurysmal bone cyst of the mandible, *Oral Surg Oral Med Oral Pathol* 64:202, 1987.

el-Mofty SK, Shannon MT, Mustoe TA: Lymph node metastasis in spindle cell carcinoma arising in an odontogenic cyst, *Oral Surg Oral Med Oral Pathol* 71:209, 1991.

Everett FG, Wescott WB: Commissural lip pits, *Oral Surg* 14:202, 1961.

Fantasia JE: Lateral periodontal cyst: an analysis of 46 cases, *Oral Surg* 48:237, 1979.

Fowler CB, Kessler HP, Kahn M: Glandular odontogenic cyst: analysis of 46 cases with special emphasis on microscopic criteria for diagnosis, *Head Neck Pathol* 5:364, 2011.

Freedman PD, Lumerman H, Gee JK: Calcifying odontogenic cyst, *Oral Surg* 40:93, 1975.

Gardner DG: An evaluation of reported cases of median mandibular cysts, *Oral Surg Oral Med Oral Pathol* 65:208, 1988.

Gardner DG: The dentinal changes in regional odontodysplasia, *Oral Surg* 38:887, 1974.

Gardner DG, Girgis SS: Taurodontism, shovel-shaped incisors and the Klinefelter syndrome, *J Can Dent Assoc* 8:372, 1978.

Gardner DG, Sapp JP: Regional odontodysplasia, *Oral Surg* 35:351, 1973.

Grahnen H, Granath LE: Numerical variations in primary dentition, *Odontol Revy* 12:342, 1961.

Grahnen H, Larsson PG: Enamel defects in deciduous dentition of prematurely born children, *Odontol Revy* 9:143, 1958.

Hamner JE III, Witko CJ, Metro PS: Taurodontism: report of a case, *Oral Surg* 18:409, 1964.

Henderson HZ: Ankylosis of primary molars: a clinical, radiographic, and histologic study, *J Dent Child* 46:117, 1979.

Hernandez GA, Castro A, Castro G, et al: Aneurysmal bone cyst versus hemangioma of the mandible, *Oral Surg Oral Med Oral Pathol* 76:790, 1993.

Holt RD, Brook AH: Taurodontism: a criterion for diagnosis and its prevalence in mandibular first molars in a sample of 1115 British school children, *J Int Assoc Dent Child* 10:41, 1979.

Howell RE, Handlers JP, Aberle AM, et al: CEA immunoreactivity in odontogenic tumors and keratocysts, *Oral Surg Oral Med Oral Pathol* 66:576, 1988.

Jasmin J, Ionesco-Benaiche N, Muller M: Latent fluorides: report of a case, *J Dent Child* 62:220, 1995.

Keith A: Problems relating to the teeth of the earlier forms of prehistoric man, *Proc R Soc Med* 6(part 3):103, 1913.

Kelly JR: Gemination, fusion, or both? *Oral Surg* 45:326, 1978.

King RC, Smith BR, Burk JL: Dermoid cyst in the floor of the mouth, *Oral Surg Oral Med Oral Pathol* 78:567, 1994.

Kitchin PC: Dens in dente, *J Dent Res* 15:1176, 1935.

Krolls SO, Donalhue AH: Double-rooted maxillary primary canines, *Oral Surg* 49:379, 1980.

Leamas R, Jimenez-Planas A: Taurodontism in premolars, *Oral Surg Oral Med Oral Pathol* 75:501, 1993.

MacDonald-Jankowski DS: Glandular odontogenic cyst: systematic review, *Dentomaxillofac Radiol* 39:127, 2010.

Mathewson RJ, Siegel MJ, McCanna DL: Ankyloglossia: a review of the literature and a case report, *J Dent Child* 33:238, 1966.

Maurette PE, Jorge J, deMoraes M: Conservative treatment protocol of the odontogenic keratocyst, *J Oral Maxillofac Surg* 64:379, 2006.

Mellor JK, Ripa LW: Talon cusp: a clinically significant anomaly, *Oral Surg* 29:224, 1970.

Milazzo A, Alexander SA: Fusion, gemination, oligodontia and taurodontism, *J Pedod* 6:194, 1982.

Mlynarczyk G: Enamel pitting: a common symptom of tuberous sclerosis, *Oral Surg Oral Med Oral Pathol* 71:63, 1991.

Morningstar CH: Effect of infection of deciduous molar on the permanent tooth germ, *J Am Dent Assoc* 24:786, 1937.

Partridge M, Towers JF: The primordial cyst (odontogenic keratocyst): its tumor-like characteristics and behavior, *Br J Oral Maxillofac Surg* 25:271, 1987.

Pendrys DG: Dental fluorosis in perspective, *J Am Dent Assoc* 122:63, 1991.

Ray GE: Congenital absence of permanent teeth, *Br Dent J* 90:213, 1951.

Reaume CE, Sofie VL: Lingual thyroid: review of the literature and a report of a case, *Oral Surg* 45:841, 1978.

Redman RS: Respiratory epithelium in an apical periodontal cyst of the mandible, *Oral Surg Oral Med Oral Pathol* 67:77, 1989.

Rushton MA: Invaginated teeth (dens in dente): contents of the invagination, *Oral Surg* 11:1378, 1958.

Rushton MA: Odontodysplasia: "ghost teeth," *Br Dent J* 119:109, 1965.

Sapp PJ, Stark M: Self-healing traumatic bone cysts, *Oral Surg Oral Med Oral Pathol* 69:597, 1990.

Shafer WG: Dens in dente, *NY Dent J* 19:220, 1953.

Suchina JA, Ludington JR Jr, Madden RM: Dens invaginatus of a maxillary lateral incisor: endodontic treatment, *Oral Surg Oral Med Oral Pathol* 68:467, 1989.

Tolson G, Czuszak CA, Billman MA, et al: Report of a lateral periodontal cyst and gingival cyst in the same patient, *J Periodontol* 67:541, 1996.

Trope M: Root resorption of dental and traumatic origin: classification based on etiology, *Pract Periodontics Anesthet Dent* 10:515, 1998.

van Gool AV: Injury to the permanent tooth germ after trauma to the deciduous predecessor, *Oral Surg* 35:2, 1973.

Vorheis JM, Gregory GT, McDonald RE: Ankylosed deciduous molars, *J Am Dent Assoc* 44:68, 1952.

Weinmann JP, Svoboda JF, Woods RW: Hereditary disturbances of enamel formation and calcification, *J Am Dent Assoc* 32:397, 1945.

Yip WK: The prevalence of dens evaginatus, *Oral Surg* 38:80, 1974.

Yoshikazu S, Tanimoto K, Wada T: Simple bone cyst: evaluation of contents with conventional radiography and computed tomography, *Oral Surg Oral Med Oral Pathol* 77:296, 1994.

Review Questions

1. Which term refers to a defect present at birth?
   A. Anomaly
   B. Inherited defect
   C. Congenital defect
   D. Developmental defect

2. Which term refers to the origin and tissue formation of teeth?
   A. Odontogenesis
   B. Dentinogenesis
   C. Amelogenesis
   D. Cementogenesis

3. Which term refers to the joining of teeth by cementum *only*?
   A. Fusion
   B. Gemination
   C. Twinning
   D. Concrescence

4. Which teeth are most often missing?
   A. Canines
   B. Deciduous second molars
   C. Third molars
   D. Premolars

5. Which tooth is the most common supernumerary tooth?
   A. Mesiodens
   B. Distomolar
   C. Paramolar
   D. Hutchinson incisor

6. Which teeth most often appear smaller than normal?
   A. Mandibular premolars
   B. Maxillary lateral incisors
   C. Mandibular lateral incisors
   D. Mandibular third molars

7. Which term refers to the developmental anomaly that arises when a single tooth germ attempts to divide and results in the incomplete formation of two teeth?
   A. Fusion
   B. Gemination
   C. Concrescence
   D. Dilaceration

8. Which term refers to the developmental anomaly that arises from the union of two normally separated adjacent tooth germs?
   A. Twinning
   B. Gemination
   C. Fusion
   D. Dilaceration

9. Which term refers to an abnormal angulation or curve in the root or crown of a tooth?
   A. Fusion
   B. Gemination
   C. Concrescence
   D. Dilaceration

10. Which term refers to a developmental anomaly in which teeth exhibit elongated, large pulp chambers and short roots?
    A. Dens in dente
    B. Dens evaginatus
    C. Taurodontism
    D. Dilaceration

11. Which *developmental* anomaly is often associated with a nonvital tooth and periapical lesions?
    A. Dens in dente
    B. Dens evaginatus
    C. Taurodontism
    D. Talon cusp

12. Which of the following teeth most often exhibit supernumerary roots?
    A. Maxillary first premolars
    B. Maxillary third molars
    C. Mandibular first molars
    D. Maxillary first molars

13. Which one of the following describes the appearance of enamel hypoplasia resulting from a febrile illness or vitamin deficiency?
    A. Pitting defects
    B. Yellowish-brown discoloration
    C. Blackish-brown staining
    D. Chalky white spots

14. Which one of the following is associated with enamel hypoplasia resulting from congenital syphilis?
    A. Turner tooth
    B. Hutchinson incisors
    C. Taurodont
    D. Dens evaginatus

15. Which one of the following describes the appearance of enamel hypocalcification?
    A. Pitting defects
    B. Yellowish-brown discoloration
    C. Blackish-brown stains
    D. Chalky white spots

16. Which term describes a tooth that has not erupted because of a lack of eruptive force?
    A. Ankylosed
    B. Impacted
    C. Embedded
    D. Fused

17. Which teeth are most often impacted?
    A. Distomolars
    B. Maxillary and mandibular first molars
    C. Mandibular cuspids
    D. Mandibular third molars

18. Which term describes a tooth in which bone has fused to cementum and dentin and prevents the eruption of an underlying permanent tooth?
    A. Concrescence
    B. Embedded
    C. Ankylosed
    D. Fused

19. Which cyst is *not* an odontogenic cyst?
    A. Dentigerous cyst
    B. Primordial cyst
    C. Median palatal cyst
    D. Lateral periodontal cyst

20. The most common cause of the radicular cyst is:
    A. Caries
    B. Trauma
    C. Malignant infiltration
    D. Food impaction

21. Which cyst is an odontogenic intraosseous cyst that forms around the crown of a developing tooth?
    A. Coronal cyst
    B. Dentigerous cyst
    C. Lateral periodontal cyst
    D. Eruption cyst

22. Which cyst develops in place of a tooth?
    A. Dentigerous cyst
    B. Primordial cyst
    C. Follicular cyst
    D. Odontogenic keratocyst

23. Which cyst is characterized by its unique microscopic appearance and frequent recurrence?
    A. Residual cyst
    B. Stafne bone cyst
    C. Odontogenic keratocyst
    D. Eruption cyst

24. The lateral periodontal cyst is defined by its location. In which area is the lateral periodontal cyst most commonly found?
    A. Mandibular third molar area
    B. Maxillary tuberosity area
    C. Between the maxillary premolars
    D. Between the mandibular cuspid and first premolar

25. The teeth are vital with all of the following cysts *except:*
    A. Nasopalatine canal cyst
    B. Cyst of the palatine papilla
    C. Dentigerous cyst
    D. Periapical cyst

26. Which cyst is characteristically pear shaped?
    A. Globulomaxillary cyst
    B. Median palatal cyst
    C. Incisal canal cyst
    D. Median mandibular cyst

27. Which of the following describes a radicular cyst left behind after extraction of the offending tooth?
    A. Periodontal cyst
    B. Gingival cyst
    C. Odontogenic cyst
    D. Residual cyst

28. With which cyst may the patient complain of dysphagia?
    A. Thyroglossal tract cyst
    B. Median palatal cyst
    C. Static bone cyst
    D. Traumatic bone cyst

29. Which cyst is considered a pseudocyst?
    A. Odontogenic keratocyst
    B. Traumatic bone cyst
    C. Lymphoepithelial cyst
    D. Primordial cyst

30. In addition to the odontogenic keratocyst, which lesion would the hygienist suspect if a radiograph revealed a multilocular radiolucency?
    A. Globulomaxillary cyst
    B. Aneurysmal bone cyst
    C. Stafne bone cyst
    D. Periapical cyst

31. Which term refers to the adhesion of the tongue to the floor of the mouth?
    A. Ankylosis
    B. Ankyloglossia
    C. Anodontia
    D. Amelogenesis

32. Which location is the most common for lip pits?
    A. Commissure
    B. Philtrum
    C. Nasolabial groove
    D. Labiomental groove

Continued

CHAPTER 5 *Synopsis—cont'd*

CONDITION/ DISEASE	CAUSE	AGE/RACE/ SEX	LOCATION
Dentigerous cyst	Developmental	Young adults	Around the crown of an unerupted, impacted, or developing tooth
Eruption cyst	Developmental	Children	Soft tissue around the crown of an erupting tooth
Primordial cyst	Developmental	Young adults	Develops in place of a tooth Mandibular third-molar area most common site
Odontogenic keratocyst (keratocystic odontogenic tumor)	Developmental (dental lamina)	Most common ages, 20-30 yr	Posterior mandible most common site
Lateral periodontal cyst (LPC) and botryoid cyst (BC)	Developmental (dental lamina)	Affects men more than women Median age, 50-60 yr	Lateral aspect of tooth root Mandibular cuspid-premolar area
Gingival cyst	Developmental (dental lamina)	Median age, 50-60 yr	Soft tissue of mandibular cuspid-premolar area
Glandular odontogenic cyst	Developmental	Median age, 40-50 yr	Most common in anterior maxilla and posterior mandible
Nasopalatine canal cyst (incisal canal cyst)	Developmental	Affects men more than women Ages, 40-60 yr	Anterior maxilla Nasopalatine canal Incisive papillae
Median palatine cyst	Developmental	*	Midline of hard palate posterior to the palatine papilla
Globulomaxillary cyst	Unclear	*	Between maxillary lateral incisor and cuspid
Median mandibular cyst	Unknown	*	Midline of mandible

N/A, Not applicable.

*Specific information not included in text.

CLINICAL FEATURES	RADIOGRAPHIC FEATURES	MICROSCOPIC FEATURES	TREATMENT	DIAGNOSTIC PROCESS
When larger, can displace teeth	Well-defined unilocular radiolucency	Cyst lined by cuboidal to squamous epithelium	Removal of cyst and associated tooth	Radiographic Microscopic
Swelling at the site of erupting tooth	N/A	Cyst lined by cuboidal to squamous epithelium	Usually none Tooth erupts though cyst	Radiographic Microscopic (erupting tooth)
Asymptomatic	Well-defined radiolucency	Cyst lined by cuboidal to squamous epithelium	Surgical removal of the cyst	Radiographic
When large, may cause buccal expansion	Well-defined, usually multilocular radiolucency	Cyst lined by thin corrugated parakeratotic squamous epithelium 8-10 cell layers thick Prominent, palisaded basal cell layer with flat interface between the epithelium and connective tissue	Surgical removal of the cyst with peripheral osseous curettage (recurrence high)	Microscopic
Asymptomatic	LPC has unilocular radiolucency BC has multilocular radiolucency	Cyst lined by thin nonkeratinized squamous epithelium with focal thickenings	Surgical removal	Microscopic Radiographic
Bulge or swelling of attached gingiva or interdental papillae	N/A	Cyst lined by thin nonkeratinized squamous epithelium that may have focal thickenings	Surgical removal	Clinical Microscopic
May cause enlargment of bone	Unilocular or multilocular radiolucency	Microscopic cyst lined by cuboidal-columnar epithelium with microcysts and focal thickenings	Surgical removal	Radiographic Microscopic
Asymptomatic Pink bulge at the incisive papillae area	Well-circumscribed radiolucency between the maxillary central incisors Open heart shaped	Cyst lined by squamous or respiratory epithelium Blood vessels and small nerves in cyst wall	Surgical removal	Radiographic Microscopic
If large, swelling at midline of hard palate	Unilocular radiolucency	Cyst lined by stratified squamous epithelium surrounded by dense fibrous connective tissue	Surgical removal	Radiographic Microscopic
Asymptomatic	Pear-shaped radiolucency	Cyst lining varies from squamous to cuboidal to respiratory epithelium	Surgical removal	Radiographic Microscopic
Asymptomatic If very large, may cause expansion of lingual aspect of mandible	Well-circumscribed radiolucency below the apices of the mandibular incisors	Cyst lined by squamous epithelium	Surgical removal	Radiographic Microscopic

Continued

CHAPTER 5 *Synopsis—cont'd*

CONDITION/ DISEASE	CAUSE	AGE/RACE/ SEX	LOCATION
Mesiodens	Developmental	*	Near/at midline between maxillary central incisors
Distomolar	Developmental	*	Distal to third molars
Microdontia	Developmental	*	Maxillary lateral incisors Peg lateral is the most common Maxillary third molars
Macrodontia	Developmental	*	Any tooth
Gemination	Developmental	*	Primary > permanent Anterior > posterior
Fusion	Developmental	*	Primary > permanent Anterior > posterior Incisors
Concrescence	Developmental	*	Maxillary molars
Dilaceration	Developmental	*	Any tooth
Enamel pearl	Developmental	*	Maxillary molars (furcation area)
Talon cusp	Developmental	*	Incisors
Taurodontism	Developmental	*	Molars

N/A, Not applicable.
*Specific information not included in text.

CLINICAL FEATURES	RADIOGRAPHIC FEATURES	MICROSCOPIC FEATURES	TREATMENT	DIAGNOSTIC PROCESS
Most common extra tooth; may be erupted or unerupted/impacted Usually appear conical and small	Extra tooth seen at the midline of the anterior maxilla	N/A	Extraction No treatment	Clinical Radiographic
Second most common supernumerary tooth May be erupted (appears small) or impacted	Extra tooth distal to third molar	N/A	No treatment Extraction	Clinical Radiographic
Affected tooth appears smaller than normal One or more teeth may be affected	Tooth smaller than normal	N/A	If erupted, restore to resemble a normal-size tooth	Clinical Radiographic
Affected tooth appears larger than normal One or more teeth may be affected	Tooth larger than normal	N/A	No treatment	Clinical Radiographic
Tooth appears larger than normal Large crown (appears bifid) Normal number of teeth present	Appears as a single tooth with a bifid crown and one common root canal	N/A	If aesthetic problems, alteration of tooth to resemble normal-size tooth	Clinical Radiographic
Adjacent teeth are fused together Large crown is seen	Appears as a single large crown with separate or fused roots and root canals	N/A	If aesthetic problem, alteration of tooth to resemble normal-size tooth	Clinical Radiographic
Cannot observe clinically	Appears as though the roots of adjacent teeth are connected	N/A	No treatment	Radiographic
Cannot observe clinically	Appears as a sharp bend in a tooth root	N/A	No treatment	Radiographic
Cannot observe clinically	Appears as a small sphere of enamel on a tooth root	N/A	No treatment	Radiographic
Crown appears normal facially An accessory cusp is located in the area of the cingulum	Appears as a tooth with abnormally short roots and low furcation area Pulp chamber is abnormally large	N/A	Removal of cusp and restoration of tooth if cusp interferes with occlusion	Clinical
Cannot observe clinically Crown appears normal	Pulp chamber is enlarged and elongated Roots are short with the furcation near the apices	N/A	No treatment	Radiographic

Continued

Chapter 6

Genetics

Heddie O. Sedano

OBJECTIVES

After studying this chapter, the student will be able to:

1. Define each of the words listed in the vocabulary for this chapter.
2. State the purpose of mitosis.
3. State the purpose of meiosis.
4. Explain what is meant by the Lyon hypothesis and give an example of its clinical significance.
5. Explain what is meant by a gross chromosomal abnormality and give three examples of syndromes that result from gross chromosomal abnormalities.
6. List the four inheritance patterns described in this chapter.
7. Explain what is meant by X-linked inheritance.
8. State the inheritance pattern and describe the oral manifestations and, if appropriate, the characteristic facies for each of the following: cyclic neutropenia, Papillon-Lefèvre syndrome, cherubism, Ellis–van Creveld syndrome (chondroectodermal dysplasia), mandibulofacial dysostosis (Treacher Collins syndrome), osteogenesis imperfecta, hereditary hemorrhagic telangiectasia (Osler-Rendu–Parkes Weber syndrome), Peutz-Jeghers syndrome, white sponge nevus (Cannon disease), hypohidrotic ectodermal dysplasia, hypophosphatasia, and hypophosphatemic vitamin D–resistant rickets.
9. State the inheritance pattern, the oral or facial manifestations, and the type and location of the malignancy associated with each of the following syndromes: Gardner syndrome; nevoid basal cell carcinoma syndrome (Gorlin syndrome); multiple mucosal neuromas, medullary carcinoma of the thyroid gland, and pheochromocytoma syndrome (multiple endocrine neoplasia type 2B [MEN 2B]); and neurofibromatosis of von Recklinghausen.
10. State the location and malignant potential of the intestinal polyps in Peutz-Jeghers syndrome and Gardner syndrome.
11. List the four types of amelogenesis imperfecta.
12. Briefly compare and contrast dentinogenesis imperfecta, amelogenesis imperfecta, and dentin dysplasia, including the inheritance patterns, the clinical manifestations, and the radiographic appearance of each.

VOCABULARY

Alleles (ə-lēlz′) Genes that are located at the same level or locus in the two chromosomes of a pair and that determine the same functions or characteristics.

Amino acid (ə-me′no as′id) Organic compound containing an amino group NH_2; amino acids are the main component of proteins.

Autosomes (aw′to-sōmz) (adjective, *autosomal*) Nonsex chromosomes, which are identical for men and women.

Barr body (bahr bod′e) Condensed chromatin of the inactivated X chromosome, which is found at the periphery of the nucleus of cells in women.

VOCABULARY—cont'd

Carrier (kar'e-ər) In genetics, a heterozygous individual who is clinically normal but who can transmit a recessive trait or characteristic; also, a person who is homozygous for an autosomal-dominant condition with low penetrance.

Centromere (sen'tro-mĕr) Constricted portion of the chromosome that divides the short arms from the long arms.

Chromatid (kro'mə-tid) Either of the two vertical halves of a chromosome that are joined at the centromere.

Chromatin (kro'mə-tin) General term used to refer to the material (deoxyribonucleic acid [DNA]) that forms the chromosomes.

Chromosome (kro'mo-sōm) Structures located in the nucleus of cells and on which genes are found.

Codon (ko'don) Sequence of three bases in DNA that encodes an amino acid.

Consanguinity (kon″san-gwin'ĭ-te) Blood relationship; in genetics the term is generally used to describe a mating or marriage between close relatives.

Deoxyribonucleic acid (de-ok″se-ri″bo-noo-kle'ik as'id) DNA; a substance composed of a double chain of polynucleotides, with both chains coiled around a central axis to form a double helix; it is the basic genetic code or template for amino acid formation.

Diploid (dip'loid) Having two sets of chromosomes; the normal constitution of somatic cells.

Dominant (dom'ĭ-nənt) In genetics, a trait or characteristic that is manifested when it is carried by only one of a pair of homologous chromosomes.

Expressivity (ek″sprĕ-siv'ĭ-te) Degree of clinical manifestation of a trait or characteristic.

Facies (fa'she-ēz) Appearance of the face.

Gamete (gam'ēt) Spermatozoon or ovum.

Gene (jēn) Hereditary units, transmitted from one generation to another, that are made up of a sequence of nucleotides and located on a chromosome.

Genetic heterogeneity (jə-net'ik het″ər-o-jə-ne'ĭ-te) Having more than one inheritance pattern.

Haploid (hap'loid) Having a single set of chromosomes; a gamete is haploid.

Heterozygote (het″ər-o-zi'gōt) (adjective, *heterozygous*) Individual with two different genes at the allele loci.

Homozygote (ho″mo-zi'gōt) (adjective, *homozygous*) Individual having identical genes at the allele loci.

Hypertelorism (hi″pər-te'lor-iz-əm) A condition in which there is greater than normal distance between two paired organs; ocular hypertelorism, a condition marked by a greater than normal distance between the eyes.

Hypodontia (hi″po-don'shə) A developmental condition marked by fewer than normal teeth; also called *partial anodontia*.

Hypohidrosis (hi′po-hi-dro'sis) Abnormally diminished secretion of sweat.

Hypotrichosis (hi′po-trĭ-ko'sis) Presence of less than the normal amount of hair.

Hypoplastic (hi″po-plas'tik) Underdeveloped.

Karyotype (kar'e-o-tīp) Photomicrographic representation of a person's chromosomal constitution arranged according to the Denver classification.

Locus (lo'kəs) (plural, *loci*) Position occupied by a gene on a chromosome.

Meiosis (mi-o'sis) Two-step cellular division of the original germ cells, which reduces the chromosomes from 4n DNA to 1n DNA.

Metaphase (met'ə-fāz) Phase of cellular division in which the chromosomes are lined up evenly along the equatorial plane of the cell and in which they are most visible.

Mitochondria (mi″to-kon'dre-ə) Cytoplasmic organelles that have their own DNA in a circular chromosome.

Mitochondrial DNA (mi″to-kon'dre-əl DNA) Unique DNA that is maternally inherited.

Mitosis (mi-to'sis) Way in which somatic cells divide so that the two daughter cells receive the same number of identical chromosomes.

Multifactorial inheritance (mul″tĭ-fak-tor'e-əl in-her'ĭ-təns) The type of hereditary pattern seen when there is more than one genetic factor involved and, sometimes, when there are also environmental factors participating in the causation of a condition.

Mutation (mu-ta'shən) Permanent change in the arrangement of genetic material.

Nondisjunction In genetics, when chromosomes that are crossing over do not separate; therefore, both migrate to the same cell.

Oligodontia (ol″ĭ-go-don'she-ə) A condition in which more that six teeth are developmentally absent.

Oogenesis (o″o-jen'ə-sis) Process of formation of female germ cells (ova).

Ovum (o'vəm) (plural, *ova*) Egg; mature feminine germ cell.

Penetrance (pen'ə-trəns) Frequency with which a heritable trait is exhibited by individuals carrying the gene or genes that determine that trait.

Phenotype (fe'noh-tīp) Entire physical, biochemical, and physiologic makeup of an individual; genotype is the genetic composition, and phenotype is its observable appearance.

Continued

chromosomes. **Meiosis** is a two-step special type of cell division in which the primitive germ cells reduce their chromosome number by half and become mature germ cells. The primitive germ cells have two chromosomes for each pair and are called **diploid.** The suffix -*ploid* refers to the number of sets of chromosomes, and its prefix refers to the degree of ploidy. In diploid *di*- indicates two. The mature germ cells (or **gametes**) have half the number of chromosomes and are called **haploid.** During the period in which the cell is not in division, the DNA content of diploid cells is designated 2n DNA; in metaphase it is double or 4n DNA. After the two stages of meiosis have been completed, the 4n DNA is reduced to 1n DNA. The two steps are called **first meiosis** and **second meiosis.** This reduction is necessary to maintain the normal number of human chromosomes. A new embryo must have 46 chromosomes per cell, as did its parents. Therefore the union of germ cells needs to result in 46 chromosomes. If two cells with 46 chromosomes were combined, the resulting cell would have 92 chromosomes.

FIRST MEIOSIS

Before the first meiosis in the primitive germ cells, a replication of DNA occurs that is similar to that observed in the S phase of somatic cells. After replication the members of each pair of chromosomes line up next to each other in an intimate point-by-point relationship (Figure 6-5, *A*). This pairing does not occur in mitosis. After pairing, the two chromosomes establish actual contact at different locations. These contacts are known as **chiasmata** (meaning X shaped) and determine points of crossing over (Figure 6-5, *B*). This crossing over achieves the exchange of chromosome segments between a chromatid of one chromosome and a chromatid of the other chromosome of a pair (between homologous chromosomes) (Figure 6-5, *C*). This special aspect of the first meiosis takes place at metaphase. After metaphase of the first meiotic division, the chromosomes separate from each other, but no splitting of the centromere occurs. The chromosomes remain intact, and each member of the pair migrates to one of the new cells, each of which contains 23 chromosomes but twice the final amount of

DNA. During this migration chromosomes of the paternal and maternal lines segregate at random, thus ensuring diversity of the species by creating a new combination of chromosomes.

On occasion, the chromosomes that were crossing over do not separate, and both migrate to the same cell. This is known as **nondisjunction** and results in the formation of a germ cell with an extra chromosome. If this occurs and that cell (either an **ovum** or a **spermatozoon**) participates in the formation of an embryo, three chromosomes **(trisomy)** instead of two result. An example of this type of abnormality is **Down syndrome**, also called **trisomy 21**, in which three of chromosome 21 are found instead of two. Trisomy has been reported for several different chromosomes.

In a female embryo **oogenesis** (ovum development) starts around the third month of prenatal life, and the future ova remain suspended, crossing over from about the time of birth until the time ovulation starts. At the beginning of ovulation the first meiosis is completed. Nondisjunction is more prevalent in female oogenesis than in male **spermatogenesis.** This is probably because of the period of prolonged crossing over; therefore the older the woman, the greater the chance of shedding a trisomic ovum and of bearing a child with Down syndrome or other trisomy.

SECOND MEIOSIS

The second stage of meiosis is essentially a mitotic division in which each chromosome splits longitudinally. No replication of DNA occurs before the second meiosis. After the splitting, two cells are formed, each containing the right amount of DNA (1n DNA) (Figure 6-6).

Nondisjunction can occur during the first and second meiosis. If it occurs in second meiosis, a chromosome does not split, and one daughter cell has a full chromosome, and the other has none.

Immediately after fertilization the chromosomes of the ovum and spermatozoon, each having 1n DNA, condense independently and form round structures, each known as a *pronucleus.* The DNA in these pronuclei replicates, forming a

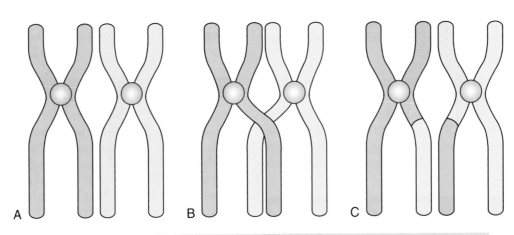

FIGURE 6-5 ■ Homologous autosomal chromosomes line up in first meiosis **(A),** cross over during metaphase of first meiosis **(B),** and exchange segments after crossing over **(C).**

set of 23 full chromosomes for each, the maternal and paternal pronuclei. When the membranes of these pronuclei break, the 46 chromosomes mix at random, initiating the first cellular division (mitosis) that starts the development of the new embryo.

FIGURE 6-6 ■ Two haploid cells after second meiosis, each having 1n DNA.

LYON HYPOTHESIS

The sex chromosomes are designated XX in women and XY in men. During the early period of embryonic development (possibly by the end of the second week), the genetic activity of one of the X chromosomes in each cell of a female embryo is inactivated. The inactivation is a random process affecting either the X chromosome derived from the mother or the X chromosome derived from the father. Activated chromosomes are dispersed in the nucleus. The inactivated chromosome remains contracted when the cell is not dividing and forms a structure known as the **Barr body.**

Barr bodies are only seen in female cells. The Barr body can be seen easily under the light microscope, especially in cytologic smears, including those obtained from the oral mucosa. The Barr body appears as a dark dot at the periphery of the nucleus (Figure 6-7).

This inactivation of one of the X chromosomes in a female embryo was postulated by Mary Lyon and is known as the **Lyon hypothesis.** This hypothesis has interesting clinical implications for female **carriers** of conditions caused by genes located on the X chromosome, which are explained later in this chapter.

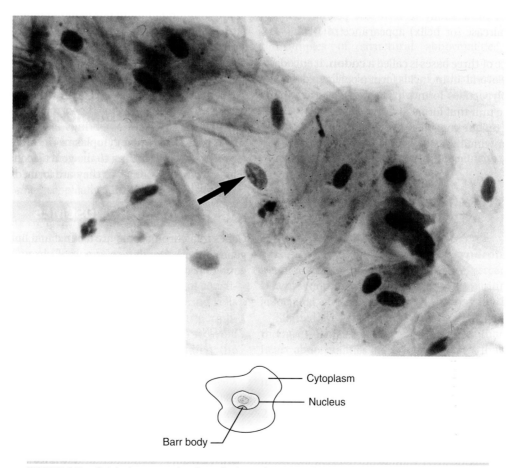

FIGURE 6-7 ■ Cytologic preparation from the buccal mucosa shows the Barr body (the small dark dot on the nuclear membrane [arrow]) at the periphery of the nucleus of a desquamated epithelial cell from a woman's buccal mucosa. (Courtesy Dr. Carl J. Witkop.)

FIGURE 6-10 ■ Karyotype from a female shows the 22 pairs of autosomal chromosomes and the pair of X chromosomes. (Courtesy Dr. Jaroslav Cervenka.)

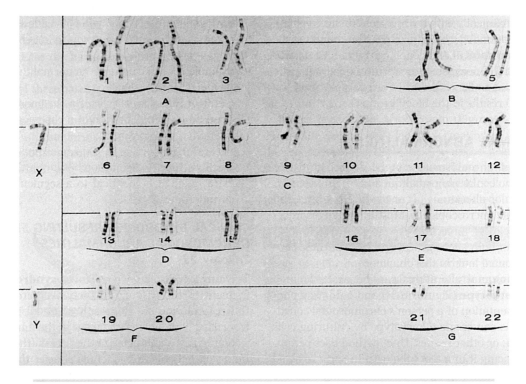

FIGURE 6-11 ■ Karyotype from a male shows the 22 pairs of autosomal chromosomes and the X and Y chromosomes. (Courtesy Dr. Jaroslav Cervenka.)

findings. Dental hygienists play an important role in the maintenance of oral health in these patients.

Trisomy 13

Trisomy 13 is characterized by multiple abnormalities in various organs. Seventy percent of live-born infants die

within the first 7 months of life. Characteristic clinical findings include bilateral cleft lip and palate, microphthalmia (small eyes) or anophthalmia (no eyes), superficial hemangioma of the forehead or nape of the neck, growth retardation, severe mental handicap, polydactyly of hands and feet (supernumerary digits), clenching of the fist with the

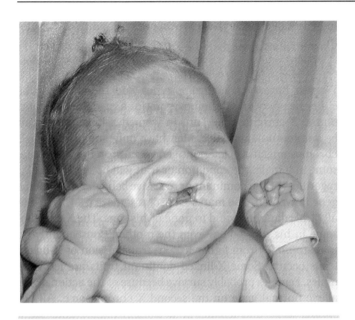

FIGURE 6-12 ■ Newborn with trisomy 13. Cleft lip, frontal hemangioma, and abnormal position of fingers should be noted.

FIGURE 6-13 ■ Patient with Turner syndrome. Note the webbing of the neck.

thumb under the fingers, rocker-bottom feet, heart malformations, and several anomalies of the external genitals. The facial appearance is quite striking because of the cleft lip, cleft palate, and ocular abnormalities (Figure 6-12).

Turner Syndrome

Patients with Turner syndrome have a female phenotype, and in the majority of cases the karyotype has the normal 44 autosomal chromosomes and only one X chromosome. A normal female would have two X chromosomes: one from the mother and one from the father. Most cases of Turner syndrome are the result of nondisjunction of the X chromosome in the paternal gamete. Clinically, these women are of short stature and have webbing of the neck and edema of the hands and feet (Figure 6-13). They frequently exhibit a low hairline on the nape of the neck. The chest is broad with wide-spaced nipples. The aorta frequently is abnormal, and body hair is sparse. The external genitals appear infantile, and generally the ovaries are not developed; therefore these individuals have primary amenorrhea (abnormal temporary or permanent cessation of the menstrual cycle). Smears taken from the oral mucosa demonstrate the lack of Barr bodies.

Klinefelter Syndrome

Klinefelter syndrome occurs when an ovum carrying two X chromosomes is fertilized by a spermatozoon with a Y chromosome; therefore the fertilized ovum will have two X chromosomes plus a Y chromosome. The majority of cases result from nondisjunction of the X chromosome, generally in the ova of older women. Affected individuals have a male phenotype, and the condition cannot be detected clinically until after puberty. These patients are taller than normal and have wide hips and female pubic hair distribution. About 50% have gynecomastia (development of female breasts), and intelligence levels are lower than normal in 10% of affected individuals. The penis appears normal, but the testes are smaller and harder than normal and lack seminiferous tubules.

The maxilla is slightly **hypoplastic** (underdeveloped). Buccal smears reveal the presence of one Barr body.

Variations of Klinefelter syndrome also occur; they are represented by karyotypes containing XXXY or XXXXY. The greater the number of X chromosomes, the more pronounced the clinical manifestations, and the lower the level of intelligence. The maxilla becomes increasingly hypoplastic with increasing number of X chromosomes. Buccal smears show one Barr body for each extra X chromosome.

Cri du Chat (Cat Cry) Syndrome and Wolf-Hirschhorn Syndrome

Cri du chat (cat cry) syndrome and Wolf-Hirschhorn syndrome are examples of abnormalities caused by deletions. The cri du chat syndrome results from a deletion on the short arm of chromosome 5, and the Wolf-Hirschhorn syndrome results from a deletion on the short arm of chromosome 4. Newborns with a chromosome 5 deletion exhibit a catlike cry at birth and are mentally retarded. No oral abnormalities occur. Most newborns with the deletion in the short arm of chromosome 4 have a cleft palate and intelligence quotients of less than 30.

PATTERNS OF INHERITANCE

Because loci are present in both **autosomal** and X chromosomes and because of a double- and single-dose effect, four possible inheritance patterns exist. Dominant genes need only a single dose, and recessive genes need a double dose. The inheritance patterns are autosomal dominant, autosomal recessive, X-linked dominant, and X-linked recessive. Autosomal chromosomes include all chromosomes antibiotic therapy to protect against secondary opportunistic infections. Over time, episodes of neutropenia and associated ulcerative gingivitis lead to severe periodontal disease, with loss of alveolar bone, tooth mobility, and exfoliation of teeth. Treatment should be initiated when the circulating neutrophil count is normal to reduce the risk of complications such as gingival hemorrhage and secondary infection. Dental hygiene care, including frequent appointments for removal of local irritants and maintenance of optimal oral hygiene, reduces the risk of opportunistic infections in patients with cyclic neutropenia.

Patients with cyclic neutropenia are treated periodically with granulocyte colony-stimulating factor (G-CSF), which reduces the symptoms and results in substantial clinical improvement.

Chronic neutropenia, also known as *Kostmann syndrome,* is another variety of neutropenia that is inherited as an autosomal-recessive condition. In this syndrome the neutropenia is constant and not cyclic. The intraoral manifestations of Kostmann syndrome may be similar to those of the cyclic variety but are constantly present and require systemic treatment The responsible gene is still unknown, and it is also treated with periodic G-CSF.

Papillon-Lefèvre Syndrome. Papillon-Lefèvre syndrome has an autosomal-recessive inheritance pattern and is characterized by marked destruction of the periodontal tissues (periodontoclasia) of both dentitions with premature loss of teeth and hyperkeratosis of the palms of the hands and soles of the feet (palmar and plantar hyperkeratosis).

The gene for this syndrome has been mapped to the long arm of chromosome 11 regions 14-21 (11q14-21). These patients are normal at birth except for a reddening of the palms of the hands and soles of the feet. Teeth erupt in normal sequence, position, and time. At about 1½ to 2 years of age, a marked gingivoperiodontal inflammatory process develops, characterized by edema, bleeding, alveolar bone resorption, and mobility of teeth with consequent exfoliation. A red, scaly keratosis develops on the palms and soles concurrent with these oral lesions and occasionally extends to the dorsal surfaces of the hands and feet. The oral lesions are complicated by superimposed inflammation, and radiographs reveal marked alveolar bone resorption with vertical pockets. Teeth are lost in the same sequence in which they erupted. When the last tooth is lost, the gingiva regains a normal appearance.

The lesions on the hands and feet remain as reddish-white, scaly, thick areas of hyperkeratinization (Figure 6-15). The permanent dentition begins to erupt at the proper time. At about 8 or 9 years of age the gingivoperiodontal destruction is repeated in the same manner as occurred in the primary dentition (Figure 6-16). All permanent teeth are lost before 14 years of age. The gingiva again resumes a normal appearance.

The peripheral blood neutrophil count is depressed in all patients with Papillon-Lefèvre syndrome. This suggests that the neutrophils may be an important factor in the pathogenesis of severe periodontal disease in these patients. Retinoid therapy markedly improves the skin condition but has no

FIGURE 6-15 ■ Areas of hyperkeratinization of the palms are exhibited in a patient with Papillon-Lefèvre syndrome. (From Sedano HO, Sauk JJ, Gorlin RJ: *Oral manifestations of inherited disorders,* Boston, 1977, Butterworths. Used with permission.)

effect on the periodontal disease in patients with this syndrome. To date all therapeutic attempts at preventing the gingival and periodontal destruction and subsequent loss of teeth have been unsuccessful. The basic defect that causes the condition is unknown. Peripheral blood neutrophil chemotaxis has been reported to be depressed in patients with Papillon-Lefèvre syndrome. This decreased chemotaxis suggests that neutrophils may play a role in periodontal destruction in patients with this syndrome. Current research suggests bacterial and viral involvement as the initiating factors for the periodontal destruction. It has been suggested that the genetic component of Papillon-Lefèvre syndrome is a predisposition rather than the main determinant of periodontal disease.

The skin manifestations remain for life, but treatment with retinoid (oral etretinate) has proven somewhat effective in controlling the hyperkeratinization. These patients do not have any other abnormalities.

Focal Palmoplantar and Gingival Hyperkeratosis. Areas of hyperkeratinization of the palms and soles and marked hyperkeratinization of the labial and lingual gingiva characterize **focal palmoplantar** and **gingival hyperkeratosis**. This syndrome has an autosomal-dominant inheritance pattern. The palmar and plantar hyperkeratosis starts at the tips of the fingers and toes and extends to the surface of the palms and soles. This process increases with age and also becomes localized, with calluses forming on the weight-bearing areas.

FIGURE 6-16 ■ Panoramic radiograph shows marked periodontal destruction with alveolar bone resorption in the patient in Figure 6-15. (From Sedano HO, Sauk JJ, Gorlin RJ: *Oral manifestations of inherited disorders*, Boston, 1977, Butterworths. Used with permission.)

FIGURE 6-17 ■ Marked hyperkeratosis follows the normal contour of the gingiva in focal palmoplantar and gingival hyperkeratosis. (From Sedano HO, Sauk JJ, Gorlin RJ: *Oral manifestations of inherited disorders*, Boston, 1977, Butterworths. Used with permission.)

FIGURE 6-18 ■ Gingival hypertrophy is shown in a patient with isolated gingival fibromatosis.

The oral hyperkeratinization is bandlike and a few millimeters in width (Figure 6-17). It follows the normal festooned contour of the gingiva. The free gingiva is not affected. Palatal and lingual mucosa occasionally can be affected with areas of hyperkeratinization. These changes start in childhood and increase with age. The rest of the oral cavity is normal.

Gingival Fibromatosis. Gingival fibromatosis is a component of several inherited syndromes. The gingival enlargement generally develops early in life, and within a few years the teeth are completely covered. The fibromatosis is composed of very firm tissue with a granular corrugated surface. In general, the color is paler than that of the normal gingiva and results from the marked collagenization of the fibrous connective tissue. The extensive gingival enlargement leads to protrusion of the lips.

In addition to isolated gingival fibromatosis (Figure 6-18), which has an autosomal-dominant inheritance pattern and no other associated abnormalities, gingival fibromatosis is a component of a number of syndromes. Because of the gingival involvement, several of these syndromes, although rare, are described here. However, only those that are well known and occur most frequently are included.

Dental hygiene care can reduce the risk of secondary inflammation and infection in patients with gingival fibromatosis.

Laband Syndrome. The inheritance pattern of **Laband syndrome** is autosomal dominant. In addition to gingival fibromatosis, patients have dysplastic or absent nails and malformed nose and ears because of soft and pliable cartilage formation, hepatosplenomegaly (enlarged liver and spleen), and hypoplasia of terminal phalanges of the fingers and toes with a resultant froglike appearance.

Gingival Fibromatosis with Hypertrichosis, Epilepsy, and Mental Retardation Syndrome. Gingival fibromatosis with hypertrichosis, epilepsy, and mental retardation syndrome has an autosomal-dominant inheritance pattern. Hypertrichosis (excessive growth of hair), especially of the eyebrows, extremities, genitals, and sacral region, characterize gingival fibromatosis with hypertrichosis, epilepsy, and mental retardation. Epilepsy and mental retardation can also occur in this syndrome but are inconsistent features.

Gingival Fibromatosis with Multiple Hyaline Fibromas. Gingival fibromatosis with multiple hyaline fibromas has an autosomal-dominant inheritance pattern

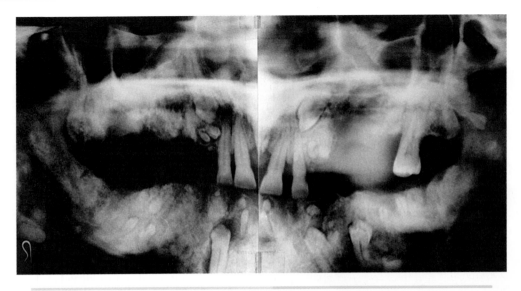

FIGURE 6-22 ■ Panoramic radiograph of a patient with Gardner syndrome shows multiple osteomas and odontomas. (Courtesy Dr. Carl J. Witkop.)

FIGURE 6-23 ■ Markedly high-arched palate and malpositioned teeth in a patient with mandibulofacial dysostosis.

with open bite is quite evident. The palate is high, or a cleft is present in about 30% of affected patients (Figure 6-23). Gingival disease is common and is related to the dental abnormalities.

Nevoid Basal Cell Carcinoma Syndrome. The **nevoid basal cell carcinoma syndrome,** also known as *Gorlin syndrome,* has an autosomal-dominant inheritance pattern with high penetrance and variable expressivity. The gene for this syndrome maps to the long arm of chromosome 9 region 22.3 (9q22.3). The facies is characterized by mild **Ocular hypertelorism** (increased distance between the eyes) and mild prognathism, with frontal and parietal bossing (enlargement) and a broad nasal root.

The cutaneous manifestations, which are called **nevi,** typically are basal cell carcinomas. The term *nevus* (plural, *nevi*), as defined here, is a congenital lesion characterized by

skin pigmentation. These basal cell carcinomas appear early in life and continue to develop over the nose, eyelids, cheeks, neck, arms, and trunk. They can be flesh colored or pale brown and develop singly or in clusters. Histologically, they are basal cell carcinomas. The palms and soles show small pits that become filled with dirt and appear as dark spots on those surfaces.

The oral manifestations of this syndrome consist of multiple cysts of the jaws (Figure 6-24) that (microscopically) are odontogenic keratocysts (keratocystic odontogenic tumor) (see Chapter 5). These cysts vary in size; they can be very large and have a marked tendency to recur after surgical removal. On occasion, an ameloblastoma arises in these cysts as part of this syndrome. The cysts develop as early as 5 to 6 years of age in some affected patients and interfere with normal development of the jawbones and teeth.

A great variety of skeletal anomalies have been reported in association with the nevoid basal cell carcinoma syndrome, the most constant being bifurcation or splaying of one or more ribs. Other frequent abnormalities of bone include shortening of the metacarpals, spina bifida occulta (defective closure of the bone encasement of the spinal cord), and kyphoscoliosis (a combination of scoliosis, which is a lateral curving of the spine, and kyphosis, which is an abnormal vertical curvature of the spine or "hunchback").

Many different neoplasms have been reported in association with this syndrome. Medulloblastoma (brain tumor) has been seen in many cases. Children surviving the medulloblastoma eventually present other manifestations of the syndrome. Other, less frequent findings include calcified ovarian fibromas and mesenteric cysts.

Osteogenesis Imperfecta. **Osteogenesis imperfecta** is known to have an autosomal-dominant inheritance pattern with variable expressivity. However, only 30% of patients have a family history of this condition. The remaining 70% represent sporadic cases and cases suggesting autosomal-recessive inheritance. The basic defect is produced by different mutations affecting the genes that encode

FIGURE 6-24 ▪ Multiple mandibular radiolucencies in a patient with nevoid basal cell carcinoma syndrome. These lesions are odontogenic keratocysts (keratocystic odontogenic tumors).

for type I collagen, resulting in abnormally formed bones that fracture easily. The genes responsible for the inherited varieties of osteogenesis imperfecta are mapped as follows: collagen type I α_2 is in the long arm of chromosome 7 region 22.1 (7q22.1); collagen type I α_1 is in the long arm of chromosome 17 region 21.31-22.05 (17q21.31-22.05). Osteogenesis imperfecta occurs in about 1 in 20,000 births, and major syndromes have been classified in four types: I, II, III, and IV.

The clinical manifestations vary markedly from patient to patient. The sporadic cases tend to be more severe than those with an autosomal-dominant inheritance pattern. The basic defect involves collagen and results in abnormally formed bones that fracture easily. Multiple spontaneous bone fractures are the main clinical complication of this syndrome. In the congenital form newborns can have several fractured bones at birth. Infants with this condition have experienced fractures just by being moved. In the most severe cases all bones can be affected, presenting a plethora of abnormalities, including bowing of the legs, curvature of the spine (kyphosis and scoliosis), deformity of the skull, shortening of arms and legs, deafness in a few cases, and other abnormalities . In the mildest cases individuals show only blue sclerae (a blue appearance of the white of the eye).

The oral manifestation of this syndrome is a dentinogenesis imperfecta–like condition (a description of dentinogenesis imperfecta follows later in this chapter). This clinical feature does not occur in all cases of osteogenesis imperfecta. Primary teeth are affected in 80% of patients, whereas permanent teeth are affected in only 35% of these individuals (Figure 6-25). The crowns, roots, and pulp chambers generally are smaller than normal. Teeth appear opalescent or translucent at the time of eruption, but they darken with age. The enamel is lost because the abnormal dentin cannot provide adequate support.

Torus Mandibularis. Mandibular tori (singular, torus) have an autosomal-dominant inheritance pattern with

FIGURE 6-25 ▪ Patient with osteogenesis imperfecta. Teeth are yellowish with chipped enamel.

variable expressivity and marked penetrance. This anomaly can be unilateral or bilateral. These tori occur on the lingual aspect of the mandible in the area of the premolar teeth (Figure 6-26). Occurrence before age 15 years is extremely rare. The size of the torus is variable, and occasionally it can be multilobulated. Mandibular tori are symptomless and generally require no treatment. Surgical removal may be necessary if the patient needs a denture. Intraoral radiographs usually show a radiopacity in the area of the mandibular premolars if mandibular tori are present. Positioning of the film or sensor may be difficult when attempting to radiograph these areas.

Torus Palatinus. Autosomal dominance with variable expressivity and almost 100% penetrance characterizes torus palatinus. A bony overgrowth occurs at the midline of the hard palate (Figure 6-27). A marked predilection exists

FIGURE 6-40 ■ Obliteration and partial lack of coronal pulp chambers and small root canals can be seen in teeth of a patient affected with coronal dentin dysplasia. (Courtesy Dr. Carl J. Witkop.)

exercise. The clinical characteristics of this condition may not be apparent until the second year of life.

The facies is quite typical, with marked frontal bossing, depressed nasal bridge (saddle nose), protuberant lips, and almost complete lack of scalp hair. The hair that is present is usually blond, short, fine, and stiff. The skin is soft, thin, and very dry. Sebaceous glands are also lacking. Linear wrinkles and increased pigmentation are seen around the eyes and mouth. The eyelashes and eyebrows are often missing entirely. After puberty the beard generally is normal, but axillary and pubic hair is scanty.

The oral manifestations of hypohidrotic ectodermal dysplasia consist of hypodontia or rarely anodontia. When present, incisors and canines have small, conical crowns (Figure 6-41). The alveolar bone is formed only when teeth are present; therefore patients lacking alveolar processes have loss of vertical dimension with markedly protruding lips. There may also be partial lack and aplasia of minor salivary glands in the buccal, labial, and lower respiratory tract mucosa.

Female carriers of the X-linked form of hypohidrotic ectodermal dysplasia have minor clinical manifestations such as thin and slightly sparse hair, cone-shaped teeth, hypodontia, and variable degrees of reduced sweating. This is in accordance with the Lyon hypothesis of variability of expression.

Hypophosphatasia. The inheritance pattern of **hypophosphatasia** is autosomal recessive. The gene for this syndrome maps to the short arm of chromosome 1 regions 36.1-34 (1p36.1-34). The basic defect in this condition is a decrease in serum alkaline phosphatase levels with increased urinary and plasma levels of phosphoethanolamine. Alkaline phosphatase participates in the process of calcification of bone and cementum; therefore these two tissues will be altered in patients with hypophosphatasia. Agenesis or abnormal formation of cementum in these patients leads to spontaneous premature shedding of primary teeth, especially mandibular incisors (Figure 6-42). Teeth are exfoliated without evidence of periodontal or gingival disease. The primary molars and permanent teeth are rarely if ever affected, which is probably associated with the greater mechanical fixation resulting from the larger size of their roots. The total lack of cementum observed in exfoliated teeth implies a lack of periodontal fiber attachment, with

FIGURE 6-41 ■ Patient with hypohidrotic ectodermal dysplasia has only three, abnormally shaped teeth.

FIGURE 6-42 ■ Histologic section of a tooth from a patient with hypophosphatasia shows only dentin. Cementum is entirely lacking.

consequent exfoliation of single-rooted teeth. The most important alteration in this syndrome is the improper formation of mature bone. Therefore individuals who survive the neonatal period experience rachitic-like changes such as bowing of legs and multiple fractures.

Hypophosphatemic Vitamin D–resistant Rickets. **Hypophosphatemic vitamin D–resistant rickets,** which

FIGURE 6-43 ■ Pegged maxillary lateral incisors. The conical shape should be noted.

FIGURE 6-44 ■ Intraoral radiograph of taurodontic teeth shows large pulp chambers and low bifurcation of the roots in this pyramid-shaped molar.

is quite common, has an X-linked dominant inheritance pattern and is the result of a mutation in the PHEX gene. It is characterized by low serum levels of phosphorus, which is caused by low absorption of inorganic phosphate in the renal tubules; rickets or osteomalacia; resistance to treatment with usual doses of vitamin D; and a lack of other abnormalities. Affected individuals generally are of short stature and have bowlegs, especially if the condition is present from childhood. Adult-onset forms also exist, and the clinical manifestations in these patients are minor or even lacking, with the exception of low serum levels of inorganic phosphate.

The characteristic radiographic oral findings are large pulp chambers with very long pulp horns. In addition, the dentin exhibits pronounced cracks that extend to the dentinoenamel junction. These cracks induce fracture of the enamel with microexposure of the pulp and subsequent pulpal infection. Eventually, infectious inflammatory pulpal disease progresses to periapical abscess formation. Gingival abscesses are also frequent. Regional lymphadenitis accompanies these processes.

Pegged or Absent Maxillary Lateral Incisors. The inheritance pattern of **pegged** or **absent maxillary lateral incisors** is generally autosomal dominant with variable expressivity. The lateral incisor can be small, peg shaped, or congenitally lacking, either unilaterally or bilaterally (Figure 6-43). Both primary and secondary dentitions can be affected, but mostly the latter. This condition has a prevalence of 1% to 3% in the white population and about 7% in Asians. In addition, the premolar teeth are congenitally lacking in 10% to 20% of affected individuals.

Taurodontism. Taurodontism is a genetic heterogeneous condition with dominant and recessive inheritance. It is characterized by very large, pyramid-shaped molars with large pulp chambers (Figure 6-44). Taurodontism is most frequent among Native Americans, including the Inuit. The furcation of the roots is displaced apically, and these teeth are classified according to the degree of furcation displacement. Taurodontism is frequently found in Klinefelter syndrome and is associated with many other syndromes as well.

SELECTED REFERENCES

Books

Cummings MR: *Human heredity: principles and issues*, ed 7, Stamford, Conn, 2006, Brooks/Cole-Cengage Learning.

Fitzgerald MJT, Fitzgerald M: *Human embryology*, London, 1994, Saunders.

Hennekam RCM, Krantz ID, Allanson JE: *Gorlin's syndromes of the head and neck*, ed 5, New York, 2010, Oxford University Press.

Neussbaum RL, McInnes RR, Willard HF: *Thompson and Thompson genetics in medicine*, ed 7, Philadelphia, 2007, Saunders.

Neville BW, Damm DD, Allen CM, et al: *Oral and maxillofacial pathology*, ed 3, St. Louis, 2009, Elsevier.

Sadler TW: *Langman's medical embryology*, ed 11, Philadelphia, 2010, Lippincott, Williams & Wilkins.

Sapp JP, Eversole LR, Wisocki GP: *Contemporary oral and maxillofacial pathology*, ed 2, St. Louis, 2004, Mosby.

Witkop CJ, Sauk JJ, Stewart R, et al: Heritable defects of enamel. In *Oral facial genetics*, St Louis, 1976, Mosby, pp 151–226.

Young WG, Sedano HO: *An atlas of oral pathology*, Minneapolis, 1981, University of Minnesota Press.

Journal Articles

Barron MJ, McDonnell ST, Mackie I, et al: Hereditary dentine disorders: dentinogenesis imperfecta and dentine dysplasia, *Orphanet J Rare Dis* 3:31, 2008.

Beriaghi S, Myers SL, Jensen SA, et al: Cleft lip and palate: association with other congenital malformations, *J Clin Pediatr Dent* 33:207, 2009.

Chaturvedi R: Idiopathic gingival fibromatosis associated with generalized aggressive periodontitis: a case report, *J Can Dent Assoc* 75:291, 2009.

Gerstenblith MR, Goldstein AM, Tucker MA: Hereditary genodermatoses with cancer predisposition, *Hematol Oncol Clin North Am* 24:885, 2010.

Hanemann JA, de Carvalho BC, Franco EC: Oral manifestations in Ellis–van Creveld syndrome: report of a case and review of the literature, *J Oral Maxillofac Surg* 68:456, 2010.

Huynh-Ba G, Brägger U, Zwahlen M, et al: Periodontal disease progression in subjects with orofacial clefts over a 25-year follow-up period, *J Clin Periodontol* 36:836, 2009.

Saeves R, Lande Wekre L, Ambjørnsen E, et al: Oral findings in adults with osteogenesis imperfecta, *Spec Care Dentist* 29:102, 2009.

Schlosser BJ, Pirigyi M, Mirowski GW: Oral manifestations of hematologic and nutritional diseases, *Otolaryngol Clin North Am* 44:183, 2011.

Senel FC, Altintas NY, Bagis B, et al: A 3-year follow-up of the rehabilitation of Papillon-Lefèvre syndrome by dental implants, *J Oral Maxillofac Surg* 70:163, 2012.

Ye Y, Carlsson G, Wondimu B, et al: Mutations in the ELANE gene are associated with development of periodontitis in patients with severe congenital neutropenia, *J Clin Immunol* 31:936, 2011.

Review Questions

1. The short and long arms of each chromosome are joined by a constriction called the:
   A. Equatorial plate
   B. Chiasmata
   C. Chromatid
   D. Centromere

2. The Lyon hypothesis is demonstrated by:
   A. Autosomal-dominant traits
   B. Autosomal-recessive traits
   C. X-linked dominant traits
   D. X-linked recessive traits

3. Trisomy is defined as:
   A. The presence of two extra X chromosomes in a male
   B. Three extra chromosomes
   C. A pair of chromosomes with an identical extra chromosome
   D. One extra chromosome in each pair

4. The process by which a primitive germ cell becomes a gamete is called:
   A. Mitosis
   B. Meiosis
   C. Haploid
   D. S phase

5. Barr bodies are seen at the:
   A. Nuclear periphery of all human cells
   B. Periphery of the cytoplasm in all human cells
   C. Nuclear periphery of cells in women
   D. Periphery of the cytoplasm in all cells from women

6. The karyotype of a patient with Turner syndrome shows:
   A. 44 autosomes and XYY
   B. 43 autosomes and XYY
   C. 44 autosomes and XXY
   D. 44 autosomes and XO

7. Hypothetically, an autosomal-dominant trait would be clinically present in:
   A. 50% of the offspring of an affected parent
   B. 75% of the offspring of an affected parent
   C. 25% of the offspring of an affected parent
   D. Only in males, never in female offspring

8. Patients with an X-linked hereditary condition:
   A. Are always men
   B. Are generally affected more severely if they are men
   C. Are always women
   D. Have cells with many Barr bodies

9. Which one of the following is associated with cyclic neutropenia?
   A. Premature loss of primary teeth
   B. Diminished number of circulating neutrophils
   C. Exfoliating teeth because of short roots
   D. Chipping away of enamel

10. In all inherited varieties of gingival fibromatosis, the gingival enlargement is characterized by a marked:
    A. Hyperplasia of the covering epithelium
    B. Chronic inflammatory cellular infiltrate
    C. Collagenization of the connective tissue
    D. Alveolar bone hypertrophy

11. A 14-year-old boy is seen in consultation because of bilateral mandibular swelling. Radiographs show a bilateral multilocular lesion in the ascending mandibular rami. The mother of this patient has similar findings. The most likely diagnosis is:
    A. Cherubism
    B. Cleidocranial dysplasia
    C. Nevoid basal cell carcinoma syndrome
    D. Ellis–van Creveld syndrome

12. A 9-year-old boy exhibits markedly swollen red and bleeding gingiva. In addition, he has tooth mobility, and the intraoral radiographs show marked alveolar bone atrophy with vertical periodontal pockets. Which of the following will be found in this child if he were to have Papillon-Lefèvre syndrome?
    A. Blue sclerae
    B. Lack of anterior vestibular sulcus
    C. Diminished sweating
    D. Palmar and plantar hyperkeratosis

13. Which of the following is the most serious component of Gardner syndrome?
    A. Mandibular odontomas
    B. Multiple osteomas
    C. Teeth hypercementosis
    D. Intestinal polyposis

14. A 19-year-old woman is diagnosed with cleidocranial dysplasia. She has absent clavicles and a mushroom-shaped skull. Which of the following conditions is she also most likely to have?
    A. Taurodontism
    B. Supernumerary teeth
    C. Pegged lateral incisors
    D. Large pulp chambers

15. Odontogenic keratocysts are a clinical component of:
    A. MEN 2B syndrome
    B. Neurofibromatosis of von Recklinghausen
    C. Nevoid basal cell carcinoma syndrome
    D. Cherubism

16. Two characteristic clinical components of mandibulofacial dysostosis are:
    A. Hypoplastic mandible and deafness
    B. Lack of clavicles and delayed teeth eruption
    C. Cleft lip and fistulas of lower lip
    D. Hypodontia and dysplastic nails

17. Torus mandibularis and torus palatinus are:
    A. Inherited as an autosomal-recessive trait
    B. More prevalent in males
    C. Inherited as an autosomal-dominant trait
    D. Sporadic traits

18. The major concern for a dental hygienist when treating a patient with Osler-Rendu–Parkes Weber syndrome should be:
    A. Gingival hemorrhage
    B. Spontaneous ulcerations
    C. Severe infections
    D. Epithelial desquamation

19. The cause of all forms of labial and palatal clefting is considered to be:
    A. Autosomal dominant
    B. Autosomal recessive
    C. Multifactorial
    D. Environmental

20. Which of the following is *true* for von Recklinghausen disease?
    A. It is inherited as an autosomal-recessive trait.
    B. Patients have multiple fibromatoses.
    C. Patients experience a generalized whitening of the oral mucosa.
    D. Patients may have gingival neurofibromas.

21. The most serious clinical manifestation of the MEN 2B syndrome is considered to be:
    A. Carcinoma of the colon
    B. Carcinoma of the thyroid gland
    C. Pheochromocytoma
    D. Basal cell carcinomas

22. Teeth in snowcapped amelogenesis imperfecta have:
    A. White hypocalcified enamel at the incisal and occlusal thirds
    B. Obliterated pulp chambers
    C. Short, blunted roots
    D. A thin, brown enamel

23. In dentinogenesis imperfecta type II, teeth have:
    A. Hard, dense dentin
    B. Dilacerated roots
    C. Markedly brittle enamel
    D. Roots that are short and thin

24. Patients with hypohidrotic ectodermal dysplasia characteristically have:
    A. Hypodontia
    B. Multiple tongue nodules
    C. Excessive amounts of hair
    D. Blue sclerae

25. Patients with hypophosphatasia characteristically have:
    A. Obliterated pulp chambers
    B. Marked gingival keratinization
    C. Increase in serum alkaline phosphatase levels
    D. Absence of root cementum

26. Taurodontic teeth:
    A. Are supernumerary
    B. Are pyramidal in shape
    C. Have long roots
    D. Have thistle-shaped pulp chambers

27. The characteristic finding in permanent teeth affected with coronal dentin dysplasia is:
    A. Crowns with amber color
    B. Markedly short roots
    C. Thistle-shaped pulp chambers on radiographs
    D. Large, square pulp chambers

28. The order of the four stages of mitosis is:
    A. Prophase, telophase, metaphase, anaphase
    B. Prophase, metaphase, anaphase, telophase
    C. Metaphase, prophase, telophase, anaphase
    D. Anaphase, metaphase, telophase, prophase

29. The so-called "enamel agenesis" is one of which type of amelogenesis imperfecta?
    A. Hypoplastic
    B. Hypocalcified
    C. Hypomaturation
    D. Hypoplastic-hypomaturation

30. The most frequent site of hemorrhage in patients with hereditary hemorrhagic telangiectasia is the
    A. Gingiva
    B. Nasal mucosa
    C. Lip mucosa
    D. Eyelids

31. The Papillon-Lefèvre syndrome is inherited according to a (an)
    A. Autosomal dominant pattern
    B. Autosomal recessive pattern
    C. X-linked dominant pattern
    D. X-linked recessive pattern

Continued

CONDITION/DISEASE	CAUSE	AGE/RACE/SEX	LOCATION
Amelogenesis imperfecta: snow-capped (hypomaturation)	AD and X-linked recessive	When teeth erupt, AD, M=F X-linked, more often men	All primary and permanent teeth
Dentinogenesis imperfecta	AD, 4q13-21	When teeth erupt	All primary and permanent teeth
Radicular dentin dysplasia	AD	When teeth erupt	All primary and permanent teeth
Coronal dentin dysplasia	AD, 4q13-21	When teeth erupt	All primary teeth
Hypohidrotic ectodermal dysplasia	X-linked recessive, Xq12-13.1 AR, 2q11-13	From birth X-linked, all males AR, M=F	Skin, sweat glands, hair, both dentitions
Hypophosphatasia	AR, 1p36.1-34	From birth M=F	Bones, teeth
Hypophosphatemic vitamin D–resistant rickets	X-linked dominant	From birth More often men	Bones, teeth

AD, Autosomal dominant; *AR*, autosomal recessive; *CL/P*, cleft lip with or without cleft palate; *M=F*, occurs in men and women equally.

CLINICAL FEATURES	RADIOGRAPHIC FEATURES	MICROSCOPIC FEATURES	TREATMENT	DIAGNOSTIC PROCESS
White discoloration of surface enamel of occlusal one third of all teeth	None	Not available	Aesthetic dentistry if the patient wants it	Clinical and family history
Bulbous crowns, opalescent brown-bluish crowns	Short pointed roots, absent pulp chambers	Abnormal globular dentin, trapped odontoblasts	Aesthetic dentistry, crowns, operative procedures	Clinical and family history
Normal crowns in size and color	Short pointed roots, absent pulp chambers	Abnormal tubular dentin and osteodentin	Prosthesis if teeth are lost	Family history Radiographic
Primary teeth amber in color, permanent teeth normal in color	Primary: absent pulp chambers Permanent molars: "bow tie" pulp Uniradicular teeth: "thistle-shaped" pulp	Abnormal dentin in primary teeth, permanent teeth with pulp stones	Regular dental and dental hygiene care	Clinical and family history Radiographic
Few teeth formed Hypotrichosis Hypohydrosis Frontal bossing Depressed nasal bridge Protuberant lips	Almost no teeth present	Reduced and abnormal sweat pores	Dental implants and/ or dental prosthesis	Clinical and family history Radiographic
Premature loss of primary anterior teeth	Large pulp chambers	Absence of root cementum	Space retainers or dental prosthesis	Clinical and family history Radiographic
Multiple periapical radiolucencies (cyst, granuloma)	Large pulp chambers, large pulp horns	Abnormal globular dentin, large cracks in dentin	Endodontics and regular dental hygiene care	Clinical and family history Radiographic

Chapter 7

Neoplasia

Anne Cale Jones, Paul D. Freedman, Joan Andersen Phelan, John E. Kacher

OBJECTIVES

After studying this chapter, the student will be able to:

1. Define each of the words in the vocabulary list for this chapter.
2. Explain the difference between a benign tumor and a malignant tumor.
3. Define leukoplakia and erythroplakia.
4. Describe the clinical and microscopic features of a calcifying odontogenic cyst and compare and contrast this lesion with an ameloblastoma.
5. Define each of the following neoplasms, describe the clinical features of each, and explain how they are treated: papilloma, squamous cell carcinoma, verrucous carcinoma, basal cell carcinoma, pleomorphic adenoma, trabecular and canalicular adenoma, adenoid cystic carcinoma, mucoepidermoid carcinoma, ameloblastoma, calcifying epithelial odontogenic tumor, adenomatoid odontogenic tumor, odontogenic myxoma, central cementifying and ossifying fibromas, benign cementoblastoma, ameloblastic fibroma, ameloblastic fibro-odontoma, odontoma, peripheral ossifying fibroma, lipoma, neurofibroma and schwannoma, granular cell tumor, congenital epulis, rhabdomyosarcoma, hemangioma, lymphangioma, Kaposi sarcoma, melanocytic nevi, malignant melanoma, torus, exostosis, osteoma, osteosarcoma, chondrosarcoma, leukemia, lymphoma, multiple myeloma, and metastatic jaw tumors.

VOCABULARY

Aberrant (ab-ar'ənt) Deviating from the usual or natural type; atypical.

Anaplastic (an″ə-plas'tik) Characterized by a loss of differentiation of cells and their orientation to one another; a characteristic of malignant tumors.

Bence Jones proteins (bens-jōnz pro'tēnz) Fragments of abnormal immunoglobulins excreted in the urine of patients with multiple myeloma.

Benign (be-nīn') A condition that is not life-threatening, not cancerous, not malignant.

Benign tumor (be-nīn' too'mor) A tumor that is not malignant and favorable for treatment and recovery.

Carcinoma (kahr″sĭ-no'mə) Malignant tumor of the epithelium.

Central (sen'trəl) In oral pathology, describing a tumor or lesion occurring within bone.

Dysplasia (dis-pla'zhə) Disordered growth; alteration in size, shape, and organization of adult cells.

Encapsulated (en-kap'su-lāt-əd) Surrounded by a dense band of fibrous connective tissue.

Enucleation (ē-noo'klē-ā'shən) Complete surgical removal without cutting into the lesion.

Excision (ek-sizh'ən) Surgical removal.

Hyperchromatic (hi″pər-kro-mat'ik) Microscopic staining that is more intense than normal.

Hyperplasia (hi″pər-pla'zhə) Abnormal increase in the number of cells in an organ or tissue.

VOCABULARY—cont'd

Immunoglobulin (im″u-no-glob′u-lin) A protein, also called an antibody, synthesized by plasma cells in response to a specific antigen.

In situ (in si′tu) Confined to the site of origin without invasion of neighboring tissues.

Invasion (in-va′shən) Infiltration and active destruction of surrounding tissues.

Leukoplakia (loo″ko-pla′ke-ə.) Clinical term used to identify a white, plaquelike lesion of the oral mucosa that cannot be wiped off or diagnosed as any other disease.

Malignant (mə-lig′nənt) Tending to produce death, able to metastasize; describing cancer.

Malignant tumor (mə-lig′nənt too′mor) Cancer; a tumor that is resistant to treatment and may cause death; a tumor that has the potential for uncontrolled growth and dissemination or recurrence, or both.

Metastasis (mə-tas′tə-sis) (plural, *metastases* [mə-tas′tə-sēz])** Transport of neoplastic cells to parts of the body remote from the primary tumor and the establishment of new tumors at those sites.

Metastatic tumor (met″ə-stat′ik too′mor) Tumor formed by cells that have been transported from the primary tumor to sites not connected with the original tumor.

Mitotic figure (mi-tot′ik fig′ər) A term, used in microscopy, to describe dividing cells caught in the process of mitosis **(mi-to′sis).**

Monoclonal spike (mon″o-klōn′əl spīk) An elevation of a single type of immunoglobulin; detected by a process called immunoelectrophoresis.

Neoplasia (ne″o-pla′zhə) New growth; the formation of tumors by the uncontrolled proliferation of cells.

Neoplasm (ne′o-plaz-əm) Tumor; a new growth of tissue in which growth is uncontrolled and progressive.

Neoplastic (ne″o-plas′tik) Pertaining to the formation of tumors by the uncontrolled proliferation of cells.

Nevus (ne′vəs) (plural, *nevi* [ne′vi]) A benign tumor consisting of melanocytes (nevus cells); also a circumscribed, usually pigmented, congenital malformation of the skin or oral mucosa.

Odontogenic (o-don″to-jen′ik) Tooth forming.

Oncology (ong-kol′ə-je) The study of tumors or neoplasms.

Pedunculated (pə-dung′ku-lāt-əd) Attached by a stalk.

Peripheral (pə-rif′ər-əl) In oral pathology, describing a lesion that occurs on the gingiva or alveolar mucosa.

Pleomorphic (ple″o-mor′fik) Occurring in various forms.

Primary tumor (pri′mar-e too′mor) Original tumor; the source of metastasis.

Sarcoma (sahr-ko′mə) Malignant tumor of the connective tissue.

Sessile (ses′il) Attached by a broad base.

Tumor (too′mor) Neoplasm; also, a swelling or enlargement.

Undifferentiated (ən-dif″ər-en′she-āt-əd) Absence of normal differentiation; anaplasia; a characteristic of some malignant tumors.

Waldeyer ring (vahl′di-er ring) A ring of lymphatic tissue formed by the two palatine tonsils, the pharyngeal tonsil, the lingual tonsil, and intervening lymphoid tissue.

DESCRIPTION OF NEOPLASIA

Neoplasia means new growth. It is a process in which cells exhibit abnormal and uncontrolled proliferation. A **neoplasm** is a mass of such cells. Although the word **tumor** means swelling, it is commonly used as a synonym for neoplasm. The study of tumors is called **oncology.** *Onco* in Greek means swelling or mass.

For neoplasia to occur, an irreversible change must take place in the cells, and this change must be passed on to new cells, resulting in uncontrolled cell multiplication. In most cases the initial stimulus that triggers the process of cell change is not known. Regulatory processes maintain the size of normal tissues. The regulatory processes that maintain the size of normal tissues do not function correctly in a neoplasm; therefore it exhibits unlimited and unregulated growth.

Unlike **hyperplasia,** neoplasia is an uncontrolled abnormal process. With hyperplasia, normal cells proliferate in a normal arrangement in response to tissue damage, and the proliferation stops when the stimulus is removed. Although the size of the tissue may be greater than normal, the growth of the tissue is still under control. Reactive lesions such as the irritation fibroma, denture-related hyperplasia (epulis fissuratum), and pyogenic granuloma are examples of hyperplasia. In contrast, neoplasia is a completely abnormal process; the cells are abnormal, and the proliferation of these cells is uncontrolled and unlimited.

CAUSES OF NEOPLASIA

Many agents—principally chemicals, viruses, and radiation—have been shown to cause **neoplastic** transformation of cells in the laboratory. Hundreds of chemicals have been shown to cause cancer in animals. In addition, certain chemicals, viruses such as Epstein-Barr virus (EBV) and human papilloma virus (HPV), and radiation have been shown to cause specific types of cancer in humans. Neoplastic transformation may also occur spontaneously secondary to a genetic mutation. Viruses that cause tumors are called **oncogenic viruses.** Radiation from sunlight (ultraviolet rays), x-rays, nuclear fission, or other sources is well established as a cancer-producing agent in humans.

FIGURE 7-1 ■ Photomicrographs of malignant tumors show pleomorphic *(P)* and hyperchromatic *(H)* nuclei and mitotic figures *(MI)*. **A,** Squamous cell carcinoma. **B,** Osteosarcoma.

CLASSIFICATION OF TUMORS

Tumors are divided into two categories: **benign** and **malignant**. A **benign tumor** or neoplasm remains localized. It may be **encapsulated,** which means that it is walled off by surrounding fibrous connective tissue. Sometimes a benign tumor can invade adjacent structures, but it does not have the ability to spread to distant sites. In contrast, a **malignant tumor** both invades and destroys surrounding tissue and has the ability to spread throughout the body. **Cancer** is synonymous with malignancy.

Benign tumors almost always resemble normal cells, whereas malignant tumors vary in their microscopic appearance. Malignant tumors composed of neoplastic cells that resemble normal cells are called *well-differentiated tumors.* Malignant tumors may also be poorly differentiated. The cells of these tumors have only some of the characteristics of the tissue from which they were derived. Still others may be **undifferentiated** or **anaplastic** and do not resemble at all the tissue from which they were derived. Malignant tumors are often composed of cells that vary in size and shape **(pleomorphic)** (Figure 7-1). The nuclei of these cells are darker than those of normal cells **(hyperchromatic)** and exhibit an increased nuclear-to-cytoplasmic ratio (Figure 7-1). Normal and abnormal **mitotic figures** are seen in the nucleus of the neoplastic cells (Figure 7-1, *A*). Abnormal mitotic figures are those that are not dividing normally; therefore the shape of the dividing nucleus does not follow the shape of a normal mitotic figure. Table 7-1 compares benign and malignant tumors.

NAMES OF TUMORS

The prefix of the name of a tumor is determined by the cell or tissue of origin. The suffix *-oma* is used to indicate a tumor. The prefix of the name of a benign or malignant tumor is also determined by the cell or tissue of origin. For example, a benign tumor of fat is called a **lipoma,** and a benign tumor of bone is called an **osteoma.** Malignant tumors are named in a similar fashion. Malignant tumors of epithelium are called **carcinomas,** and malignant tumors of connective tissue are

TABLE 7-1

Comparison of Benign and Malignant Tumors

BENIGN	MALIGNANT
Usually well differentiated	Well differentiated to anaplastic
Usually slow growth	Slow to rapid growth
Mitotic figures are rare	Mitotic figures may be numerous
Usually encapsulated	Invasive and unencapsulated
No metastasis	Metastasis likely

TABLE 7-2

Names of Tumors

TISSUE OF ORIGIN	BENIGN TUMOR	MALIGNANT TUMOR
Epithelium		
Squamous cells	Papilloma	Squamous cell or epidermoid carcinoma
Basal cells		Basal cell carcinoma
Glands or ducts	Adenoma	Adenocarcinoma
Neuroectoderm		
Melanocytes	Nevus	Melanoma
Connective Tissue		
Fibrous	Fibroma	Fibrosarcoma
Cartilage	Chondroma	Chondrosarcoma
Bone	Osteoma	Osteosarcoma
Fat	Lipoma	Liposarcoma
Endothelium		
Blood vessels	Hemangioma	Angiosarcoma
Lymphatic vessels	Lymphangioma	Lymphangiosarcoma
Muscle		
Smooth muscle	Leiomyoma	Leiomyosarcoma
Striated muscle	Rhabdomyoma	Rhabdomyosarcoma

called **sarcomas.** Therefore a malignant tumor of squamous epithelium is called a **squamous cell carcinoma** or an **epidermoid carcinoma,** and a malignant tumor of bone is called an **osteosarcoma** (osteogenic sarcoma). Carcinomas are about 10 times more common than sarcomas. Table 7-2 lists tumors according to their tissue or cell of origin.

TREATMENT OF TUMORS

Benign tumors generally are treated by surgical **excision,** which can be accomplished through **enucleation** or by wide local excision. Malignant tumors are treated by surgery, chemotherapy, or radiation therapy; a combination is often used.

Because many different types of tissue are present in the oral cavity, many different types of tumor can arise in this location. These neoplasms can be either benign or malignant. In this chapter the neoplasms are classified according to their tissue of origin. Benign tumors are described first, followed by their malignant counterparts.

EPITHELIAL TUMORS

Three different types of **epithelial tumor** occur in the oral cavity: (1) tumors derived from squamous epithelium, (2) tumors derived from salivary gland epithelium, and (3) tumors derived from **odontogenic** epithelium. A few of the lesions included in this section are not true tumors. The reasons for their inclusion are explained in their descriptions.

TUMORS OF SQUAMOUS EPITHELIUM

PAPILLOMA

The **papilloma** is a benign tumor of squamous epithelium that presents as a small, exophytic, **pedunculated** or **sessile** growth. These tumors are composed of numerous papillary projections that may be either white or the color of normal mucosa (Figure 7-2). The color of the lesion depends on the amount of surface keratin; the more keratin, the whiter the lesion appears clinically.

They are often described as cauliflower-like in appearance. Most cases arise on the soft palate or tongue. A papilloma may occur at any age, and an equal sex predilection

is noted. Microscopic examination demonstrates numerous fingerlike or papillary projections composed of normal stratified squamous epithelium surfaced by a thickened layer of keratin. A central core of fibrous connective tissue supports each papillary projection.

Other oral lesions that may resemble a papilloma clinically are a verruca vulgaris (common wart) and condyloma acuminatum (venereal wart). These two lesions are caused by human papillomaviruses and are described in Chapter 4. They are differentiated from the papilloma by microscopic examination. Special procedures can be used to identify specific viral particles within these lesions. Evidence suggests that low-risk types of HPV are involved in the etiology of oral squamous papillomas, but microscopic evidence of HPV infection is generally not present in squamous papillomas.

A papilloma is treated by surgical excision, which must include the base of the growth. With adequate excision, the papilloma usually does not recur.

PREMALIGNANT LESIONS

LEUKOPLAKIA

In any discussion of premalignant lesions of the oral mucosa, it is important to define the term **leukoplakia.** Leukoplakia is a clinical term and does not refer to a specific microscopic appearance. It is defined as a white plaquelike lesion of the oral mucosa that cannot be rubbed off and cannot be diagnosed clinically as a specific disease (Figure 7-3, *A* and *B*).

Leukoplakia is sometimes referred to as *idiopathic leukoplakia* to emphasize that the specific cause of the lesion is not known. The white lesion illustrated in Figure 7-4 is more accurately called **smokeless tobacco–associated keratosis** rather than a leukoplakia because the direct cause of the lesion is known.

The microscopic appearance of leukoplakia varies; therefore a biopsy is essential to establish a definitive diagnosis. Most leukoplakias are the result of hyperkeratosis (thickening of the keratin layer) or a combination of epithelial

FIGURE 7-2 ▪ **A,** Clinical appearance of a papilloma of the oral mucosa shows a cauliflower-like appearance and rough surface resulting from finger-like projections. **B,** Microscopic appearance of a papilloma shows fingerlike projections surfaced by squamous epithelium and supported by thin cores of fibrous connective tissue.

FIGURE 7-3 ▪ Clinical appearance of leukoplakia. **A,** Floor of the mouth. **B,** Maxillary alveolar mucosa and palate. The cause of these lesions could not be identified. **C,** Erythroplakia in this case diagnosed microscopically as squamous cell carcinoma. (**C,** Reprinted with permission from SAVVY SUCCESS: Volume II: Patient Care, Flanders, NJ.)

FIGURE 7-4 ▪ Clinical appearance of a white lesion that was associated with smokeless tobacco (smokeless tobacco–associated keratosis). This lesion developed on the lower labial mucosa at the site where the tobacco was held.

hyperplasia (thickening of the prickle cell or spinous layer) and hyperkeratosis. When examined microscopically, a leukoplakia may also show epithelial **dysplasia,** a premalignant condition, or even squamous cell carcinoma, a malignant tumor of the squamous epithelium. Depending on the study, approximately 5% to 25% of leukoplakias examined microscopically demonstrate epithelial dysplasia. Studies have also revealed that leukoplakia found on the floor of the mouth, ventrolateral tongue, soft palate, and lip is more likely to represent epithelial dysplasia or squamous cell carcinoma than leukoplakia occurring in other areas of the oral cavity.

When a white lesion is identified in the oral cavity, the first goal is to identify the cause. Any associated irritation should be removed. If the lesion does not resolve, a biopsy and microscopic examination of the tissue must be performed. Any white lesion that is diagnosed as epithelial dysplasia or that cannot be diagnosed as a specific disease should be removed completely. When leukoplakia is found on the floor of the mouth, ventrolateral tongue, soft palate, or lip, the lesion should be removed regardless of the microscopic appearance because there is an increased risk of squamous cell carcinoma developing in these areas.

The treatment of leukoplakia depends on the microscopic diagnosis. The treatment of epithelial dysplasia and squamous cell carcinoma is discussed in the sections that follow.

ERYTHROPLAKIA

Erythroplakia is a clinical term used to describe an oral mucosal lesion that appears as a smooth red patch or a granular red and velvety patch (see Figure 7-3, C). A lesion that shows a mixture of red and white areas is generally called **speckled leukoplakia** rather than erythroplakia. Most cases of erythroplakia occur in the floor of the mouth, tongue, and soft palate. Erythroplakia is much less common than leukoplakia. In one study 60 cases of leukoplakia were seen for every 1 case of erythroplakia. When examined microscopically, 90% of cases of erythroplakia demonstrate epithelial dysplasia or squamous cell carcinoma. Because of these microscopic findings, erythroplakia is considered a more serious clinical finding than leukoplakia (a biopsy must be performed to establish a definitive diagnosis).

Treatment of erythroplakia depends on the microscopic diagnosis.

EPITHELIAL DYSPLASIA

Epithelial dysplasia is a microscopic diagnosis that indicates disordered growth. It is considered a premalignant condition. Lesions that microscopically exhibit epithelial dysplasia frequently precede squamous cell carcinoma. Unlike squamous cell carcinoma, the cellular changes in epithelial dysplasia may revert to normal if the stimulus such as tobacco smoking is removed. Epithelial dysplasia may present clinically as an erythematous (red) lesion (erythroplakia), a white lesion (leukoplakia), or a mixed erythematous and white lesion (speckled leukoplakia). Lesions often arise in the floor of the mouth or tongue. The term **dysplasia** may also be used to describe lesions that occur in tissues other than epithelium. These lesions are developmental and characterized by disordered growth. They are not considered premalignant lesions.

Microscopic examination of epithelial dysplasia demonstrates abnormal maturation of epithelial cells with disorganization of the epithelial layers; hyperplasia of the basal cells; and epithelial cells with enlarged and hyperchromatic nuclei, increased nuclear-to-cytoplasmic ratios, abnormal keratinization, and increased numbers of normal and abnormal mitotic figures (Figure 7-5). Microscopically, epithelial dysplasia differs from squamous cell carcinoma in that there is no **invasion** of the abnormal epithelial cells through the basement membrane into the underlying tissue. Severe dysplasia involving the full thickness of the epithelium is called carcinoma **in situ.**

All dysplastic lesions should be excised surgically. Close long-term follow-up examinations are indicated because of the potential for recurrence.

FIGURE 7-5 ■ Microscopic appearance of epithelial dysplasia. Loss of the normal stratification of the epithelium, hyperplasia of the basal cells, and enlarged, hyperchromatic nuclei are seen.

SQUAMOUS CELL CARCINOMA

Squamous cell carcinoma, or epidermoid carcinoma, is a malignant tumor of the squamous epithelium. It is the most common primary malignancy of the oral cavity and, like other malignant tumors, can infiltrate adjacent tissues and metastasize to distant sites. Squamous cell carcinoma usually metastasizes to lymph nodes of the neck and then to more distant sites such as the lungs and liver. Clinically, squamous cell carcinoma usually presents as an exophytic ulcerative mass (Figure 7-6), but early tumors may be white and plaquelike (leukoplakia), erythematous (red) and plaquelike (erythroplakia), or a mixture of erythematous and white areas (speckled leukoplakia). Squamous cell carcinoma can infiltrate and destroy bone (Figure 7-6, D).

The essential microscopic feature of a squamous cell carcinoma is the invasion of tumor cells through the epithelial basement membrane into the underlying connective tissue (Figure 7-7, A). Invasive sheets and nests of neoplastic squamous cells characterize this tumor. Although squamous cell carcinoma is a malignant tumor, it exhibits features that allow the cells to be recognized as squamous epithelial cells. In well-differentiated tumors these features are easily recognized; however, they may not be easily seen in a poorly differentiated squamous cell carcinoma. Because keratin is a product of squamous epithelium, well-differentiated tumors show keratin formation. In addition to normal surface keratin, the keratin may be seen in individual cells within the tumor and as structures called **keratin pearls** (Figure 7-7, B). The neoplastic cells are not normal cells. They contain large hyperchromatic nuclei and numerous mitotic figures. Some of the mitotic figures appear normal, whereas others are bizarre (Figure 7-7, B).

Squamous cell carcinomas may occur anywhere in the oral cavity, but most tumors arise on the floor of the mouth, ventrolateral tongue, soft palate, and tonsillar pillar. The clinical appearance of squamous cell carcinoma occurring in several different locations may be seen in Figure 7-6.

Squamous cell carcinomas may occur on the vermilion border of the lips and skin of the face (Figure 7-8). In this location they are associated with sun exposure (actinic cheilitis and actinic keratosis) and tend to be more common in individuals with fair skin. The prognosis for squamous cell carcinoma of the lips and skin is much better than that for squamous cell carcinoma of the oral mucosa. Sun exposure causes recognizable changes of the vermilion border of the lips. The color changes from dark and uniform to mottled grayish-pink. The interface of the vermilion border and the skin becomes blurred, and linear fissures are seen at right angles to the line of the interface. Microscopically, damage from ultraviolet rays as a result of sun exposure is seen as changes that range from degeneration of the collagen under the epithelium to a condition called **solar** or **actinic cheilitis,** in which mild-to-severe epithelial dysplasia occurs. Avoidance of sun exposure and the use of a sun-blocking agent are important in preventing the damaging effects of sunlight.

FIGURE 7-6 ■ **A,** Clinical appearance of a squamous cell carcinoma of the posterolateral tongue shows an exophytic, ulcerated mass. **B,** Clinical appearance of a squamous cell carcinoma on the left side of the soft palate and fauces. **C,** Clinical appearance of a squamous cell carcinoma on the floor of the mouth. **D,** Left side of a panoramic radiograph shows destruction of the mandible by a squamous cell carcinoma. (**C,** Courtesy Dr. Edward V. Zegarelli.)

FIGURE 7-7 ■ **A,** Microscopic appearance (low power) of a squamous cell carcinoma shows infiltration of the tumor into the connective tissue. **B,** High-power photomicrograph shows abnormal keratinization and keratin pearls (K).

FIGURE 7-8 ▪ **A** and **B,** Clinical appearance of squamous cell carcinoma of the lower lip. Squamous cell carcinoma (*arrow*) is seen with actinic (solar) cheilitis in **(A).** (Courtesy Dr. Edward V. Zegarelli.)

The majority of squamous cell carcinomas occur in patients over 40 years of age. In the past, more men than women have developed squamous cell carcinoma; however, in the last 30 years there has been an increased incidence of squamous cell carcinoma in women. This is most likely a result of the increased number of women who smoke and the fact that women outnumber men in older age groups.

RISK FACTORS

Several risk factors have been associated with the development of squamous cell carcinoma. The most significant is tobacco—including cigar, pipe, and cigarette smoking; snuff dipping; and tobacco chewing. Alcohol consumption appears to add to the risk of oral squamous cell carcinoma, especially in individuals who also use tobacco products. High-risk types of human papillomavirus (HPV) have been identified in squamous cell carcinomas of the oropharynx and have been suggested to be important factors in the pathogenesis of these cancers... There is evidence that HPV contributes to the transformation of normal epithelial cells into malignant epithelial cells (HPV infection is discussed in Chapter 4). There is no evidence that chronic irritation (i.e., an ill-fitting denture) is an initiating factor in the development of oral cancer.

TREATMENT AND PROGNOSIS

Squamous cell carcinoma generally is treated by surgical excision. Radiation therapy or chemotherapy may be used in combination with surgery. On occasion, radiation therapy is used alone. The prognosis of squamous cell carcinoma is related to the size and location of the tumor and the presence or absence of metastases. The smaller the tumor is at the time of treatment, the better the prognosis. For oral squamous cell carcinoma, determining the size of the tumor and the presence or absence of cervical lymph node involvement and distant **metastasis** is important in predicting the patient's prognosis. These are assessed using a system called the **TNM staging system;** the higher the stage, the worse the prognosis (Box 7-1 and Table 7-3). Metastasis to cervical lymph nodes is associated with a much poorer prognosis, as is the presence of distant metastasis. Therefore, it

---

Box 7-1

TNM Staging System for Oral Squamous Cell Carcinoma

T: Tumor

T_1: Tumor less than 2 cm in diameter
T_2: Tumor 2-4 cm in diameter
T_3: Tumor greater than 4 cm in diameter
T_4: Tumor invading adjacent structures

N: Node

N_0: No palpable nodes
N_1: Ipsilateral (same side as primary tumor) palpable nodes (same side as tumor)
N_2: Contralateral (opposite side from primary tumor) or bilateral nodes
N_3: Fixed palpable nodes

M: Metastasis

M_0: No distant metastasis
M_1: Clinical or radiographic evidence of metastasis

Adapted from International Union against Cancer: *TNM classification of malignant tumours* (Sobin LH, Wittekind C, editors), ed 6, New York, 2002, Wiley-Liss.

TABLE 7-3

TNM Staging System

STAGE	TUMOR	NODE	METASTASIS
I	T_1	N_0	M_0
II	T_2	N_0	M_0
III	T_3	N_0	M_0
	T_1	N_1	M_0
	T_2	N_1	M_0
	T_3	N_1	M_0
IV	T_1	N_2	M_0
	T_2	N_2	M_0
	T_3	N_2	M_0
	T_1	N_3	M_0
	T_2	N_3	M_0
	T_3	N_3	M_0
	T_4	N_0	M_0
Stage IV includes any patients with M_1.			

Adapted from International Union against Cancer: *TNM classification of malignant tumours* (Sobin LH, Wittekind C, editors), ed 6, New York, 2002, Wiley-Liss.

FIGURE 7-9 ■ **A,** Clinical appearance of a verrucous carcinoma occurring on the commissure and anterior buccal mucosa. **B,** Maxillary alveolar ridge.

is important to clinically identify asymptomatic areas of leukoplakia and erythroplakia while they are small and to remove all potentially premalignant lesions.

Patients who have undergone radiation therapy for malignant tumors of the head and neck often experience severe xerostomia (dry mouth) as a result of radiation damage to the salivary gland tissue. These patients require preventive dental care consisting of nutritional counseling, topical fluoride application, and meticulous home care. Oral manifestations of therapy for oral cancer are included in Chapter 9.

VERRUCOUS CARCINOMA

Verrucous carcinoma is a specific type of squamous cell carcinoma that is separated from other squamous cell carcinomas because it has a much better prognosis. Clinically, it appears as a slow-growing exophytic tumor with a pebbly white and red surface (Figure 7-9). Most cases occur in men over 55 years of age and involve the vestibule and buccal mucosa. The use of smokeless tobacco products has been associated with the development of verrucous carcinoma. Microscopic examination demonstrates a tumor composed of numerous papillary epithelial proliferations. The spaces between these papillary projections are filled with keratin (keratin plugging). The epithelium is well differentiated, does not contain atypical cells, and exhibits broad-based rete pegs that penetrate deeply into the connective tissue. The epithelial basement membrane is intact, and the tumor does not show invasion of tumor cells through the basement membrane, as is seen in squamous cell carcinoma.

Verrucous carcinoma is treated by surgical excision. Although it is a carcinoma, it usually does not metastasize; therefore the prognosis is better for verrucous carcinoma than for squamous cell carcinoma. If it is not treated, it can cause extensive local damage. Close long-term follow-up is necessary for patients with this condition.

BASAL CELL CARCINOMA

Basal cell carcinoma is a malignant skin tumor associated with sun exposure. This particular neoplasm does not occur in the oral cavity. Basal cell carcinoma frequently arises on the skin of the face and appears as a nonhealing ulcer with characteristic rolled borders (Figure 7-10). Most cases arise in white adults, and no sex predilection is seen.

A basal cell carcinoma is composed of a proliferation of basal cells derived from the surface stratified squamous epithelium. Microscopic examination demonstrates nests and

FIGURE 7-10 ■ Clinical appearance of a basal cell carcinoma *(arrow)*, illustrating the characteristic "rolled" borders.

islands of basal epithelial cells in the underlying connective tissue. In most cases the tumor cells are well differentiated.

Basal cell carcinoma is a locally invasive tumor that can become quite large and disfiguring if it is not removed. Surgical excision is the treatment of choice, and radiation therapy may be used to treat large lesions. Only rarely does a basal cell carcinoma metastasize. As a general rule, a patient should be referred to an oral and maxillofacial surgeon or dermatologist to have a biopsy performed on any nonhealing ulcer of the skin or lips that has been present for more than 10 days.

SALIVARY GLAND TUMORS

Benign and malignant tumors may arise in either the major or minor salivary glands. Tumors may occur within the parotid, submandibular, or sublingual glands; or they may involve any of the minor salivary glands located throughout the oral cavity. Intraorally, minor salivary gland tumors are located most commonly at the junction of the hard and soft palates. They can also occur on the labial and buccal mucosa, the retromolar area, the floor of the mouth, and rarely the tongue (Figure 7-11). Tumors of minor salivary

FIGURE 7-11 ■ **A,** Benign salivary gland tumor of the palate (pleomorphic adenoma). **B,** Malignant salivary gland tumor of the palate (adenoid cystic carcinoma). Biopsy site should be noted. **C,** Benign salivary gland tumor of the upper lip (pleomorphic adenoma). **D,** Malignant salivary gland tumor of the buccal mucosa (mucoepidermoid carcinoma). **E,** Malignant salivary gland tumor of the tongue (adenoid cystic carcinoma).

FIGURE 7-12 ■ Microscopic appearance of a pleomorphic adenoma. **A,** Low-power photomicrograph shows a capsule (C). **B,** High-power photomicrograph shows a mixture of epithelium (E) and connective tissue (CT).

gland origin are much more common in the upper lip than in the lower lip.

Because the origin of these tumors is glandular epithelium, benign tumors of salivary gland origin are called **adenomas.** Although some malignant salivary gland tumors are called **adenocarcinomas,** most have more specific names such as adenoid cystic carcinoma and mucoepidermoid carcinoma. All salivary gland tumors are diagnosed on the basis of their microscopic appearance. A biopsy and microscopic examination of the tissue are required to establish a specific diagnosis.

PLEOMORPHIC ADENOMA (BENIGN MIXED TUMOR)

The **pleomorphic adenoma** is a benign salivary gland tumor. It is the most common salivary gland neoplasm and accounts for about 90% of all benign salivary gland tumors. Microscopic examination reveals an encapsulated tumor composed of tissue that appears to be a mixture of both epithelium and connective tissue (Figure 7-12). For this reason this tumor is often called a **benign mixed tumor.** The connective tissue–like part can vary from loose and dense fibrous connective tissue to cartilage. The tissue that looks like connective tissue is derived from a salivary gland cell called a **myoepithelial cell.**

The most common extraoral location for the pleomorphic adenoma is the parotid gland. The most common intraoral site is the palate. However, these tumors can occur wherever salivary gland tissue is present. Clinically, the pleomorphic adenoma appears as a slowly enlarging, nonulcerated, painless, dome-shaped mass (see Figure 7-11, *A* and *C*). The surface can be ulcerated if traumatized. Its size can range from a few to several centimeters. Most pleomorphic adenomas occur in individuals over 40 years of age, and a female predilection has been noted. Pleomorphic adenomas have also been reported in children.

A pleomorphic adenoma is treated by surgical excision. The extent of the surgery depends on the location of the

FIGURE 7-13 ■ Microscopic appearance (low power) of a portion of a monomorphic adenoma shows a capsule and a uniform pattern of epithelial cells.

tumor. Clinicians treat parotid gland tumors by removing the part of the parotid gland (partial parotidectomy) containing the tumor, whereas minor salivary gland tumors are treated by more conservative surgical excision. A pleomorphic adenoma grows by extension of projections of tumor into the surrounding tissue. Therefore, some tumors are difficult to remove completely. Recurrence rates vary and are related to the adequacy of the initial surgical removal. Pleomorphic adenomas have been known to undergo malignant transformation; this occurrence is known as a **carcinoma arising in a pleomorphic adenoma.**

MONOMORPHIC ADENOMAS

Monomorphic adenomas are benign encapsulated salivary gland tumors that occur less frequently than the pleomorphic adenoma. They are composed of a uniform pattern of epithelial cells (Figure 7-13). These tumors do not have the connective tissue–like component seen in a pleomorphic adenoma. Several specific types of monomorphic adenoma have been identified on the basis of their microscopic patterns. Trabecular adenoma and canalicular adenoma are monomorphic-type adenomas that are named for the microscopic pattern of the tumor. These tumors occur most commonly in adult women, with a predilection for the upper lip and buccal mucosa. A **papillary cystadenoma lymphomatosum** is another type of monomorphic adenoma. It is also called a *Warthin tumor*. Microscopic examination of this particular variant demonstrates an encapsulated tumor composed of two types of tissue: epithelial and lymphoid (Figure 7-14). The epithelial component is neoplastic. It lines papillary projections that protrude from cystic structures. Sheets of lymphocytes surround the cystic structures. In some cases the lymphoid component demonstrates germinal center formation. A Warthin tumor presents as a painless, soft, and compressible or fluctuant mass, usually located in the parotid gland. This tumor often

develops bilaterally and occurs predominantly in adult men. Intraoral examples are very rare.

All monomorphic adenomas are treated by surgical excision. Recurrence is rare.

MUCOEPIDERMOID CARCINOMA

Mucoepidermoid carcinoma is a malignant salivary gland tumor. It is an unencapsulated, infiltrating tumor composed of a combination of mucous cells interspersed with squamous-like epithelial cells called **epidermoid cells** (Figure 7-15). Most studies show the mucoepidermoid carcinoma to be the most commonly occurring malignant salivary gland tumor of intraoral minor salivary gland origin.

Mucoepidermoid carcinomas involving the major glands occur most often in the parotid gland, whereas minor gland tumors are most common on the palate. They appear clinically as slowly enlarging masses (see Figure 7-11, *D*). On occasion, a mucoepidermoid carcinoma may arise **centrally** within bone (Figure 7-15, *B*), usually in the mandibular premolar and molar region. In this location it appears as either a unilocular or multilocular radiolucency (Figure 7-15, *B*). A central mucoepidermoid carcinoma is derived from either salivary gland tissue trapped within bone or the transformed epithelial lining of a dentigerous cyst (a developmental odontogenic cyst that forms around the crown of an unerupted or impacted tooth; see Chapter 5).

A mucoepidermoid carcinoma may occur over a wide age range. Although it usually occurs in adults after middle age, this tumor is the most common malignant salivary gland tumor in children. A female predilection is noted.

Treatment of a mucoepidermoid carcinoma consists of complete surgical excision, with close, long-term follow-up for signs of recurrence and metastasis. The behavior of any one tumor is difficult to predict and is related to the microscopic appearance of the tumor. Low-grade tumors have a

FIGURE 7-14 ■ Microscopic appearance of a portion of a papillary cystadenoma lymphomatosum (Warthin tumor) shows spaces lined by epithelium and surrounded by sheets of lymphocytes.

A

B

FIGURE 7-15 ■ **A,** Microscopic appearance (low power) of a mucoepidermoid carcinoma shows cystic structures, mucous cells, and epidermoid cells. **B,** Radiograph of a central mucoepidermoid carcinoma shows a multilocular radiolucency.

Ameloblastomas are treated by complete surgical removal. Recurrence is common. On occasion, these tumors occur in the gingiva and do not involve bone, in which case they are called **peripheral ameloblastomas.** These are also treated by surgical excision and differ from the central ameloblastomas in that they generally do not recur.

CALCIFYING EPITHELIAL ODONTOGENIC TUMOR

The **calcifying epithelial odontogenic tumor,** also known as a *Pindborg tumor,* is a benign epithelial odontogenic tumor that occurs much less frequently than the ameloblastoma. It is a unique odontogenic tumor because the proliferating cells do not resemble odontogenic epithelium. The tumor is composed of islands and sheets of polyhedral (multisided) epithelial cells. Deposits similar to amyloid are

FIGURE 7-19 ■ Radiograph of an ameloblastoma that formed in association with an impacted tooth and dentigerous cyst.

seen in the tumor, and calcifications are seen within these deposits. The amyloid-like material is thought to represent a form of abnormal enamel protein (Figure 7-20, *A*). Radiographically, a calcifying epithelial odontogenic tumor appears as a unilocular or multilocular radiolucency (Figure 7-20, *B*). Calcifications that form within the tumor appear as radiopacities within the radiolucency.

The majority of patients affected with this tumor are adults. However, the calcifying epithelial odontogenic tumor affects a broad age range that extends from young adults to elderly individuals. No sex predilection is noted. Reports of this tumor occurring in the mandible are twice as common as reports of it occurring in the maxilla. Although it can occur anywhere in the maxilla or mandible, the bicuspid and molar areas are the most common locations.

Treatment of a calcifying epithelial odontogenic tumor depends on the size and location of the tumor and involves complete surgical excision. Recurrence has been reported, but the recurrence rate is lower than that for an ameloblastoma.

ADENOMATOID ODONTOGENIC TUMOR

The **adenomatoid odontogenic tumor** (AOT), also known as the **odontogenic adenomatoid tumor** (OAT), is an encapsulated, benign epithelial odontogenic tumor that has a distinctive age, sex, and site distribution. It also differs from other epithelial odontogenic tumors in that it does not recur. Approximately 70% of AOTs occur in females less than 20 years of age, and 70% involve the anterior part of the jaws. The maxilla is more commonly involved than the mandible. Many AOTs are associated with impacted teeth. Although a localized swelling may be present, most are asymptomatic and are discovered on routine radiographic examination.

FIGURE 7-20 ■ Calcifying epithelial odontogenic tumor. **A,** Microscopic appearance (low power) of a calcifying epithelial odontogenic tumor shows sheets of epithelial cells *(E),* amorphous material *(A),* and calcifications *(C).* **B,** Radiograph of a calcifying epithelial odontogenic tumor shows a multilocular radiolucency.

Radiographically, an AOT appears as a well-circumscribed radiolucency (Figure 7-21, *B*). Because of the frequent association with an impacted tooth, an adenomatoid odontogenic tumor often simulates a dentigerous cyst. However, unlike the dentigerous cyst, the adenomatoid odontogenic tumor extends beyond the cementoenamel junction and can involve 50% to 60% of the root. As calcifications form within the tumor, radiopaque areas of varying size are visible on radiographs. Microscopic examination reveals a dense, fibrous connective tissue capsule surrounding ductlike structures, whorls, and large masses of cuboidal and spindle-shaped epithelial cells (Figure 7-21, *A*). The ductlike structures are one of the distinctive features of this tumor and are the reason for the name **adenomatoid**, or glandlike.

These structures are not ducts but actually ameloblast-like cells that resemble ducts because of their circular arrangement. Eosinophilic material is seen in the centers of these structures, and calcifications also form in this tumor.

The clinician should treat an adenomatoid odontogenic tumor conservatively by enucleation. The tumor is removed in its entirety because it is easily separated from the surrounding bone. Recurrence is rare.

CALCIFYING ODONTOGENIC CYST

The **calcifying odontogenic cyst** is a nonaggressive cystic lesion that affects a broad age range but is most commonly seen in individuals younger than 40 years of age. No sex predilection has been noted. A solid variant of the calcifying odontogenic cyst has been reported and has been suggested to represent a neoplasm rather than a cyst.

Microscopic examination reveals a cystic structure lined by odontogenic epithelium with an associated and characteristic ghost cell keratinization (Figure 7-22, *A*). The epithelium resembles that seen in an ameloblastoma, consisting of ameloblast-like cells and stellate reticulum–like areas. The ghost cells that are characteristic of this lesion exhibit

FIGURE 7-21 ■ Adenomatoid odontogenic tumor. **A,** Microscopic appearance of a portion of an adenomatoid odontogenic tumor shows the capsule *(C)*, epithelial cells, and ductlike structures *(D)*. **B,** Radiograph of an adenomatoid odontogenic tumor shows a unilocular radiolucency surrounding the crown of an unerupted maxillary cuspid. (Note that the radiolucency extends beyond the cemento-enamel junction.)

FIGURE 7-22 ■ Calcifying odontogenic cyst. **A,** Microscopic appearance of a calcifying odontogenic cyst shows a cystic structure lined by odontogenic epithelium *(E)* with associated ghost cells *(G)*. **B,** Radiograph of a calcifying odontogenic cyst shows a unilocular radiolucency of the mandible.

Treatment of the benign cementoblastoma consists of enucleation of the tumor and removal of the involved tooth. It does not recur.

MIXED ODONTOGENIC TUMORS

AMELOBLASTIC FIBROMA

The **ameloblastic fibroma** is a benign, mixed odontogenic tumor that consists of both epithelium and mesenchymal tissue. It occurs in young children and adults. Most cases occur in individuals younger than 20 years of age. A male sex predilection is noted. The most common location is the mandibular bicuspid and molar region. Most patients are asymptomatic, but bone expansion or swelling may be noted. Radiographically, the ameloblastic fibroma appears as either a well-defined or poorly defined unilocular or multilocular radiolucency (Figure 7-26, *B*).

Histologic examination demonstrates a nonencapsulated odontogenic tumor composed of strands and small islands of ameloblast-like epithelial cells and tissue that resembles the dental papilla (Figure 7-26, *A*).

An ameloblastic fibroma is treated by surgical excision, and recurrence rate is low.

ODONTOMA

The **odontoma** is an odontogenic tumor composed of mature enamel, dentin, cementum, and pulp tissue. The odontoma is the most common of the odontogenic tumors. Two types of odontomas are recognized: compound and complex. A **compound odontoma** consists of a collection of numerous small teeth. Although compound odontomas may consist of many small teeth, they do not exhibit unlimited growth potential and therefore are more accurately described as developmental lesions rather than true tumors. A **complex odontoma** consists of a mass of enamel, dentin, cementum, and pulp that does not resemble a normal tooth.

Most odontomas are detected in adolescents and young adults. No sex predilection is noted. The compound odontoma is usually located in the anterior maxilla, and the complex odontoma most commonly occurs in the posterior mandible. The most common clinical manifestation of an odontoma is the failure of a permanent tooth to erupt. Most odontomas are small, but large lesions can cause swelling, displacement of teeth, and prevention of eruption of a permanent tooth. Odontomas can be associated with impacted or unerupted teeth, and with odontogenic cysts and tumors.

Radiographically, compound odontomas appear as a cluster of numerous miniature teeth surrounded by a radiolucent halo (Figure 7-27). A complex odontoma appears as a radiopaque mass surrounded by a thin radiolucent halo (Figure 7-28).

Treatment of an odontoma consists of surgical excision. They generally do not recur.

FIGURE 7-26 ■ **A,** Microscopic appearance of an ameloblastic fibroma shows a combination of odontogenic epithelium (*E*) and mesenchymal tissue (*M*). **B,** Radiograph of an ameloblastic fibroma shows a poorly defined unilocular radiolucency.

FIGURE 7-27 ■ Radiograph of a compound odontoma shows a collection of numerous, small, toothlike radiopacities surrounded by a radiolucent halo.

AMELOBLASTIC FIBRO-ODONTOMA

The **ameloblastic fibro-odontoma** is a benign odontogenic tumor that has features of both an ameloblastic fibroma and an odontoma. Most cases occur in young adults, with an average age of 10 years. No sex predilection is noted. The ameloblastic fibro-odontoma typically arises in the posterior jaws and is often asymptomatic. However, some patients may experience swelling of the affected area.

Radiographic examination reveals a well-delineated radiolucent lesion that may be unilocular or multilocular. Calcifications of various size and shape are noted within the radiolucency. These calcifications represent tooth formation.

Microscopic examination demonstrates features similar to those described for the ameloblastic fibroma combined with structures that resemble teeth. Therefore various amounts of enamel, dentin, cementum, and pulp tissue are produced.

FIGURE 7-28 ■ Radiograph of a complex odontoma shows a radiopaque mass surrounded by a radiolucent halo.

The ameloblastic fibro-odontoma is a well-circumscribed lesion that usually separates easily from the surrounding bone. It is treated by conservative surgical excision, and recurrence is unusual.

PERIPHERAL ODONTOGENIC TUMORS

PERIPHERAL OSSIFYING FIBROMA

The peripheral ossifying fibroma is usually a well-demarcated sessile or pedunculated lesion that appears to originate from the gingival interdental papilla and is most likely derived from cells of the periodontal ligament (Figure 7-29, A). It is more common in females than in males and often occurs in young individuals. It has been reported in both children and adults.

It is composed of cellular fibrous connective tissue interspersed with scattered bone and cementum-like calcifications (Figure 7-29, B). Microscopically, the peripheral ossifying fibroma is similar to the central cementifying fibroma and central ossifying fibroma.

Treatment of a peripheral ossifying fibroma consists of surgical excision with thorough scaling of the adjacent teeth to remove any irritants that can induce regrowth of the lesion. The recurrence rate for the peripheral ossifying fibroma is about 16%.

OTHER PERIPHERAL ODONTOGENIC TUMORS

Several other odontogenic tumors have been reported to occur in the gingiva without underlying bone involvement. Although rare, these lesions are important to the dental hygienist because of their gingival location. The peripheral odontogenic fibroma is much rarer than the peripheral ossifying fibroma. It is composed of a combination of fibrous tissue and islands or strands of odontogenic epithelium, and calcifications may also be present. The peripheral ameloblastoma (described earlier in this chapter) and the peripheral calcifying epithelial odontogenic tumor have been reported to occur in this location.

FIGURE 7-29 ■ **A,** Clinical appearance of a peripheral ossifying fibroma shows an exophytic lesion involving the palatal gingiva of the maxillary anterior teeth. **B,** Photomicrograph of a peripheral ossifying fibroma shows bonelike calcifications (B) in cellular fibrous connective tissue (CT). A small amount of surface epithelium (E) is also visible.

FIGURE 7-30 ■ **A,** Clinical appearance of a lipoma. **B,** Photomicrograph of a lipoma shows mature fat cells. (**A,** Courtesy Dr. Edward V. Zegarelli.)

Treatment for the tumors described previously is surgical excision. After appropriate treatment recurrence is rare.

TUMORS OF SOFT TISSUE

Tumors of soft tissue include benign and malignant tumors of adipose (fat) tissue, nerve, muscle, blood, and lymphatic vessels.

LIPOMA

The lipoma is a benign tumor of mature fat cells (adipose tissue). Clinically, it appears as a yellowish mass that is surfaced by a thin layer of epithelium (Figure 7-30, *A*). Because of this thin epithelium, a delicate pattern of blood vessels is usually seen on its surface. The majority of lipomas occur in individuals over 40 years of age, and no sex predilection is noted. The most common intraoral locations are the buccal mucosa and the vestibule. Microscopic examination reveals a well-delineated tumor composed of lobules of mature fat cells that are uniform in size and shape (Figure 7-30, *B*).

The lipoma is treated by surgical excision and generally does not recur.

TUMORS OF NERVE TISSUE

NEUROFIBROMA AND SCHWANNOMA

The **neurofibroma** (Figure 7-31, *A*) and the **schwannoma** are benign tumors derived from nerve tissue. The schwannoma is also called a *neurilemmoma.* The schwannoma is derived from Schwann cells, and the neurofibroma is derived from Schwann cells and perineural fibroblasts. Both of these cells are components of the connective tissue surrounding a nerve. Although the neurofibroma and schwannoma are distinct tumors microscopically, they are quite similar in their clinical presentation and behavior and, therefore, are discussed together. The tongue is the most common intraoral location. On occasion, macroglossia (tongue enlargement) may occur as a result of growth of these tumors in this location. Schwannomas have been reported to occasionally cause a complaint of pain. Neurofibromas and

FIGURE 7-31 ■ **A,** Clinical appearance of a neurofibroma shows a nonulcerated mass on the lateral border of the tongue. **B,** Photomicrograph of a neurofibroma.

schwannomas may occur at any age, and no sex predilection is noted. Microscopic examination of a neurofibroma reveals a fairly well-delineated but unencapsulated proliferation of spindle-shaped Schwann cells and perineural fibroblasts (Figure 7-31, *B*). A schwannoma is composed of spindle-shaped Schwann cells arranged in palisaded whorls around a central pink zone. A connective tissue capsule surrounds the schwannoma.

A neurofibroma and a schwannoma are both treated by surgical excision. They generally do not recur. Malignant tumors of nerve tissue occur but are extremely rare.

Multiple neurofibromas occur in a genetically inherited disorder known as **neurofibromatosis of von Recklinghausen** or *von Recklinghausen disease*. Patients with this syndrome have numerous neurofibromas on the skin and other sites, including the mandible, in addition to other abnormalities. This syndrome is genetically inherited and is described in detail in Chapter 6.

GRANULAR CELL TUMOR

The **granular cell tumor** is a benign tumor composed of large cells with a granular cytoplasm. This tumor most likely arises from a neural or primitive mesenchymal cell. The granular cell tumor most often occurs on the tongue, followed by the buccal mucosa. It appears as a painless, nonulcerated nodule (Figure 7-32, *A*). Most cases occur in adults, and a female sex predilection is noted. Microscopic examination reveals large oval-shaped cells with a granular cytoplasm. The granular cells are found in the connective tissue and between striated muscle fibers (Figure 7-32, *B*). The overlying surface epithelium

may exhibit pseudoepitheliomatous hyperplasia, which is a benign proliferation of epithelium into the connective tissue (Figure 7-32, *C*).

This tumor is treated by surgical excision and does not recur.

CONGENITAL EPULIS

The **congenital epulis,** or congenital epulis of the newborn, is a benign neoplasm composed of cells that closely resemble those seen in the granular cell tumor. The neoplasm most likely arises from a primitive mesenchymal cell. This tumor is present at birth and appears as a sessile or pedunculated mass on the gingiva. It usually occurs on the anterior maxillary gingiva and almost always occurs in girls.

The congenital epulis is treated by surgical excision and does not recur. Occasional examples have regressed without treatment.

TUMORS OF MUSCLE

Tumors of muscle are extremely uncommon in the oral cavity. The **rhabdomyoma,** a benign tumor of striated muscle, has been reported to occur on the tongue. The **leiomyoma,** a benign tumor of smooth muscle, may occur in

FIGURE 7-32 ▪ A, Clinical appearance of a granular cell tumor of the tongue shows a nonulcerated mass. **B,** Photomicrograph of a granular cell tumor showing granular cell(s) *(G)* between striated muscle fiber(s) *(M)*. **C,** Photomicrograph of a granular cell tumor, showing overlying pseudoepitheliomatous hyperplasia. **(A,** Courtesy Dr. Sidney Eisig.)

association with blood vessels. These tumors are called **vascular leiomyomas** and occasionally occur in the oral cavity.

The **rhabdomyosarcoma**, a malignant tumor of striated muscle, is the most common malignant soft tissue tumor of the head and neck in children. It typically occurs in individuals under 10 years of age and has a male sex predilection. It is a rapidly growing, destructive tumor. The rhabdomyosarcoma is an aggressive malignant tumor that is best treated by a combination of multidrug chemotherapy, radiation therapy, and surgery. Despite treatment, the prognosis is poor.

VASCULAR TUMORS

HEMANGIOMA

The **hemangioma** is a benign proliferation of capillaries (Figure 7-33, A and B). It is a common vascular lesion considered by many to represent a developmental lesion rather than a tumor because hemangiomas generally do not exhibit unlimited growth potential. Some contain numerous small capillaries and are called **capillary hemangiomas**. Others contain larger blood vessels and are called **cavernous hemangiomas** (Figure 7-33, C).

Most are present at birth or arise shortly thereafter. More than half of the hemangiomas that occur in the body occur in the head and neck area. The tongue is the most common intraoral location. Involvement of the tongue often leads to marked enlargement. Hemangiomas are more common in girls than in boys. They also occur in adults as a response to trauma and represent an abnormal proliferation of blood vessels during the healing process. They appear as variably sized, deep-red or blue lesions that frequently blanch when pressure is applied.

Many hemangiomas undergo spontaneous remission. Others can enlarge rapidly because of hemorrhage, thrombosis, or inflammation. Treatment is variable and includes surgery or the injection of a sclerosing solution into the lesion. Injection of a sclerosing solution into the lesion will cause it to shrink in size or resolve.

LYMPHANGIOMA

The **lymphangioma** is a benign tumor of lymphatic vessels. It is less common than the hemangioma. Most lymphangiomas are congenital (present at birth), and half arise in the head and neck area. No sex predilection is noted. The most common intraoral location is the tongue, where a lymphangioma presents as an ill-defined mass with a pebbly surface. Involvement of the tongue may lead to macroglossia. A cystic lymphangioma in the neck is called a *cystic hygroma*. It is usually present at birth or develops shortly thereafter.

Lymphangiomas are generally treated by surgical excision and tend to recur.

MALIGNANT VASCULAR TUMORS

Malignant vascular tumors such as *angiosarcoma* may occur in the oral cavity but are rare. **Kaposi sarcoma** is a

FIGURE 7-33 ■ Clinical appearance of a hemangioma of the lower lip **(A)** and of the buccal mucosa **(B). C,** Microscopic appearance of a cavernous hemangioma showing large dilated blood vessels (*B*) filled with red blood cells (*RBC*).

malignant vascular tumor and may arise in multiple sites, including the skin and oral mucosa. Classic Kaposi sarcoma occurs as multiple purplish tumors of the lower extremities in older men. The neoplasm progresses slowly, usually resolves with low doses of radiation, and rarely causes death.

With the advent of the human immunodeficiency virus (HIV) epidemic in the 1980s, Kaposi sarcoma appeared in a much more aggressive form. In HIV-positive patients these lesions are often seen in the oral cavity, where they present as purple macules, plaques, or exophytic tumors. The hard palate and gingiva are the most common intraoral sites. Kaposi sarcoma associated with HIV infection is described in Chapter 4 (see Figure 4-37). It may also occur in patients with other forms of immunodeficiency, specifically patients who have received immunosuppressive drug therapy as a result of organ transplantation.

Kaposi sarcoma is caused by a human herpesvirus (HHV) that is called both *human herpesvirus type 8* and *Kaposi sarcoma–associated herpesvirus.* Men are affected more often than women. Microscopic examination reveals a neoplasm composed of spindle-shaped cells mixed with slitlike spaces containing red blood cells.

Kaposi sarcoma is treated by surgical excision, radiation therapy, chemotherapy, or a combination of these therapies. In HIV-positive patients recurrence is common, and the disease may progress rapidly.

TUMORS OF MELANIN-PRODUCING CELLS

MELANOCYTIC NEVI

The word **nevus** (plural, *nevi*) has two meanings. Here the word is used to mean a benign tumor of melanocytes (melanin-producing cells), which are called **nevus cells.** Nevus also refers to a pigmented congenital lesion (a lesion present at birth). A hemangioma present at birth is an example of this second type of nevus.

Melanocytic nevi can arise on the skin or the oral mucosa. Intraoral tumors consist of tan-to-brown macules or papules that occur most often on the hard palate. The buccal mucosa is the second most common intraoral location (Figure 7-34). They occur twice as often in women as in men and are usually first identified in individuals between 20 and 50 years of age. Most pigmented lesions that occur in the oral cavity are benign. Pigmented lesions that exhibit ulceration, an increase in size, or a change in shape or color may be malignant.

The ABCDEs (*Asymmetry, Border, Color, Diameter, Evolving*) of malignant melanoma should be considered when assessing pigmented lesions of skin. Lesions that show these characteristics should be further evaluated to rule out melanoma. These include lesions that are **A**symmetric (that is, one half is different from the other), lesions that have irregular **B**orders, lesions in which the **C**olor varies from tan to black and possibly red or blue, lesions that have **D**iameters greater than 6 mm, and lesions that are **E**volving, (that is, changing in size, shape, or color).

A biopsy followed by microscopic examination is indicated for pigmented lesions of unknown cause, unknown duration, or recent onset. Surgical excision is the treatment of choice for intraoral melanocytic nevi. Recurrence is rare.

MALIGNANT MELANOMA

Malignant melanoma is a malignant tumor of melanocytes (Figure 7-35). Although the name malignant melanoma suggests that a benign counterpart exists, all melanomas are malignant. Most malignant melanomas arise on the skin as a result of prolonged exposure to sunlight. Primary malignant melanoma of the oral cavity is rare. However, malignant melanomas that arise on the skin may metastasize to the oral cavity.

Malignant melanoma usually presents as a rapidly enlarging blue-to-black mass. Malignant melanoma is a very aggressive tumor that exhibits unpredictable behavior and early metastasis. The most common intraoral locations

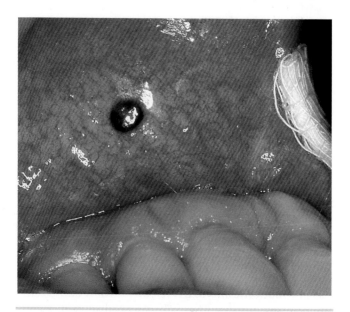

FIGURE 7-34 ■ Clinical appearance of a melanocytic nevus shows a well-defined pigmented lesion on the labial mucosa.

FIGURE 7-35 ■ Clinical appearance of a malignant neoplasma shows a darkly pigmented lesion in the area of the fauces. (Courtesy Dr. Edward V. Zegarelli.)

FIGURE 7-36 ■ **A,** Clinical appearance of bilateral lobulated mandibular tori. **B,** Clinical appearance of a lobulated torus palatinus.

are the palate and maxillary gingiva. These neoplasms usually occur in adults older than 40 years of age.

Malignant melanomas are treated by surgical excision. Chemotherapy may be used in conjunction with surgery. The prognosis for oral malignant melanoma is poor.

TUMORS OF BONE AND CARTILAGE

TORUS

A **torus** (plural, *tori*) is a benign lesion composed of normal compact bone. Tori are located in the midline of the palate (**torus palatinus** or **palatal torus**) or the lingual aspect of the mandible in the area of the premolars (**torus mandibularis** or **mandibular torus**) (Figure 7-36, *A* and *B*). Tori are not true tumors. They are described in this chapter because of their resemblance to an osteoma, a benign tumor of bone. Tori occur in adults and are more common in women than in men. They present as an asymptomatic, bony hard, lobulated mass covered by epithelium with very little underlying fibrous connective tissue. Surface ulceration may occur if a torus is traumatized. Palatal or mandibular tori may result in radiopaque areas superimposed on tooth roots. The diagnosis is confirmed by the presence of a torus on clinical examination.

No treatment is necessary unless they interfere with the fabrication of a prosthetic appliance. If a prosthetic appliance needs to be constructed, a torus should be excised surgically.

EXOSTOSIS

An **exostosis** (plural, *exostoses*) is a small nodular excrescence of normal compact bone (Figure 7-37). Exostoses present as asymptomatic, bony hard nodules on the buccal

FIGURE 7-37 ■ Clinical appearance of exostoses on the labial and buccal aspect of the maxilla. Less prominent exostoses are noted on the labial and buccal aspect of the mandible.

aspect of the maxillary or mandibular alveolar ridges. Most cases occur in adults, and no sex predilection is noted. An increased incidence is noted in individuals who have a grinding or bruxing habit.

No treatment is indicated unless they interfere with the fabrication of a prosthetic appliance. If a prosthetic appliance needs to be constructed, an exostosis should be excised surgically. Tori are examples of exostoses that occur in specific locations.

OSTEOMA

An osteoma is an asymptomatic benign tumor composed of normal compact bone. It is a slow-growing tumor that appears radiographically as either a sharply defined radiopaque mass within bone (endosteal) or a delineated mass attached to the outer surface of the bone (periosteal) (Figure 7-38). A large osteoma within bone may cause expansion of the involved bone. No sex predilection is noted. The most common location within the jaws is the posterior mandible.

FIGURE 7-38 ■ Radiograph of an osteoma shows a radiopacity of the posterior mandible. (Courtesy Dr. Sidney Eisig.)

Osteomas are a component of Gardner syndrome, which is transmitted genetically and described in Chapter 6.

Osteomas are treated by surgical excision and generally do not recur.

OSTEOSARCOMA

Osteosarcoma (osteogenic sarcoma) is a malignant tumor of bone-forming tissue. It is the most common primary malignant tumor of bone in patients under 40 years of age. Tumors that involve the long bones occur at an average age of 27 years, whereas the average age of occurrence for tumors that involve the jaws is about 37 years of age. These tumors occur in the mandible twice as frequently as in the maxilla and are more common in men than in women. Patients may experience a diffuse swelling or mass that is often painful (Figure 7-39, *A*). Some patients present

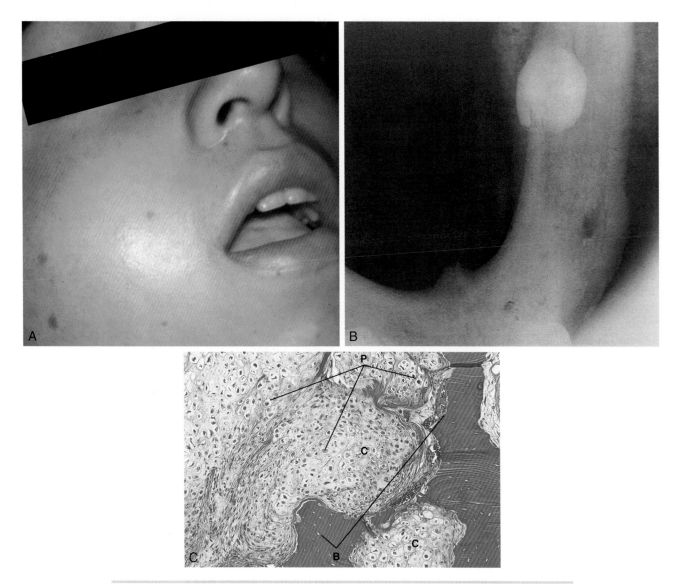

FIGURE 7-39 ■ **A,** Clinical appearance of an osteogenic sarcoma shows swelling. **B,** Radiograph of an osteogenic sarcoma in the left molar area shows a poorly defined radiopaque lesion. **C,** Microscopic appearance of an osteogenic sarcoma shows pleomorphic *(P)* and hyperchromatic cells, abnormal cartilage *(C)*, and bone formation *(B)*.

FIGURE 7-40 ■ Clinical appearance of a chondrosarcoma shows an exophytic mass in the anterior mandible.

FIGURE 7-41 ■ Clinical appearance of a patient with leukemic infiltration of the gingiva, resulting in diffuse enlargement. (Courtesy Dr. Edward V. Zegarelli.)

initially with a toothache or exhibit tooth mobility. Paresthesia of the lip is common in tumors involving the mandible.

The radiographic appearance of an osteosarcoma varies from radiolucent to radiopaque (Figure 7-39, *B*). It is usually a destructive, poorly defined lesion and may or may not involve the adjacent soft tissue. Asymmetric widening of the periodontal ligament space and a sunburst pattern may be seen radiographically in some cases. Microscopic examination of this tumor shows pleomorphic and hyperchromatic cells and abnormal bone formation. Abnormal cartilage formation may also be present (Figure 7-39, *C*).

At present, osteosarcomas are treated with preoperative multiagent chemotherapy followed by surgery. Jaw tumors frequently recur after treatment. Only about 20% of patients with osteosarcoma of the jaws survive 5 years.

TUMORS OF CARTILAGE

Cartilaginous tumors of the jawbones are extremely rare and are more likely to be malignant than benign. A **chondroma** is a benign tumor of cartilage. A **chondrosarcoma** is a malignant tumor of cartilage (Figure 7-40). A chondrosarcoma may occur in either the maxilla or the mandible and is more common in men than in women. Most patients have enlargement of the affected bone.

Chondrosarcomas are treated by wide surgical excision. Radiation therapy and chemotherapy are not effective. The prognosis is poor. Only about 30% of patients with chondrosarcoma involving the jaws survive 5 years after the diagnosis.

TUMORS OF BLOOD-FORMING TISSUES
LEUKEMIA

Leukemia comprises a broad group of disorders characterized by an overproduction of atypical white blood cells. The atypical white blood cells proliferate in the bone marrow and then spill into the circulating blood and tissues. Several types of leukemia are classified according to the kind of cells that are proliferating: myelocytes, lymphocytes, or monocytes.

Leukemias are divided into two forms: acute and chronic. Acute leukemia is most common in children and young adults and is characterized by a proliferation of immature white blood cells (blasts). Chronic leukemia is characterized by an excess proliferation of mature white blood cells and most frequently occurs in middle-aged adults. Leukemia occurs more often in men than in women.

Although oral involvement may occur in any type of leukemia, the monocytic variant most often exhibits oral lesions. A common oral manifestation of monocytic leukemia is diffuse gingival enlargement with persistent bleeding (Figure 7-41). (Leukemia is further described in Chapter 9.)

The treatment of leukemia consists of chemotherapy, radiation therapy, and corticosteroids. The prognosis depends on the type of leukemia and the extent of disease.

LYMPHOMA (NON-HODGKIN LYMPHOMA)

Lymphoma is a malignant tumor of lymphoid tissue. Numerous types of lymphoma exist, each of which is differentiated on the basis of microscopic findings with immunohistochemical and genetic testing to identify the specific types of malignant lymphocytes. The characteristic clinical presentation is gradual enlargement of the involved lymph nodes. Rarely, a lymphoma may present as a primary lesion in the oral soft tissues or bone. However, most lymphomas involve either lymph nodes or aggregates of lymphoid tissue that are located in the digestive tract from the oral cavity to the anus. In the oral cavity lymphoid tissue is located at the base of the tongue, soft palate, and pharynx (Waldeyer ring). The most common location for intraoral lymphoma is the tonsillar area. Lymphomas usually occur in adults and are more common in men than in women.

Lymphoma is treated by radiotherapy, surgery, chemotherapy, or a combination of these therapies. The prognosis depends on the type of lymphoma and the extent of involvement.

MULTIPLE MYELOMA

Multiple myeloma is a systemic, malignant proliferation of plasma cells that causes destructive lesions in bone. The neoplastic plasma cells produce large amounts of

FIGURE 7-42 ▪ Multiple myeloma. **A,** Microscopic appearance of multiple myeloma shows a proliferation of plasma cells. **B,** Radiograph shows multiple radiolucent lesions of the mandible in a patient with multiple myeloma.

immunoglobulin. Most patients are older than 40 years of age, and the disease occurs most commonly in the seventh decade of life. Men are affected more often than women. Patients usually experience bone pain and swelling. Pathologic fracture of an involved bone is common and typically occurs in bones weakened as a result of their destruction by the proliferation of neoplastic plasma cells (Figure 7-42, *A*).

Radiographically, the involved bones show multiple radiolucent lesions. The disease can involve the skull, spine, ribs, pelvis, long bones, and jaws. The mandible is affected more often than the maxilla (Figure 7-42, *B*). Most patients have an elevation of a single type of immunoglobulin, which is detected by a process called immunoelectrophoresis. This elevation is called a **monoclonal spike.** Patients may have fragments of immunoglobulins in the urine. These fragments are called **Bence Jones proteins.**

The tumors are composed of sheets of well to poorly differentiated plasma cells.

A localized tumor of plasma cells in soft tissue is called an **extramedullary plasmacytoma.** Although these are rare tumors, they are more common in the head and neck region than anywhere else in the body. Many patients with extramedullary plasmacytoma will eventually develop multiple myeloma. Therefore, patients with a single tumor of plasma cells must be evaluated to determine whether the lesion is solitary or part of multiple myeloma.

Patients with multiple myeloma are treated with chemotherapy, radiation therapy, and autologous stem cell transplantation. New treatment modalities have dramatically improved the prognosis for patients with multiple myeloma. Systemic bisphosphonate medication is used to prevent bone destruction in patients with multiple myeloma. Oral complications related to this treatment are discussed in Chapter 9.

METASTATIC TUMORS OF THE JAWS

Metastatic tumors of the jaws from primary sites elsewhere in the body are rare. Most of these tumors arise from the thyroid, breast, lungs, prostate gland, and kidneys. The most frequent intraoral site for metastatic tumors of the jaws is the mandible. Patients display various signs and symptoms, including pain, paresthesia or anesthesia of the lip, swelling, expansion of the affected bone, and loosening of the teeth in the involved area. Metastatic lesions usually appear several years after the primary lesion is discovered. On occasion, the oral metastatic tumor is the first manifestation of a **primary tumor** elsewhere. Most patients are adults, and men are affected more often than women.

The radiographic appearance of metastatic tumors varies (Figure 7-43). Lesions are usually poorly defined and radiolucent. The roots of the involved teeth may show a spiked

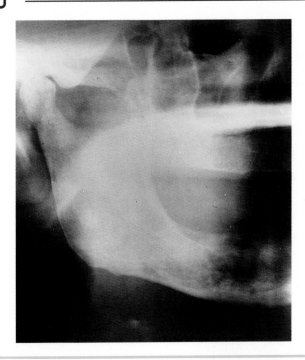

FIGURE 7-43 ■ Radiograph shows diffuse radiolucent and radiopaque changes resulting from metastatic carcinoma of the prostate gland.

appearance. Metastatic tumors from the breast, prostate gland, and lungs may form bone and, therefore, may show areas of radiopacity.

Microscopically, a metastatic tumor resembles the primary malignancy. Most metastatic tumors in the jaws are epithelial in origin, and most are adenocarcinomas.

Chemotherapy and radiation therapy are used to alleviate the discomfort of metastatic tumors in the jaws. The prognosis for patients with tumors that have metastasized to the jaws is poor. Systemic bisphosphonate medication is used to prevent bone destruction in patients with tumors such as breast and prostate cancer that metastasize to bone. Oral complications related to this treatment are discussed in Chapter 9.

SELECTED REFERENCES

Books

Kumar V, Cotran RS, Robbins SL: *Robbins basic pathology*, ed 8, St. Louis, 2013, Saunders.

Neville BW, Damm DD, Allen CM, et al: *Oral and maxillofacial pathology*, ed 3, St. Louis, 2009, Saunders.

Regezi JA, Sciubba JJ, Jordan RCK: *Oral pathology: clinical-pathologic correlations*, ed 6, St. Louis, 2012, Saunders.

Journal Articles
Tumors of Squamous Epithelium

Abbey LM, Page DG, Sawyer DR: The clinical and histopathologic features of a series of 464 oral squamous cell papillomas, *Oral Surg Oral Med Oral Pathol* 49:419, 1980.

Cleveland JL, Junger ML, Saraiya M, et al: The connection between human papillomavirus and oropharyngeal squamous cell carcinomas in the United States: implications for dentistry, *J Am Dent Assoc* 142:915, 2011.

Fantasia JE, Damm DD: Oral diagnosis: exophytic lesion of palatal mucosa: papilloma, *Gen Dent* 181:183, 2004.

Freitas MD, Blanco-Carrión A, Gándara-Vila P, et al: Clinicopathologic aspects of oral leukoplakia in smokers and nonsmokers, *Oral Surg Oral Med Oral Pathol Oral Radiol Endod* 102:199, 2006.

Gillison ML, Broutian T, Pickard RK, et al: Prevalence of oral HPV infection in the United States, 2009-2010, *JAMA* 307:693, 2012.

Kaugars GE, Pillion T, Svirsky JA, et al: Actinic cheilitis: a review of 152 cases, *Oral Surg Oral Med Oral Pathol Oral Radiol Endod* 88:181, 1999.

Krutchkoff DF, Chen JK, Eisenberg E, et al: Oral cancer: a survey of 566 cases from the University of Connecticut Oral Pathology Biopsy Service 1975-1986, *Oral Surg Oral Med Oral Pathol* 70:192, 1990.

Medina JE, Dichtel W, Luna MA: Verrucous-squamous carcinomas of the oral cavity: a clinicopathologic study of 104 cases, *Arch Otolaryngol* 110:437, 1984.

Warnakulasuriya KA, Ralhan R: Clinical, pathological, cellular and molecular lesions caused by oral smokeless tobacco—a review, *J Oral Pathol Med* 36:63, 2007.

Leukoplakia and Erythroplakia

Shafer WG, Waldron CA: Erythroplakia of the oral cavity, *Cancer* 36:1021, 1975.

Silverman S Jr, Gorsky M, Lozada F: Oral leukoplakia and malignant transformation: a follow-up study of 257 patients, *Cancer* 53:563, 1984.

Sugiyama M, Bhawal UK, Dohmen T, et al: Detection of human papillomavirus-16 and HPV-18 DNA in normal, dysplastic, and malignant oral epithelium, *Oral Surg Oral Med Oral Pathol Oral Radiol Endod* 95:594, 2003.

Waldron CA, Shafer WG: Leukoplakia revisited: a clinicopathologic study of 3256 oral leukoplakias, *Cancer* 36:1386, 1975.

Salivary Gland Tumors

Eveson JW, Cawson RA: Tumours of the minor (oropharyngeal) salivary glands: a demographic study of 336 cases, *J Oral Pathol* 14:500, 1985.

Pires FR, Pringle GA, de Almeida OP, et al: Intra-oral minor salivary gland tumors: a clinicopathological study of 546 cases, *Oral Oncol* 43:463, 2007.

Waldron CA, El-Mofty SK, Gnepp DR: Tumors of the intraoral minor salivary glands: a demographic and histologic study of 426 cases, *Oral Surg Oral Med Oral Pathol* 66:323, 1988.

Odontogenic Tumors

Ai-Ru L, Zhen L, Jian S: Calcifying epithelial odontogenic tumors: a clinicopathologic study of 9 cases, *J Oral Pathol* 11:399, 1982.

Buchner A, Ficarra G, Hansen LS: Peripheral odontogenic fibroma, *Oral Surg Oral Med Oral Pathol* 64:432, 1987.

Courtney RM, Kerr DA: The odontogenic adenomatoid tumor: a comprehensive study of 20 new cases, *Oral Surg Oral Med Oral Pathol* 39:424, 1975.

Kaugars GE, Miller ME, Abbey LM: Odontomas, *Oral Surg Oral Med Oral Pathol* 67:172, 1989.

Ritwik P, Brannon RB: Peripheral odontogenic fibroma: a clinicopathologic study of 151 cases and review of the literature with special emphasis on recurrence, *Oral Surg Oral Med Oral Pathol Oral Radiol Endod* 110:357, 2010.

Shamaskin RG, Svirsky JA, Kaugars GE: Intraosseous and extraosseous calcifying odontogenic cyst (Gorlin cyst), *J Oral Maxillofac Surg* 47:562, 1989.

Ulmansky M, Hjørting-Hansen E, Praetorius F, et al: Benign cementoblastoma, *Oral Surg Oral Med Oral Pathol* 77:48, 1994.

Waldron CA, El-Mofty SK: A histopathologic study of 116 ameloblastomas with special reference to the desmoplastic variant, *Oral Surg Oral Med Oral Pathol* 63:441, 1987.

Zomosa X, Müller S: Calcifying cystic odontogenic tumor, *Head Neck Pathol* 4:292, 2010.

Lipoma

Furlong MA, Fanburg-Smith JC, Childers ELB: Lipoma of the oral and maxillofacial region: site and subclassification of 125 cases, *Oral Surg Oral Med Oral Pathol* 98:441, 2004.

Neurogenic Tumors

Cunha KS, Barboza EP, Dias EP, et al: Neurofibromatosis type I with periodontal manifestations: a case report and literature review, *Br Dent J* 196:457, 2004.

Vascular Tumors

Greene AK: Current concepts of vascular anomalies, *J Craniofac Surg* 23:220, 2012.

Hernandez GA, Castro A, Castro G, et al: Aneurysmal bone cyst versus hemangioma of the mandible, *Oral Surg Oral Med Oral Pathol* 76:790, 1993.

Tumors of Melanin-producing Cells

Kaugars GE, Heise AP, Riley WT, et al: Oral melanotic macules, *Oral Surg Oral Med Oral Pathol* 76:59, 1993.

Kerr EH, Hameed O, Lewis JS Jr, et al: Head and neck mucosal malignant melanoma: clinicopathologic correlation with contemporary review of prognostic indicators, *Int J Surg Pathol* 20:37, 2012.

Web Site: http://www.melanoma.org/learn-more/melanoma-101/abcdes-melanoma

Tumors of Bone

Canadian Society of Otolaryngology—Head and Neck Surgery Oncology Study Group: Osteogenic sarcoma of the mandible and maxilla: a Canadian review (1980-2000), *J Otolaryngol* 33:139, 2004.

Ottaviani G, Jaffe N: The epidemiology of osteosarcoma, *Cancer Treat Res* 152:3, 2009.

Tumors of Blood-forming Tissues

Lambertenghi-Deliliers G, Bruno E, Cortelezzi A, et al: Incidence of jaw lesions in 193 patients with multiple myeloma, *Oral Surg Oral Med Oral Pathol* 65:533, 1988.

Mhaskar R, Redzepovic J, Wheatley K, et al: Bisphosphonates in multiple myeloma, *Cochrane Database Syst Rev* 3:CD003188, 2010. Update in: *Cochrane Database Syst Rev* 5:CD003188, 2012.

Raubenheimer EJ, Dauth J, van Wilpe E: Multiple myeloma: a study of 10 cases, *J Oral Pathol* 16:383, 1987.

Metastatic Tumors

Hashimoto N, Kurihara K, Yamasaki H, et al: Pathological characteristics of metastatic carcinoma in the human mandible, *J Oral Pathol* 16:362, 1987.

Khalili M, Mahboobi N, Shams J: Metastatic breast carcinoma initially diagnosed as pulpal/periapical disease: a case report, *J Endod* 36:922, 2010.

Review Questions

1. All of the following are associated with the neoplastic transformation of cells *except*:
   A. Chemicals
   B. Sunlight
   C. Repeated trauma
   D. Viruses

2. Neoplasia involves all of the following *except*:
   A. Normal arrangement of cells
   B. Irreversible cellular changes
   C. Abnormal process
   D. Uncontrolled cell multiplication

3. Which of the following statements concerning leukoplakia is *true*?
   A. Most cases have a history of radiation damage.
   B. Sites that are at high risk for epithelial dysplasia include the buccal mucosa and gingiva.
   C. A biopsy should be performed to establish a diagnosis.
   D. Leukoplakia is less common than erythroplakia.

4. Which of the following is a characteristic of benign tumors?
   A. Abnormal mitotic figures
   B. Anaplastic cells
   C. Slow growth
   D. Metastasis likely

5. A small white exophytic lesion on the palate is a benign lesion composed of squamous epithelium. Papillary projections are arranged in a cauliflower-like appearance. It is most likely a:
   A. Peripheral ossifying fibroma
   B. Neurofibroma
   C. Granular cell tumor
   D. Papilloma

6. Which of the following is *not* a microscopic characteristic of squamous cell carcinoma?
   A. Invasion of tumor cells into the connective tissue
   B. Cells with very small nuclei
   C. Cells with hyperchromatic nuclei
   D. Keratin pearls

7. Which of the following are the most common locations for intraoral squamous cell carcinoma?
   A. Upper labial mucosa, frenum, and lingual gingiva
   B. Lower labial mucosa, maxillary gingiva, and buccal mucosa
   C. Floor of the mouth, ventrolateral tongue, and soft palate
   D. Anterior tongue, mandibular gingiva, and retromolar area

8. A patient with squamous cell carcinoma of the lateral tongue exhibits metastatic disease in the liver. What clinical stage correlates with these findings?
   A. Stage I
   B. Stage II
   C. Stage III
   D. Stage IV

9. Which of the following represents the earliest clinical example of squamous cell carcinoma?
   A. Nonhealing ulceration
   B. Exophytic lesion
   C. Pigmented area
   D. Destructive radiolucency

10. The most appropriate treatment for epithelial dysplasia is:
    A. Radiation therapy
    B. Chemotherapy
    C. Surgical excision
    D. Observation

Continued

Review Questions—cont'd

11. Verrucous carcinoma is differentiated from squamous cell carcinoma because it:
    A. Occurs primarily in the nasal passages
    B. Responds to chemotherapy
    C. Often mestastasizes
    D. Has a better prognosis

12. The most common intraoral location for salivary gland tumors is the:
    A. Upper lip
    B. Anterior buccal mucosa
    C. Junction of the hard and soft palate
    D. Posterior lateral tongue

13. Which of the following is *not* an example of a malignant salivary gland tumor?
    A. Pleomorphic adenoma
    B. Mucoepidermoid carcinoma
    C. Cylindroma
    D. Adenoid cystic carcinoma

14. Which of the following statements concerning an ameloblastoma is *false*?
    A. It can present as a multilocular radiolucency.
    B. It is a benign and locally aggressive lesion.
    C. It often occurs in the mandibular molar and ramus area.
    D. It should be treated with radiation therapy.

15. The odontogenic tumor that characteristically appears as a well-circumscribed radiolucency located in the anterior maxilla of an adolescent girl is a(n):
    A. Ameloblastic fibro-odontoma
    B. Adenomatoid odontogenic tumor
    C. Peripheral ossifying fibroma
    D. Odontogenic myxoma

16. Which odontogenic tumor most closely resembles the mesenchyme of the dental follicle?
    A. Benign cementoblastoma
    B. Odontogenic myxoma
    C. Compound odontoma
    D. Ameloblastoma

17. Which one of the following best describes a benign cementoblastoma?
    A. It is a well-circumscribed radiopaque lesion with a radiolucent halo fused to the root of a vital tooth.
    B. It has a radiolucent multilocular appearance.
    C. It is a radiolucent lesion surrounding the crown of an impacted tooth.
    D. It is composed of numerous toothlike structures.

18. Which of the following lesions characteristically occurs on the alveolar mucosa in newborn girls?
    A. Granular cell tumor
    B. Congenital epulis
    C. Lymphangioma
    D. Plasmacytoma

19. Human herpesvirus 8 is associated with:
    A. Herpangina
    B. Rhabdomyosarcoma
    C. Kaposi sarcoma
    D. Schwannoma

20. A compound odontoma differs from a complex odontoma in that a compound odontoma:
    A. Is composed of several toothlike structures
    B. Has unlimited growth potential
    C. Presents as a radiopaque mass
    D. Is located in the posterior mandible

21. Peripheral odontogenic tumors are located on the:
    A. Palate
    B. Gingiva
    C. Lower lip
    D. Buccal mucosa

22. A benign tumor of adipose tissue is called a:
    A. Lipoma
    B. Neurofibroma
    C. Hemangioma
    D. Lymphangioma

23. The most common malignant soft tissue tumor of the head and neck in children is:
    A. Squamous cell carcinoma
    B. Lymphangioma
    C. Rhabdomyosarcoma
    D. Osteosarcoma

24. Malignant melanoma of the oral cavity is rare; however, the most common intraoral location is the:
    A. Lateral tongue
    B. Anterior buccal mucosa
    C. Palate and maxillary gingiva
    D. Retromolar area

25. Which of the following neoplasms often occurs in the buccal mucosa or vestibule?
    A. Lipoma
    B. Congenital epulis
    C. Lymphangioma
    D. Rhabdomyoma

26. A malignant tumor of bone-forming tissue is called:
    A. Chondrosarcoma
    B. Neurofibroma
    C. Osteosarcoma
    D. Rhabdomyosarcoma

27. An overproduction of atypical white blood cells in the bone marrow that results in an increase white blood cells in the circulating blood is called:
    A. Lymphoma
    B. Leukemia
    C. Malignant melanoma
    D. Leukopenia

28. Which of the following is a malignant tumor of lymphocytes?
    A. Multiple myeloma
    B. Lymphoma
    C. Malignant melanoma
    D. Rhabdomyosarcoma

29. The cell type involved in multiple myeloma is a(n):
    A. Lymphocyte
    B. Neutrophil
    C. Eosinophil
    D. Plasma cell

30. The most frequent intraoral site for metastatic tumors is the:
    A. Gingiva
    B. Mandible
    C. Soft palate
    D. Floor of the mouth

31. Which of the following tumors is associated with von Recklinghausen disease?
    A. Monomorphic adenoma
    B. Lipoma
    C. Fibroma
    D. Neurofibroma

32. Which of the following is the most common odontogenic tumor?
    A. Odontoma
    B. Peripheral ossifying fibroma
    C. Ameloblastic fibroma
    D. Odontogenic myxoma

33. Which of the following salivary gland tumors often occurs in adult men?
    A. Pleomorphic adenoma
    B. Monomorphic adenoma
    C. Papillary cystadenoma lymphomatosum
    D. Mucoepidermoid carcinoma

34. A benign tumor composed of a proliferation of capillaries is called a:
    A. Neurofibroma
    B. Hemangioma
    C. Rhabdomyoma
    D. Lymphangioma

35. A white plaquelike lesion that cannot be rubbed off or diagnosed clinically as a specific disease is called:
    A. Squamous cell carcinoma
    B. Erythroplakia
    C. Leukoplakia
    D. Epithelial dysplasia

36. All of the following are benign lesions that histologically contain bone or bonelike material except a(n):
    A. Torus
    B. Odontoma
    C. Exostosis
    D. Peripheral ossifying fibroma

37. Which of the following malignant tumors may present as diffuse gingival enlargement with persistent bleeding?
    A. Leukemia
    B. Multiple myeloma
    C. Chondrosarcoma
    D. Neurofibroma

38. Which of the following malignancies is characterized by a monoclonal spike on immunoelectrophoresis?
    A. Osteosarcoma
    B. Squamous cell carcinoma
    C. Multiple myeloma
    D. Leukemia

39. Which of the following malignant tumors has been reported to show a characteristic sunburst pattern on radiographic examination?
    A. Malignant melanoma
    B. Osteosarcoma
    C. Lymphoma
    D. Rhabdomyosarcoma

40. All of the following neoplasms arise from squamous epithelium except a(n):
    A. Squamous cell carcinoma
    B. Verrucous carcinoma
    C. Adenoid cystic carcinoma
    D. Papilloma

41. Which one of the following concerning solar cheilitis is false?
    A. There is distinct demarcation between vermilion border and skin.
    B. It appears as mottled grayish-pink discoloration of lower lip.
    C. Linear fissures are seen at right angles to the vermilion border.
    D. It is caused by excessive exposure to sunlight.

42. Which of the following has the best long-term prognosis?
    A. Basal cell carcinoma
    B. Intraoral squamous cell carcinoma
    C. Rhabdomyosarcoma
    D. Malignant melanoma

43. Which of the following does not arise in the oral cavity?
    A. Squamous cell carcinoma
    B. Malignant melanoma
    C. Basal cell carcinoma
    D. Verrucous carcinoma

44. Which of the following may undergo malignant transformation?
    A. Granular cell tumor
    B. Pleomorphic adenoma
    C. Torus
    D. Hemangioma

Continued

CHAPTER 7 *Synopsis—cont'd*

CONDITION/DISEASE	CAUSE	AGE/RACE/SEX	LOCATION
Basal cell carcinoma	Neoplastic Associated with sun exposure	Age: over 40 M=F Whites	Skin of face
Pleomorphic adenoma	Neoplastic	Age: over 40 F>M	Parotid gland Most common intraoral site: palate
Monomorphic adenoma Trabecular adenoma Canalicular adenoma Warthin tumor	Neoplastic	Adults F>M	Most common oral sites: upper lip and buccal mucosa; Warthin tumor: parotid
Mucoepidermoid carcinoma	Neoplastic	F>M	Parotid gland Most common oral site: palate Some are central in mandible
Adenoid cystic carcinoma	Neoplastic	Adults F>M	Parotid gland Most common oral site: palate
Ameloblastoma	Neoplastic	Adults M=F	Intraosseous Peripheral tumors also occur Mandible>maxilla Posterior>anterior
Calcifying epithelial odontogenic tumor	Neoplastic	Adults M=F	Posterior mandible
Adenomatoid odontogenic tumor	Neoplastic	Age: 70% under 20 F>M	70% involve anterior maxilla and mandible Maxilla>mandible
Calcifying odontogenic cyst	Cyst with neoplastic variant	Age: Under 40 M=F	Maxilla and mandible
Odontogenic myxoma	Neoplastic	Age: 10-29 M=F	Mandible>maxilla
Central cementifying and ossifying fibromas	Neoplastic	Age: adults F>M	Mandible (90%)

N/A, Not applicable.

CLINICAL FEATURES	RADIOGRAPHIC FEATURES	MICROSCOPIC FEATURES	TREATMENT	DIAGNOSTIC PROCESS
Nonhealing ulcer; rolled borders	N/A	Proliferation of basal epithelial cells Broad rete pegs penetrate deeply into the connective tissue	Surgical excision Radiation therapy	Microscopic
Nonulcerated, dome-shaped	N/A	Encapsulated tumor Mixture of epithelium and tissue that resembles various forms of connective tissue	Surgical excision	Microscopic
Smooth-surfaced mass	N/A	Encapsulated epithelial tumor with a uniform pattern of epithelial cells	Surgical excision	Microscopic
Asymptomatic swelling or mass	When intraosseous, unilocular or multilocular radiolucency	Unencapsulated, infiltrating tumor composed of a combination of mucous cells and squamous-like epithelial cells	Surgical excision	
Mass, often painful Surface may be ulcerated	N/A	Unencapsulated, infiltrating tumor composed of small, deeply staining, uniform epithelial cells arranged in perforated round-to-oval islands	Surgical excision Radiation therapy	Microscopic
				Microscopic
Slow-growing Expansion of bone	Unilocular or multilocular radiolucency	Unencapsulated, infiltrating tumor composed of ameloblast-like epithelial cells surrounding areas resembling stellate reticulum	Surgical excision	Microscopic
Asymptomatic; slow-growing expansion of bone	Unilocular or multilocular radiolucency with scattered calcifications	Unencapsulated, infiltrating tumor composed of islands and sheets of polyhedral epithelial cells Calcifications and eosinophilic deposits in tumor	Surgical excision	Microscopic
Asymptomatic swelling	Well-defined radiolucency associated with an impacted tooth Radiopacities within the radiolucency	Encapsulated tumor composed of ductlike epithelial structures, masses of cuboidal and spindle-shaped epithelial cells with eosinophilic material and calcifications	Surgical excision	Microscopic
Asymptomatic swelling Root resorption	Unilocular or multilocular radiolucency Radiopacities within the radiolucency	Cyst lined with odontogenic epithelium with associated ghost cell keratinization Ameloblast-like cells and stellate reticulum-like areas	Enucleation	Microscopic
Asymptomatic expansion of bone	Multilocular, honeycombed radiolucency	Unencapsulated, infiltrating tumor composed of pale-staining substance containing widely dispersed cells with small nuclei	Surgical excision	Microscopic
Asymptomatic expansion, facial asymmetry	Wide-defined unilocular lesion, varying degrees of opacities	Well-circumscribed tumor composed of fibrous connective tissue and rounded globular calcifications, bone trabeculae, or both	Surgical excision	Radiographic Microscopic

Continued

CHAPTER 7 *Synopsis—cont'd*

CONDITION/DISEASE	CAUSE	AGE/RACE/SEX	LOCATION
Lymphangioma	Neoplastic/developmental	Congenital M=F	Most common oral site: tongue
Kaposi sarcoma	Neoplastic Human herpesvirus 8	M>F	Most common oral sites: hard palate and gingiva
Melanocytic nevi	Developmental	Age: 20-50 F>M	Most common oral sites: hard palate and buccal mucosa
Malignant melanoma	Neoplastic	Age: over 40	Most common oral sites: hard palate and maxillary
Torus	Genetic	Age: adults F>M	Midline of hard palate Lingual aspect of mandible
Exostosis	Possibly reactive	Age: adults M=F	Buccal aspect of maxillary and mandibular ridges
Osteoma	Neoplastic	M=F	Intraosseous
Osteosarcoma	Neoplastic	Most common primary malignant tumor of bone in patients younger than 40 M>F	Twice as frequent in mandible as in maxilla
Chondrosarcoma	Neoplastic	M>F	Maxilla and mandible
Leukemia	Neoplastic	M>F	Gingiva
Lymphoma	Neoplastic	Adults M>F	Most common oral site: tonsillar area
Multiple myeloma	Neoplastic	Adults M>F	Mandible>maxilla
Metastatic tumors	Neoplastic	Adults M>F	Mandible>maxilla

*Not covered in text.
N/A, Not applicable.

CLINICAL FEATURES	RADIOGRAPHIC FEATURES	MICROSCOPIC FEATURES	TREATMENT	DIAGNOSTIC PROCESS
Ill-defined mass with a pebbly surface	N/A	Lesion composed of lymphatic vessels	Surgical excision	Clinical Microscopic
Purple macules, plaques, or exophytic tumors	N/A	Unencapsulated tumor composed of spindle-shaped cells mixed with slitlike spaces containing red blood cells	Surgical excision Radiation therapy Chemotherapy	Clinical Microscopic
Tan/brown macules or papules	N/A	Benign tumor composed of nevus cells	Surgical excision	Clinical Microscopic
Rapidly enlarging blue-and-black mass	N/A	Malignant tumor	Surgical excision	Microscopic
Asymptomatic, bony hard, lobulated mass	Radiopaque mass superimposed on tooth roots	Benign, compact bone	None unless necessary for fabrication of prosthetic appliance	Clinical
Asymptomatic, bony hard nodules	Occasionally seen radiopacity	Benign, compact bone	None unless necessary for fabrication of prosthetic appliance	Clinical
Asymptomatic	Sharply defined radiopaque mass	Benign, compact bone	None unless necessary for fabrication of prosthetic appliance	Microscopic
Painful, diffuse swelling or mass Expansion of involved bone	Destructive, poorly defined radiolucency to radiopacity Asymmetric widening of the periodontal ligament space Sunburst pattern	Malignant tumor of bone*	Surgical excision Multiagent chemotherapy	Microscopic
Enlargement of involved bone	*	Malignant tumor of cartilage*	Wide surgical excision	Microscopic
Diffuse gingival enlargement with persistent bleeding	N/A	Atypical white blood cells in circulating blood and tissues	Chemotherapy Radiation therapy Corticosteroids	Laboratory Microscopic
Enlargement of involved tissue	N/A	Malignant tumor of lymphoid tissue	Radiation therapy Chemotherapy	Laboratory Microscopic
Bone pain, swelling	Multiple radiolucent lesions	Malignant proliferation of plasma cells	Chemotherapy	Laboratory Microscopic
Pain Paresthesia Swelling Expansion of bone	Variable Usually poorly defined and radiolucent Tooth roots may show spiked appearances Some may show area of radiopacity	Resemble primary malignancy	Chemotherapy Radiation	Microscopic

FIGURE 8-5 ■ Radiographs of central giant cell granulomas showing multilocular radiolucencies in the mandible (**A**) and maxilla (**B**). **C,** Microscopic appearance of a central giant cell granuloma showing the same features as a peripheral giant cell granuloma except for the absence of surface mucosa.

results in an aneurysmal bone cyst. Surgical excision and supplemental cryotherapy are the recommended treatments for an aneurysmal bone cyst.

OSTEOMALACIA

Osteomalacia is a disease of bone that develops over a long period of time as the result of a calcium deficiency. When this disease occurs in young children, it is usually caused by a nutritional deficiency of vitamin D, and the associated disease is termed *rickets.* An inherited form of vitamin D deficiency called **hypophosphatemic vitamin D–resistant rickets** is included in Chapter 6. In adults the disease may be related to various problems such as a malabsorption syndrome, drugs, liver or kidney disease, and the chronic use of antacids. Osteomalacia may also be induced by certain tumors.

Delayed tooth eruption and periodontal disease have been associated with osteomalacia. Changes in bone trabeculation that occur in patients with osteomalacia may be subtle and difficult to detect. Pathologic fractures may also occur.

Treatment is based on identification of the cause of the vitamin D deficiency and includes nutritional supplementation with vitamin D and dietary calcium.

SELECTED REFERENCES

Books

Neville BW, Damm DD, Allen CM, et al: *Oral and maxillofacial pathology,* ed 3, St. Louis, 2009, Saunders.

Regezi JA, Sciubba JJ, Jordan RCK: Oral pathology: clinical-pathologic correlations, ed 6, St. Louis, 2012, Saunders.

Journal Articles

Alsufyani NA, Lam EW: Cemento-osseous dysplasia of the jaw bones: KEY radiographic features, *Dentomaxillofac Radiol* 40:141, 2011.

Bessho K, Tagawa T, Murata M, et al: Monostotic fibrous dysplasia with involvement of the mandibular canal, *Oral Surg Oral Med Oral Pathol* 68:396, 1989.

Beylouni I, Farge P, Mazoyer JF, et al: Florid cemento-osseous dysplasia: report of a case documented with computed tomography and 3D imaging, *Oral Surg Oral Med Oral Pathol Oral Radiol Endod* 85:707, 1998.

Cohen MM Jr, Howell RE: Etiology of fibrous dysplasia and McCune-Albright syndrome, *Int J Oral Maxillofac Surg* 28:366, 1999.

Collins MT: Spectrum and natural history of fibrous dysplasia of bone, *J Bone Miner Res* 21(Suppl 2):99, 2006.

Hadjipavlou AG, Gaitanis IN, Kontakis GM: Paget disease of the bone and its management, *J Bone Joint Surg* 84:160, 2002.

MacDonald-Jankowski DS: Fibro-osseous lesions of the face and jaws, *Clin Radiol* 59:11, 2004.

Ozek C, Gundogan H, Bilkay U, et al: Craniomaxillofacial fibrous dysplasia, *J Craniofac Surg* 13:382, 2002.

Polyzos SA, Anastasilakis AD, Makras P, et al: Paget's disease of bone and calcium homeostasis: focus on bisphosphonate treatment, *Exp Clin Endocrinol Diabetes* 119:519, 2011.

Regezi JA: Odontogenic cysts, odontogenic tumors, fibro-osseous, and giant cell lesions of the jaws, *Mod Pathol* 15:331, 2002.

Singer SR, Mupparapu M, Rinaggio J: Florid cemento-osseous dysplasia and chronic diffuse osteomyelitis: report of a simultaneous presentation and review of the literature, *J Am Dent Assoc* 136:927, 2005.

Siris ES, Lyles KW, Singer FR, et al: Medical management of Paget's disease of bone: indications for treatment and review of current therapies, *J Bone Miner Res* 21(Suppl 2):4, 2006.

Summerlin Don-John, Tomich CE: Focal cemento-osseous dysplasia: a clinicopathologic study of 221 cases, *Oral Surg Oral Med Oral Pathol* 78:611, 1994.

Sun ZJ, Zhao YF, Yang RL, et al: Aneurysmal bone cysts of the jaws: analysis of 17 cases, *J Oral Maxillofac Surg* 68:2122, 2010.

Triantafillidou K, Venetis G, Karakinaris G, et al: Central giant cell granuloma of the jaws: a clinical study of 17 cases and a review of the literature, *Ann Otol Rhinol Laryngol* 120:167, 2011.

Whyte MP: Clinical practice: Paget disease of bone, *N Engl J Med* 355:593, 2006.

Zacharin M: The spectrum of McCune Albright syndrome, *Pediatr Endocrinol Rev* 4(Suppl):412, 2007.

Review Questions

1. A 48-year-old black woman has multiple asymptomatic, radiopaque masses in the mandible and maxilla. No expansion of bone is noted. The most likely diagnosis is:
   A. Central cementifying fibromas
   B. Florid cemento-osseous dysplasia
   C. Periapical cemento-osseous dysplasia
   D. Fibrous dysplasia

2. All of the following are examples of benign fibro-osseous lesions *except*:
   A. Fibrous dysplasia
   B. Periapical cemento-osseous dysplasia
   C. Central ossifying fibroma
   D. Osteoma

3. Which of the following is characterized by precocious puberty in females?
   A. Monostotic fibrous dysplasia
   B. Jaffe-Lichtenstein–type fibrous dysplasia
   C. Albright-McCune–type fibrous dysplasia
   D. Focal cemento-osseous dysplasia

4. Periapical cemento-osseous dysplasia is located in the:
   A. Posterior mandible
   B. Posterior maxilla
   C. Craniofacial bones
   D. Anterior mandible

5. Periapical cemento-osseous dysplasia has also been known as a(n):
   A. Cementoma
   B. Odontoma
   C. Cementoblastoma
   D. Fibrous dysplasia

6. Which of the following diseases is associated with café au lait spots?
   A. Polyostotic fibrous dysplasia
   B. Paget disease
   C. Monostotic fibrous dysplasia
   D. Periapical cemento-osseous dysplasia

7. What is the name of the type of fibrous dysplasia that involves the maxilla and adjacent bones?
   A. Periapical
   B. Jaffe
   C. Craniofacial
   D. Monostotic

8. Which one of the following is not a feature of Paget disease?
   A. Deposition of amorphous material
   B. Resorption and osteoblastic repair
   C. Chronic metabolic bone disease
   D. Hypercementosis

9. The most characteristic radiographic appearance of fibrous dysplasia is described as a:
   A. "Cotton-wool" appearance
   B. Well-circumscribed radiopacity
   C. "Ground glass" appearance
   D. Well-circumscribed multilocular radiolucency

10. All of the following are histologic features seen in Paget disease except one. Which one is the exception?
    A. Osteoblasts and osteoclasts
    B. Bone with prominent irregular dark lines
    C. Well-vascularized fibrous connective tissue
    D. Hyperchromatic nuclei and atypical mitotic figures

11. All of the following have a characteristic radiographic appearance *except*:
    A. Paget disease
    B. Osteomalacia
    C. Florid cemento-osseous dysplasia
    D. Periapical cemento-osseous dysplasia

12. In patients with fibrous dysplasia, which of the following is the only recommended treatment modality?
    A. Surgery
    B. Radiation therapy
    C. Chemotherapy
    D. Sclerosing agent

13. Which of the following is helpful in the diagnosis of Paget disease?
    A. Immunoelectrophoresis
    B. Serum alkaline phosphatase
    C. Serum calcium
    D. Urinalysis

Continued

Chapter 9

Oral Manifestations of Systemic Diseases

Olga A.C. Ibsen, Joan Andersen Phelan, Anthony T. Vernillo

OBJECTIVES

After studying this chapter, the student will be able to:

1. Define each of the words in the vocabulary list for this chapter.
2. Describe the difference between gigantism and acromegaly and list the physical characteristics of each.
3. State the oral manifestations of hyperthyroidism and hypothyroidism.
4. Describe the difference between primary and secondary hyperparathyroidism.
5. List the oral and systemic manifestations that occur in the uncontrolled diabetic state.
6. List the major clinical characteristics of type 1 and type 2 diabetes.
7. Define Addison disease and describe the changes that occur on the skin and oral mucosa in a patient with Addison disease.
8. Compare and contrast the cause, laboratory findings, and oral manifestations of each of the following: iron deficiency anemia, pernicious anemia, folic acid deficiency, and vitamin B_{12} deficiency.
9. Compare and contrast the definitions and oral manifestations of thalassemia major and sickle cell anemia.
10. Define celiac disease.
11. Describe the difference between primary and secondary aplastic anemia.
12. Compare and contrast primary and secondary polycythemia and describe the oral manifestations of polycythemia.
13. Explain why platelets may be deficient in polycythemia vera.
14. Describe the most characteristic oral manifestations of agranulocytosis.
15. Describe and contrast acute and chronic leukemia.
16. State the purpose of each of the following laboratory tests: platelet count, bleeding time, prothrombin time, partial thromboplastin time, and international normalized ratio.
17. List two causes of thrombocytopenic purpura.
18. Describe the oral manifestations of thrombocytopenia and nonthrombocytopenic purpura.
19. Define hemophilia and describe its oral manifestations and treatment.
20. Describe the difference between primary and secondary immunodeficiency.
21. Describe the oral problems that would be expected to occur in a patient with radiation-induced xerostomia.
22. List two drugs that are associated with gingival enlargement.
23. Describe the criteria used to define bisphosphonate-associated osteonecrosis of the jaw.

VOCABULARY

Agranulocytosis (a-gran″u-lo-si-to′sis) Marked decrease in the number of granulocytes, particularly neutrophils.

Anemia (ə-ne′me-ə) Reduction of the number of red blood cells, quantity of hemoglobin, or volume of packed red blood cells to less than normal.

Apertognathia (ə-per″tog-na′the-ə) Anterior open bite

Aplasia (ə-pla′zhə) (adjective, *aplastic*) Lack of development.

Arthralgia (ahr-thral′jə) Severe pain in a joint.

Atherosclerosis (ath″ər-o-sklə-ro′sis) The process by which lipid accumulates within the walls of large and medium-sized arteries. It leads to reduced blood flow to and death of vital organs.

Autoimmunity (aw″to-ĭ-mun′ĭ-te) Immune-mediated destruction of the body's own cells and tissues; immunity against self.

Catabolism (kə-tab′o-liz-əm) Component of metabolism that involves the breakdown of tissues.

Coagulation (ko-ag″u-la′shən) Formation of a clot.

Dysphagia (dis-fa′zhə) Difficulty swallowing.

Ecchymosis (ek″ĭ-mo′sis) Small, flat, hemorrhagic patch larger than a petechia on the skin or mucous membrane.

Exophthalmos (ek″sof-thal′mos) An abnormal protrusion (bulging) of one or both eyes.

Fibrin (fi′brin) Insoluble protein that is essential to the clotting of blood.

Hematocrit (he-mat′ə-krit) Volume percentage of red blood cells in whole blood.

Hemolysis (he-mol′ə-sis) Release of hemoglobin from red blood cells by destruction of the cells.

Hemostasis (he″mo-sta′sis) Stoppage or cessation of bleeding.

Hepatomegaly (hep″ə-to-meg′ə-le) Enlargement of the liver.

Hormone (hor′mōn) Secreted molecules produced in the body that have a specific regulatory action on target cells that are distant from their sites of synthesis; an endocrine hormone is frequently carried by the blood from its site of release to its target.

Hypercalcemia (hi″pər-kal-se′me-ə) Excess calcium in the blood.

Hyperglycemia (hi″pər-gli-se′me-ə) Excess glucose in the blood.

Hypochromic (hi″po-kro′mik) Stained less intensely than normal.

Hypophosphatemia (hi″po-fos″fə-te′me-ə) Deficiency of phosphates in the blood.

Insulin (in′sə-lin) Hormone produced in the pancreas by beta cells in the islets of Langerhans; insulin regulates glucose metabolism and is the major fuel-regulating hormone.

Insulin shock (in′sə-lin shok) Profound hypoglycemia, or low blood sugar, that necessitates emergency intervention.

Ketoacidosis (ke″to-as″ĭ-do′sis) Accumulation of acid in the body resulting from the accumulation of ketone bodies.

Macrovascular disease (mak″ro-vas′ku-lər dĭ-zēz′) Atherosclerosis of large and medium-size blood vessels

Microcyte (mi′kro-sīt) Red blood cell that is smaller than normal.

Microvaseular disease (mi″kro-vas′ku-lər dĭ-zēz′) Damage to small blood vessels.

Myalgia (mi-al′jə) Muscle pain.

Neutropenia (noo″tro-pe′ne-ə) Decreased number of neutrophils in the blood.

Osteoporosis (os″te-o-pə-ro′sis) Abnormal rarefaction of bone.

Pancytopenia (pan″si-to-pe′ne-ə) A dramatic decrease in all types of circulating blood cells.

Parathormone (par″ə-thor′mōn) Parathyroid hormone.

Petechia (pə-te′ke-ə) Minute red spot on the skin or mucous membrane caused by escape of a small amount of blood.

Platelet (plāt′lət) Disk-shaped structure, also called a thrombocyte, found in the blood; it plays an important role in blood coagulation.

Polycythemia (pol″e-si-the′me-ə) Increase in the total red blood cell mass in the blood.

Polydipsia (pol″e-dip′se-ə) Chronic excessive thirst and intake of fluid.

Purpura (pur′pu-rə) Blood disorders characterized by purplish or brownish-red discolorations caused by bleeding into the skin or tissues.

Receptor (re-sep′tər) Cell surface protein to which a specific molecule (e.g., a hormone) can bind; such binding leads to biochemical events.

Splenomegaly (sple″no-meg′ə-le) Enlargement of the spleen.

Thrombocyte (throm′bo-sīt) Platelet.

Thrombocytopenia (throm″bo-si′to-pe′ne-ə) Decrease in the number of platelets in circulating blood.

Xerostoma (zēr″o-sto′me-ə) Dry mouth.

Many diseases that affect the body as a whole are associated with alterations of the oral mucosa, maxilla, and mandible. Systemic diseases can cause mucosal changes such as ulceration or mucosal bleeding. Generalized immunodeficiency can lead to the development of opportunistic diseases such as infection and neoplasia. Bone disease can affect the maxilla and mandible, and systemic disease can cause dental and periodontal changes. Drugs prescribed for a systemic disease can affect the oral tissues.

Local factors are frequently involved in manifestations of systemic disease in the oral mucosa. In some systemic diseases the mucosa is more easily injured; therefore mild irritation and chronic inflammation can cause lesions that would not occur without the presence of the systemic disease.

This chapter includes systemic diseases that have oral manifestations. Some overlap may occur among the diseases included in this chapter and those included in other chapters in this text. Included here are endocrine disorders, blood disorders including those of red and white blood cells, disorders of **platelets** and bleeding and clotting disorders, and immunodeficiency disorders. Oral changes can be similar for several different systemic diseases, and similar oral lesions can occur without the presence of systemic disease.

ENDOCRINE DISORDERS

The endocrine system consists of a group of integrated glands and cells that secrete **hormones.** The secretion of hormones by these glands is controlled by feedback mechanisms in which the amount of hormone circulating in blood triggers factors that control production. Diseases of this system can result from (1) conditions in which too much or too little hormone is produced, and (2) from either dysfunction of the glands themselves or a problem in the mechanism that controls hormone production. Some of the endocrine gland diseases in which oral changes occur are included here.

HYPERPITUITARISM

Hyperpituitarism is excess hormone production by the anterior pituitary gland. It is caused most often by a benign tumor **(pituitary adenoma)** that produces growth hormone. If the increase in growth hormone production occurs during development before the closure of the long bones, **gigantism** results. Endocrine disturbances associated with genetic conditions are responsible for close to 20% of the cases of gigantism. Treatment involves surgical removal of the pituitary adenoma.

Acromegaly is a rare condition that results when the hypersecretion occurs in adult life after closure of the long bones. The occurrence rate is about 65 patients per million. A pituitary adenoma is also thought to be the cause.

CLINICAL FEATURES AND ORAL MANIFESTATIONS

Gigantism includes excessive growth of the overall skeleton. Affected individuals can be more than 8 feet tall and weigh several hundred pounds; and as adults they experience headaches, chronic fatigue, and muscle and joint pain.

Acromegaly affects both men and women and most commonly occurs in the fourth decade of life. The onset is slow and insidious. Patients experience poor vision, sensitivity to light, enlargement of the hands and feet, and an increase in rib size. The facial changes include enlargement of the maxilla and mandible, frontal bossing (an enlargement of the bones of the forehead), and enlargement of the

FIGURE 9-1 ■ Enlarged tongue (macroglossia) in a patient with acromegaly.

nasal bones. An enlargement of the maxillary sinus also occurs, which causes a characteristically deep voice. The enlargement of the maxilla and mandible results in separation of teeth and malocclusion. **Apertognathia** (anterior open bite) has also been reported. Mucosal changes such as thickened lips and macroglossia (enlarged tongue) have also been described in patients with acromegaly (Figure 9-1).

DIAGNOSIS AND TREATMENT

Laboratory tests may be performed to evaluate serum growth hormones by giving the patient an oral dose of glucose. Normally, growth hormone measured after intake of glucose would decrease. If the patient has acromegaly, the growth hormone will not decrease. Treatment for acromegaly involves surgical removal of the pituitary adenoma. Medical management may be attempted if the cause is not a tumor. Radiation therapy is also an option, but results are not as rapid or successful. In the untreated patient, other conditions such as diabetes, cardiovascular diseases, respiratory diseases, and colon cancer have been reported, increasing the patient's morbidity.

HYPERTHYROIDISM (THYROTOXICOSIS, GRAVES DISEASE)

Hyperthyroidism is a condition characterized by excessive production of thyroid hormone. It is 10 times more common in women than in men, and patients are typically diagnosed in their 30s or 40s. Hyperthyroidism has several different causes. The most common cause (60% to 90%) is a condition called *Graves disease.* Graves disease is an autoimmune disorder in which antibodies called thyroid-stimulating immunoglobulins (THIs) stimulate the thyroid cells, and as a result the thyroid gland enlarges and too much thyroid hormone is produced. This increase in hormone causes an increase in the patient's metabolism. In children hyperactivity is observed. Other causes of hyperthyroidism include hyperplasia of the gland, benign and malignant tumors of the thyroid, pituitary gland disease, and metastatic tumors.

CLINICAL FEATURES

The clinical features of hyperthyroidism include thyroid enlargement (goiter), rosy complexion, erythema of the palms, excessive sweating, fine hair, and softened nails. **Exophthalmos** (protrusion of the eyeballs) is a significant clinical characteristic and is often seen in patients with Graves disease. Weight loss, anxiety, weakness, restlessness, and cardiac problems (tachycardia) may be associated with this condition.

ORAL MANIFESTATIONS

Hyperthyroidism in children may lead to premature exfoliation of deciduous teeth and premature eruption of permanent teeth. In adults **osteoporosis** may occur, which may affect alveolar bone. Dental caries and periodontal disease appear to develop and progress more rapidly in these patients than in other patients. Burning discomfort of the tongue has also been reported.

TREATMENT

Treatment of hyperthyroidism depends on the cause and may include surgery, medications to suppress thyroid activity, or the administration of radioactive iodine. The treatment of hyperthyroidism is the most common cause of hypothyroidism. Clinical mismanagement of hyperthyroidism may lead to hypothyroidism and is thus described as iatrogenic or clinician-caused disease.

HYPOTHYROIDISM (CRETINISM; MYXEDEMA)

Hypothyroidism is characterized by decreased output of thyroid hormone. When hypothyroidism is present during infancy and childhood it is called **cretinism.** In older children and adults the condition is known as **myxedema.** Causes include developmental disturbances, autoimmune destruction of the thyroid gland (also known as Hashimoto's thyroiditis), iodine deficiency, drugs, and pituitary treatments for hyperthyroidism. In infants facial and oral changes include thickened lips, enlarged tongue, and delayed eruption of teeth. Adults with hypothyroidism may have dry skin, swelling of the face, weakness, fatigue, and an enlarged tongue (macroglossia). Laboratory tests are done to determine the diagnosis of primary or secondary hypothyroidism. Free thyroxine (T_4) and thyroid-stimulating hormone (TSH) levels are measured. In primary hypothyroidism TSH levels are increased. In secondary hypothyroidism TSH levels are normal.

HYPERPARATHYROIDISM

Hyperparathyroidism results from excessive secretion of parathyroid hormone (**parathormone** [PTH]), which is secreted by the parathyroid glands. The four parathyroid glands are located near the thyroid gland. PTH plays an important role in calcium and phosphorus metabolism. Elevated blood levels of calcium (**hypercalcemia**), low blood levels of phosphorus (**hypophosphatemia**), and abnormal bone metabolism characterize primary

hyperparathyroidism. Secondary hyperparathyroidism results when there is an overproduction of PTH in response to long-term decreased levels of serum calcium often associated with chronic renal disease.

Primary hyperparathyroidism may be the result of hyperplasia of the parathyroid glands, a benign tumor of one or more of the parathyroid glands (parathyroid adenoma), or (less commonly) a malignant parathyroid tumor. Because of elevated serum calcium, these patients often have kidney stones. The disease is found in adults over 60 years of age and is far more common in women than in men.

Calcium is obtained mainly from dairy products and plays an important role in the contraction of all types of muscle. PTH maintains normal blood levels of calcium through its effects on the kidney, gastrointestinal tract, and bone. It increases the uptake of dietary calcium from the gastrointestinal tract and is able to move calcium from bone to circulating blood when necessary. The hormone appears to be able to remove calcium from bone through the action of osteoclasts.

Hyperparathyroidism that results from an abnormality of the parathyroid glands is called *primary hyperparathyroidism.* Secondary hyperparathyroidism occurs when calcium is abnormally excreted by the kidneys and the parathyroid glands increase their production of PTH to maintain adequate blood levels of calcium. The most common cause of secondary hyperparathyroidism is kidney failure. Problems with absorption of nutrients and fat-soluble vitamins such as vitamin D through the gut or small intestine are also an important cause of secondary hyperparathyroidism.

CLINICAL FEATURES

The clinical manifestations of hyperparathyroidism are varied. Patients with mild cases can be asymptomatic. Joint pain or stiffness may be present. The disease can affect the kidneys, skeletal system, and gastrointestinal system. In severe disease lethargy, dementia, and coma can occur.

ORAL MANIFESTATIONS

The oral manifestations of hyperparathyroidism include changes in the bone of the mandible and maxilla. The chief oral manifestation is the appearance of well-defined unilocular or multilocular radiolucencies (Figure 9-2, *A*). Microscopically, these lesions appear indistinguishable from central giant cell granulomas (described in Chapter 2) (Figure 9-2, *B*). Although rare, there have been reports of a few cases of peripheral giant cell granulomas associated with hyperparathyroidism. Other radiographic changes that occur in secondary hyperparathyroidism include a generalized "ground-glass" appearance of the trabeculae and loss of the lamina dura. Loosening of teeth can also occur (Figure 9-2, *C*).

DIAGNOSIS AND TREATMENT

The diagnosis of hyperparathyroidism involves the measurement of PTH blood levels and can also include serum calcium and phosphorus measurements. Treatment is infection is increased. Therefore elimination of infection is extremely important in patients with diabetes. Antibiotic medication, calculus and plaque removal, effective oral hygiene care, and adequate nutrition are especially important in the management of the patient with diabetes. One final point deserves mention here. People with well-controlled diabetes of either type can lead long, productive lives. However, diabetes control is not an "in-between." A patient either controls his or her diabetes, or does not—there is also no such thing as "mild" diabetes. Good control of diabetes represents a synthesis of effort between the physician, nurse, nutritionist, dentist, and dental hygienist. It is truly a team effort.

ADDISON DISEASE

Addison disease, also known as **primary adrenal cortical insufficiency,** is characterized by an insufficient production of adrenal steroids. A malignant tumor and infections (including tuberculosis, deep fungal infections, and human immunodeficiency virus [HIV] infection) may be responsible for destruction of the adrenal gland. However, in most cases the cause of the destruction of the adrenal cortex is unknown. In these patients the condition may be an autoimmune disease.

As a result of the decreased production of adrenal steroids, the pituitary gland increases its production of adrenocorticotropic hormone, which would normally increase the production of adrenal steroids. This hormone is similar to melanin-stimulating hormone and causes stimulation of

melanocytes. Brown pigmentation (bronzing) of the skin occurs, and melanotic macules can develop on the oral mucosa. Treatment of Addison disease involves corticosteroid replacement therapy.

BLOOD DISORDERS

The **complete blood count (CBC)** is important in the diagnosis of blood disorders. The CBC is a series of tests that examine the red blood cells, white blood cells, and platelets. It provides information about the number of each type of cell, the ratio of types of cells, and the appearance of the cells. The information included in a CBC and normal values are listed in Box 9-1.

DISORDERS OF RED BLOOD CELLS AND HEMOGLOBIN

ANEMIA

Anemia is defined as a reduction in the oxygen-carrying capacity of the blood that in most cases is related to a decrease in the number of circulating red blood cells. There are many different types and causes of anemia.

FIGURE 9-4 ■ Periapical radiograph of a patient with diabetes mellitus shows severe alveolar bone loss.

BOX 9-1

Complete Blood Count: Normal Adult Values

Red Blood Cells

Count: The total number of red blood cells (RBCs) per mm^3 of whole blood
  Males: $4.7\text{-}6.1 \times 10^6$
  Females: $4.2\text{-}5.4 \times 10^6$
Hemoglobin: The amount of hemoglobin contained in 100 ml of whole blood
  Males: 13.8-17.2 gm/deciliter (dL)
  Females: 12.1-15.1 gm/deciliter (dL)
Hematocrit: The volume of packed RBCs in a sample of whole blood
  Males: 40.7%-50.3%
  Females: 36.1%-44.3%

Indices

Mean corpuscular (cell) volume: Describes the average size of an individual RBC: 80-95 femtoliter (fm)
Mean corpuscular (cell) hemoglobin: Indicates the amount of hemoglobin present in an RBC by weight: 27-31 picograms/cell (pg/cell)
Mean corpuscular (cell) hemoglobin concentration: Indicates the proportion of each cell occupied by hemoglobin: 32-36 gm/deciliter (dL)

White Blood Cells (WBC)

Count: 4,500-10,000 cells/microliter of whole blood
Differential count: The number of each type of WBC expressed as a percentage of the total number of WBCs:

Mature neutrophils (granulocytes)	40%-60%
Immature neutrophils (bands)	0%-3%
Lymphocytes	20%-40%
Monocytes	2%-8%
Basophils	0.5%-1%
Eosinophils	1%-4%

From www.nlm.nih.gov/medlineplus/ency/article/003642.htm and www.nlm.nih.gov/medlineplus/ency/article/003657.htm

Nutritional anemias occur when a substance necessary for the normal development of red blood cells is in scant supply in the bone marrow. The most common deficiencies are of iron, folic acid, or vitamin B_{12}. These deficiencies can occur when the intake of the nutrient is insufficient or when disorders of absorption prevent its uptake. Anemia can also occur when suppression of the bone marrow stem cells takes place, resulting in an inability of the bone marrow to produce red blood cells.

Oral manifestations are similar for all types of anemia and include skin and mucosal pallor, angular cheilitis, erythema and atrophy of the oral mucosa, and loss of filiform and fungiform papillae on the dorsum of the tongue. Circumvallate papillae and foliate papillae are not affected.

IRON DEFICIENCY ANEMIA

Iron deficiency anemia occurs when an insufficient amount of iron is supplied to the bone marrow for red blood cell development. It is the most common cause of anemia in the United States. This type of anemia can occur as a result of a deficiency of iron intake, excessive blood loss from heavy menstrual bleeding or chronic gastrointestinal bleeding, poor iron absorption, or an increased requirement for iron as in pregnancy or infancy.

Plummer-Vinson syndrome is rare and can develop as a result of long-standing iron deficiency anemia. This syndrome includes **dysphagia** (difficulty swallowing), glossitis (inflammation of the tongue, causing a burning sensation), angular cheilitis, atrophy of the papilla on the dorsal tongue, atrophy of the upper alimentary tract, and a predisposition to the development of esophageal and oral cancer. In Plummer-Vinson syndrome evaluation of the esophagus is performed by endoscopy or esophageal barium, which will help to identify esophageal webs. These abnormal bands of tissue in the esophagus contribute to the diagnosis.

Clinical Features and Oral Manifestations

Iron deficiency anemia is most often asymptomatic. When significant enough to show systemic symptoms, patients experience weakness (tiring easily), fatigue, low energy, shortness of breath, and sometimes cardiac palpitations. Oral mucosal signs in severe cases include angular cheilitis; pallor of the oral tissues; and an erythematous, depapillated, smooth, painful burning tongue (Figure 9-5). The changes in the oral mucosa occur as a result of a lack of nutrients to the epithelium. The filiform papillae on the dorsum of the tongue disappear first because they have the highest metabolic requirements. Disappearance of the fungiform papillae can also occur in chronic and severe cases. Some researchers have suggested that iron deficiency anemia places the patient at risk for oral candidiasis, which exacerbates angular cheilitis and depapillation of the tongue.

Diagnosis and Treatment

The diagnosis of iron deficiency anemia is made by laboratory tests, which show a low hemoglobin content of red blood cells and a reduced **hematocrit** (the volume of red blood cells in blood) value. Iron is needed for hemoglobin

FIGURE 9-5 ■ Iron deficiency anemia. The tongue is devoid of filiform papillae. Angular cheilitis was also present in this patient.

synthesis; therefore in iron deficiency anemia the red blood cells appear smaller than normal (microcytic) and lighter in color than normal **(hypochromic).** Increasing the intake of iron is the treatment for iron deficiency anemia; dietary supplements are usually used. The oral lesions resolve when the deficiency is corrected.

PERNICIOUS ANEMIA

Pernicious anemia is a vitamin B_{12} deficiency that is caused by a deficiency of intrinsic factor, a substance secreted by the parietal cells of the stomach. Intrinsic factor is necessary for the absorption of vitamin B_{12}. Normally vitamin B_{12} is transported across the intestinal mucosa by intrinsic factor. An autoimmune mechanism is the most likely cause of this type of pernicious anemia. Antibodies to components of gastric mucosa have been identified in patients with pernicious anemia. Other causes include surgical removal of the stomach (gastrectomy), gastric cancer, or gastritis. Vitamin B_{12} is needed for DNA synthesis; when it is lacking, the development of rapidly dividing cells such as bone marrow cells and epithelial cells is affected.

Clinical Features and Oral Manifestations

The clinical signs of pernicious anemia are weakness, pallor, fatigue, and shortness of breath on exertion. Other constitutional signs can include nausea, dizziness, diarrhea, abdominal pain, loss of appetite, and weight loss. Neurologic changes such as severe paresthesia may also occur in patients with pernicious anemia.

Oral manifestations of pernicious anemia include angular cheilitis; mucosal pallor; painful, atrophic, and erythematous mucosa; mucosal ulceration; loss of papillae on the dorsum of the tongue; and burning and painful tongue (Figure 9-6).

Diagnosis and Treatment

The diagnosis of pernicious anemia is made by laboratory testing. The diagnostic features include low serum vitamin

FIGURE 9-6 ■ Pernicious anemia. **A,** Angular cheilitis and depapillation of the tongue in a patient with pernicious anemia. **B,** The mucosa becomes atrophic in pernicious anemia and easily ulcerated. Note ulcer on left lateral aspect of tongue.

B_{12} levels and gastric achlorhydria (lack of hydrochloric acid). Pernicious anemia is a megaloblastic anemia. **Megaloblastic anemia** is characterized by red blood cells that are immature, abnormally large, and have nuclei **(megaloblasts).** Immature neutrophils and platelets are also seen in both the bone marrow and the circulating blood. The Schilling test, which detects an inability to absorb an oral dose of vitamin B_{12} (cyanocobalamin), is another method used to diagnose pernicious anemia. Another test used more frequently today that is specific for pernicious anemia is one that identifies the presence of serum antibodies directed against intrinsic factor. Treatment consists of injections of vitamin B_{12}. The oral mucosa improves in time, but the papillae on the dorsum of the tongue may not regenerate completely.

FOLIC ACID AND VITAMIN B_{12} DEFICIENCY ANEMIA

Dietary deficiencies of **folic acid** and **vitamin B_{12}** can result in anemia and can occur in association with malnutrition and increased metabolic requirements. Malnutrition can occur in association with alcoholism, and pregnant women can experience a deficiency because of increased metabolic demands. Folic acid and vitamin B_{12} are essential for DNA synthesis.

Oral Manifestations

The oral manifestations are indistinguishable from those of pernicious anemia.

Diagnosis and Treatment

The diagnosis of these anemias is based on laboratory test results that include serum assays of folic acid and vitamin B_{12}. These are also megaloblastic anemias. Thus, as in pernicious anemia, the red blood cells are immature, abnormally large, and nucleated (megaloblasts). Treatment involves dietary supplements.

THALASSEMIA

Thalassemia, also called *Mediterranean* or **Cooley anemia,** is the name of a group of inherited disorders of hemoglobin synthesis (see Chapter 6). It has an autosomal inheritance pattern and both heterozygous and homozygous forms; no predilection for either sex is seen. The heterozygous form in which only one gene at a locus is involved, is called **thalassemia minor** and can be asymptomatic or only mildly symptomatic. The homozygous form, in which the genes on both chromosomes are involved, is called **thalassemia major** and is associated with severe hemolytic anemia, which results from damage to the red blood cell membranes and destruction of the red blood cells.

Clinical Features and Oral Manifestations

The severe form of the disease begins early in life. The child has a yellowish skin pallor, fever, malaise, and weakness. An enlarged liver and spleen are common. The characteristic facies includes prominent cheekbones, depression of the bridge of the nose, an unusual prominence of the premaxilla, and protrusion or flaring of the maxillary anterior teeth. Intraoral radiographs show a peculiar trabecular pattern, showing reduced trabeculation of the maxilla and mandible. There is a prominence of some trabeculae and a blurring and disappearance of others, resulting in a "salt and pepper" effect. Thinning of the lamina dura and circular radiolucencies in the alveolar bone have also been described. Lateral skull radiographs may demonstrate the characteristic "hair-on-end" appearance.

Treatment

Treatment of thalassemia major is experimental. Blood transfusions and splenectomy have provided periods of remission. The prognosis is poor. However, these supportive therapies have extended life from early childhood to about 20 years of age. Multiple and frequent blood transfusions can lead to death due to deposition of excessive iron throughout the body (hemochromatosis).

SICKLE CELL ANEMIA

Sickle cell anemia is an inherited significant disorder of the blood that is found predominantly in black individuals and those of Mediterranean or Asian origin. Persons who are heterozygous for the disease are generally asymptomatic. This is called **sickle cell trait.** Those who are homozygous are much more severely affected. The disease presents before age 30 years. Sickle cell anemia occurs as a result of an abnormal type of hemoglobin in red blood cells. Because of this abnormal hemoglobin, the cells develop a sickle shape in the presence of decreased oxygen; hence the name *sickle cell anemia*. Exercise, exertion, administration of a general anesthetic, pregnancy, or even sleep can trigger a sickling of the red blood cells. Because of the change in their shape, the red blood cells are no longer able to pass through small blood vessels and are destroyed more rapidly than normal.

Clinical Features and Oral Manifestations

The patient with sickle cell anemia experiences weakness, shortness of breath, fatigue, joint pain, and nausea. Two severe systemic characteristics of sickle cell anemia include sickle cell crisis (severe sickling of erythrocytes) and acute chest syndrome (in which there is pulmonary involvement). Abnormalities in kidney function, the eyes, the cardiovascular system, and the central nervous system have all been reported. All organs and tissues of the body can be affected by sickle cell anemia. Oral manifestations are seen on dental radiographs (Figure 9-7). A loss of trabeculation takes place, with the appearance of large, irregular marrow spaces. This change is most prominent in the alveolar bone. Changes in the skull have been described as a "hair-on-end" pattern because the trabeculae radiate outward.

Diagnosis and Treatment

The sickle-shaped cells may be seen on a blood smear (Figure 9-8). The number of red blood cells is usually low, as is the hemoglobin content. Management of sickle cell anemia is largely symptomatic and supportive and involves the administration of oxygen and intravenous and oral fluids. Sickle cell anemia can result in profound changes of the heart, such as enlargement, and lead to cardiac failure.

FIGURE 9-7 ■ Sickle cell anemia. Radiograph shows abnormal trabeculation. (Courtesy Dr. Edward V. Zegarelli.)

of agranulocytosis have been described. The cause of the primary form is unknown; it may be an immunologic disorder. The secondary form of agranulocytosis is most commonly produced by chemotherapeutic drugs and other immunologic reactions. Secondary agranulocytosis is most commonly seen in women.

Clinical Features and Oral Manifestations

After ingesting the offending drug, clinically patients experience a sudden onset of high fever, chills, jaundice **(icterus)**, weakness, and sore throat. Orally the most characteristic feature is the presence of ulcerations and infection. Necrotizing ulcerations, excessive bleeding from the gingiva, and rapid destruction of the supporting tissue of the teeth have been described. Regional lymphadenopathy can accompany the oral problems.

Diagnosis and Treatment

The diagnosis is made by laboratory testing. The white blood cell count, which is normally 4,500 to 10,000 cells/microliter is dramatically reduced to less than 1,000 cells/microliter. Treatment includes transfusions; antibiotics to control infection; and, in the secondary form, removal of the causative agent. Infections can become overwhelming and cause death. All surgical procedures, including dental hygiene procedures, are contraindicated.

CYCLIC NEUTROPENIA

Cyclic neutropenia is a form of agranulocytosis. A severe depression of granulocytes (neutrophils) occurs at periodic intervals. The main cause is a mutation of the gene *ELA-2*. This disorder is characterized by cycles every 21 to 27 days, when there is a sharp decrease in the neutrophil count that lasts 2 to 3 days. This decrease in neutrophils causes gingival inflammation, and ulceration of the tongue and mucosal tissues. The ulcerations vary in size, are very painful and usually become infected until the neutrophils return to normal. Cyclic neutropenia is described in greater detail in Chapter 6.

LEUKEMIA

Leukemias are malignant neoplasms of the hematopoietic (blood-forming) stem cells. They are disorders that primarily originate in the stem cells of the bone marrow. The most dramatic feature of leukemias is the excessive number of abnormal white blood cells in the circulating blood. The pathogenesis is unknown. However, current investigations are focusing on oncogenic viruses (see Chapter 7). Many different types of leukemia exist. They are classified on the basis of the cell type involved and the maturity of the neoplastic cells (Box 9-2). Leukemias are described in this chapter with other abnormalities of the blood. They also have been included in Chapter 7, together with other white blood cell neoplasms. Many different types of leukemia are known; this text gives only an overview of the two general categories, acute and chronic, with focus on the oral manifestations. Oral lesions are most common in acute leukemias but may also occur in chronic forms.

BOX 9-2

Classification of Leukemias

Acute Leukemias
Acute lymphoblastic (lymphocytes) leukemia
Acute nonlymphoblastic leukemia (granulocytes, monocytes, erythrocytes)

Chronic Leukemias
Chronic lymphocytic leukemia
Chronic myelogenous (myeloid, granulocytic) leukemia

Acute Leukemias

Acute leukemias are characterized by the presence of very immature cells (blast cells) and by a rapidly fatal course if not treated. They can involve immature lymphocytes (acute lymphoblastic leukemia) or immature granulocytes (acute myelogenous or myeloid leukemia). Acute lymphoblastic leukemia primarily affects children and young adults and has a good prognosis. Acute myeloblastic leukemia involves adolescents and young adults (age range, 15 to 39 yr), and the prognosis is not as good. The onset of acute leukemia is sudden and dramatic.

Clinical Features. Clinically, patients experience weakness, fever, enlargement of lymph nodes, and bleeding. The lymph node enlargement can include cervical lymphadenopathy (enlargement of the lymph nodes in the neck) and is typically seen earlier in the course of disease, with the leukemias involving immature lymphocytes. A general loss of cells produced by the bone marrow occurs. The fatigue results mainly from anemia, the fever from infection, and the bleeding from a decrease in platelets (thrombocytopenia). In advanced disease enlargement of the spleen **(splenomegaly)** and liver **(hepatomegaly)** occurs when these organs are infiltrated by the leukemic cells.

Oral Manifestations. Oral manifestations can include gingival enlargement (which can be severe) caused by infiltration of leukemic cells (Figure 9-11) and oral infections (including necrotizing ulcerative gingivitis) because the white blood cells are not functioning. In addition, if a decrease in platelets occurs, bleeding gums, petechiae, and ecchymoses may be present. Toothache as the result of invasion of the pulp by leukemic cells has been reported.

Diagnosis and Treatment. In acute leukemia laboratory findings include an elevated white blood cell count with the presence of many immature cells, anemia, and a low platelet count. In young children with acute lymphocytic leukemia, the prognosis with treatment is very good. In adolescents and adults with acute myelogenous (myeloid) leukemia the prognosis is poor. Remissions occur with chemotherapy, and then relapses occur. Bone marrow transplantation is a treatment for this form of leukemia.

Chronic Leukemias

In addition, several different types of chronic leukemia exist. They are all characterized by a slow onset, and they all primarily affect adults. The disease can be present for months before a diagnosis is made, and occasionally the diagnosis is

FIGURE 9-11 ■ Generalized gingival hyperplasia in a patient with leukemia. (Courtesy Dr. Edward V. Zegarelli.)

made during a routine physical examination based on laboratory testing. One of the forms of chronic leukemia, chronic myeloid leukemia, is associated with a distinctive chromosomal abnormality, the Philadelphia chromosome. Another form of chronic leukemia, chronic lymphocytic leukemia, is the most common form and accounts for about one quarter of the total cases of leukemia. It may be asymptomatic for a long time. About half the patients with this type of leukemia have abnormal karyotypes; however, the abnormality is different from the Philadelphia chromosome.

Clinical Features and Oral Manifestations. The clinical onset is slow. The symptoms are nonspecific and include easy fatigability, weakness, weight loss, and anorexia. Oral manifestations include pallor of the lips and gingiva, gingival enlargement, petechiae and ecchymoses, gingival bleeding, and atypical periodontal disease. Cervical lymphadenopathy may be an early manifestation of chronic leukemia.

Diagnosis and Treatment. The normal white blood cell count is 4000 to 11,000/mm³. The white blood cell count in leukemia can increase to 500,000/mm³, and most of the total cells can be leukemia cells. Remissions occur with chemotherapy. High doses of chemotherapy over a short time is called *induction chemotherapy*. This type of therapy results in multiple unpleasant side effects for the patient. Cryotherapy (sucking on crushed ice during the administrations of intravenous chemotherapy) decreases the oral ulceration. After induction chemotherapy, once remission has started, low-dose chemotherapy over a longer period of time, referred to as *maintenance chemotherapy*, is the standard protocol. Bone marrow transplantation is used to treat both chronic and acute leukemia.

CELIAC DISEASE

Celiac disease (celiac sprue, gluten-sensitive enteropathy) is a chronic disorder associated with sensitivity to dietary gluten, a protein found in wheat and wheat products. When gluten is ingested, there is injury to the intestinal mucosa. Malabsorption of other nutrients such as vitamin B₁₂ and folic acid occurs because of mucosal injury and anemia develops as a result.

CLINICAL FEATURES AND ORAL MANIFESTATIONS

Systemic symptoms include diarrhea, nervousness, and paresthesia of the extremities.

Oral manifestations are the same as those that occur in anemia due to other causes. These include a painful burning tongue (glossitis), atrophy of the papillae of the tongue, and ulceration of the oral mucosa.

DIAGNOSIS AND TREATMENT

Patients should adhere to a gluten-free diet. Oral manifestations resolve when the systemic disease is under control.

BLEEDING DISORDERS

HEMOSTASIS

Patients with bleeding disorders can have one of a number of different defects.

Hemostasis (the cessation of bleeding) is a complex process that involves a number of events (Figure 9-12). When a blood vessel is damaged, marked constriction of the vessel (vasoconstriction) occurs in an attempt to stop the flow of blood. Platelets **(thrombocytes)** that are produced by the bone marrow and circulating in blood adhere to the damaged surface and aggregate to form a temporary clot. To stop the bleeding permanently, it is necessary for **fibrin** to be produced. Fibrin tightly binds the aggregating platelets to form a clot. A cascade of circulating plasma proteins that are made almost exclusively in the liver and called **clotting factors** or **coagulation factors** is necessary to convert the precursor fibrinogen to fibrin (Table 9-1 and Figure 9-13).

Finally, anticlotting mechanisms are activated to prevent the spread of more clots and to allow the clot to dissolve so that the damaged vessel can be repaired. This complexity is necessary to prevent inappropriate clotting. Successful hemostasis depends on the walls of the blood vessels, adequate numbers of functioning platelets, and adequate levels of properly functioning clotting factors.

Defects in hemostasis are caused by abnormalities of either platelets or coagulation factors. These defects can be diagnosed with a few laboratory tests (Table 9-2). Normal values may differ according to the specific test used and the individual laboratory.

Platelet Count

The **platelet count,** which is usually requested with a CBC, provides a quantitative or numeric evaluation of platelets. A normal platelet count should be 200,000 to 400,000/mm³. A platelet count less than 100,000/mm³ is considered thrombocytopenia. Spontaneous gingival bleeding can occur when a patient's platelet count is less than 20,000/mm³. In addition, a physician can request specific clotting factor assays, which can also be performed in

FIGURE 9-20 ■ Osteonecrosis associated with bisphosphonate therapy involving the mandible.

condition in patients receiving bisphosphonate medications include dentoalveolar surgery, history of inflammatory dental disease, and trauma to areas such as tori and exostoses where minimal soft tissue protects the bone. At present, there is no well-defined treatment for this condition. The medication remains in the bone for many years and therefore, discontinuation of the medication is not indicated to prevent or manage the condition.

SELECTED REFERENCES

Books

Greenberg MS, Glick M, Ship JA: *Burket's oral medicine*, ed 11, Hamilton, 2008, BC Dekker.

Kumar V, Abbas AK, Fausto N, et al: *Robbins and Cotran pathologic basis of disease*, ed 8, Philadelphia, 2010, Saunders Elsevier.

Little JW, Falace D, Miller C, et al: *Dental management of the medically compromised patient*, ed 8, St. Louis, 2012, Mosby.

Neville BW, Damm DD, Allen CM, et al: *Oral and maxillofacial pathology*, ed 3, St. Louis, 2009, Saunders.

Sciubba JJ, Regezi JA, Jordan RCK: *Oral pathology: clinical-pathologic correlations*, ed 6, Philadelphia, 2012, Saunders.

Wynn RL, Meiller TF, Crossley HL: *Drug information handbook for dentistry*, ed 18, Hudson, Ohio, 2012, Lexi-Comp.

Journal Articles

Avcu N, Avcu F, Beyan C, et al: The relationship between gastric-oral *Helicobacter pylori* and oral hygiene in patients with vitamin B_{12}-deficiency anemia, *Oral Surg Oral Med Oral Pathol Oral Radiol Endod* 92:166, 2001.

Barclay L: HbA1c may be useful for diabetes screening, diagnosis in routine clinical practice, *Medscape Today News*, January 22, 2010. Available at: http://www.medscape.com/viewarticle/715565

Centers for Disease Control and Prevention: Iron deficiency—United States, 1999-2000, *MMWR Morb Mortal Wkly Rep* 51:89, 2002.

Chávez EM, Borrell LN, Taylor GW, et al: A longitudinal analysis of salivary flow in control subjects and older adults with type 2 diabetes, *Oral Surg Oral Med Oral Pathol Oral Radiol Endod* 91:166, 2001.

Collin HL, Niskanen L, Uusitupa M, et al: Oral symptoms and signs in elderly patients with type 2 diabetes mellitus, *Oral Surg Oral Med Oral Pathol Oral Radiol Endod* 90:299, 2000.

Couri CE, Voltarelli JC: Stem cell therapy for type 1 diabetes mellitus: a review of recent clinical trials, *Diabetol Metab Syndr* 1:19, 2009. Available at: http://www.dmsjournal.com/content/1/1/19

Fletcher PD, Scopp IV, Hersh RA: Oral manifestations of secondary hyperparathyroidism related to long-term hemodialysis therapy, *Oral Surg Oral Med Oral Pathol* 43:218, 1977.

Garg AK, Malo M: Manifestations and treatment of xerostomia and associated oral effects secondary to head and neck radiation therapy, *J Am Dent Assoc* 128:1128, 1997.

Hardin DS: Screening for type 2 diabetes in children with acanthosis nigricans, *Diabetes Educ* 32:547, 2006.

Hess LM, Jeter JM, Benham-Hutchins M, et al: Factors associated with osteonecrosis of the jaw among bisphosphonate users, *Am J Med* 121:475, 2008.

Inokuchi T, Sano K, Kamingo M: Osteoradionecrosis of the sphenoid and temporal bones in a patient with maxillary sinus carcinoma: a case report, *Oral Surg Oral Med Oral Pathol* 70:278, 1990.

Khocht A, Schneider LC: Periodontal management of gingival overgrowth in the heart transplant patient: a case report, *J Periodontol* 68:1140, 1997.

Kong AS, Williams RL, Smith M, et al; RIOS Net Clinicians: Acanthosis nigricans and diabetes risk factors: prevalence in young persons seen in southwestern US primary care practices, *Ann Fam Med* 5:202, 2007.

McDonough RJ, Nelson CL: Clinical implications of factor XII deficiency, *Oral Surg Oral Med Oral Pathol* 68:264, 1989.

Miranda J et al: Prevalence and risk of gingival enlargement in patients treated with nifedipine, *J Periodontol* 72:605, 2001.

Moore PA, Weyant RJ, Etzel KR, et al: Type 1 diabetes mellitus and oral health: assessment of coronal and root caries, *Community Dent Oral Epidemiol* 29:183, 2001.

Moore PA, Guggenheimer J, Etzel KR, et al: Type 1 diabetes mellitus, xerostomia and salivary flow rates, *Oral Surg Oral Med Oral Pathol Oral Radiol Endod* 92:281, 2001.

Ohishi M, Oobu K, Miyanoshita Y, et al: Acute gingival necrosis caused by drug-induced agranulocytosis, *Oral Surg Oral Med Oral Pathol* 66:194, 1988.

Redding SW, Luce EB, Boren MW: Oral herpes simplex virus infection in patients receiving head and neck radiation, *Oral Surg Oral Med Oral Pathol* 69:578, 1990.

Ruggiero SL, Drew SJ: Osteonecrosis of the jaws and bisphosphonate therapy, *J Dent Res* 86:1013, 2007.

Shanshan L, Paige LW, Douglass CW: JADA continuing education: development of a clinical guideline to predict undiagnosed diabetes in dental patients, *J Am Dent Assoc* 142:28, 2011.

Sreebny LM, Valdini A, Yu A: Xerostomia. II. Relationship to nonoral symptoms, drugs and diseases, *Oral Surg Oral Med Oral Pathol* 68:419, 1989.

Teeuw NJ, Gerdes VE, Loos BG: Effect of periodontal treatment in glycemic control of diabetic patients: a systematic review and meta-analysis, *Diabetes Care* 33:421, 2010.

Vernillo AT: Dental considerations for the treatment of patients with diabetes mellitus, *J Am Dent Assoc* 134:24S, 2003.

Wahlin YB: Effects of chlorhexidine mouth rinse on oral health in patients with acute leukemia, *Oral Surg Oral Med Oral Pathol* 68:279, 1989.

Wu J, Fantasia JE, Kaplan R: Oral manifestations of acute myelomonocytic leukemia: a case report and review of the classification of leukemias, *J Periodontol* 73:664, 2002.

Newspaper Articles

Kleinfield NR: Diabetes and its awful toll quietly emerge as a crisis, *The New York Times*, January 9, 2006, pp A1, A18-A19.

Kleinfield NR: Living at an epicenter of diabetes: defiance and despair, *The New York Times*, January 10, 2006, pp A1, A20-A21.

Santora M: East meets West, adding pounds and peril, *The New York Times*, January 12, 2006, pp A1, A22-A23.

Urbina I: In the treatment of diabetes, success often does not pay, *The New York Times*, January 11, 2006, pp A1, A22-A23.

Websites

Mayo Clinic: Gestational diabetes. Available at: http://www.mayoclinic.com/health/gestational-diabetes/DS00316/DSECTION=symptoms

http://www.diabeteseducator.org/export/sites/aade/resources/pdf/Insulin_Pump_White_Paper.pdf.

Review Questions

1. Hyperpituitarism results from an excessive production of growth hormone. Which of the following most often causes it?
   A. Pituitary adenoma
   B. Pituitary sarcoma
   C. Carcinoma in situ
   D. Ameloblastoma

2. Hyperthyroidism in children can lead to:
   A. Partial anodontia
   B. Amelogenesis imperfecta
   C. Ankylosis
   D. Early exfoliation of the deciduous dentition and early eruption of the permanent teeth

3. Hypercalcemia, hypophosphatemia, and abnormal bone metabolism are characteristic of which of the following conditions?
   A. Hyperthyroidism
   B. Hypothyroidism
   C. Hyperparathyroidism
   D. Hyperpituitarism

4. Which of the following is typically an acute metabolic complication of uncontrolled diabetes mellitus?
   A. Eye damage
   B. Ketoacidosis
   C. Atherosclerosis
   D. End-stage kidney failure

5. Polydipsia, polyuria, and polyphagia are all characteristic of which of the following?
   A. Hyperparathyroidism
   B. Hyperthyroidism
   C. Type 1 diabetes mellitus
   D. Addison disease

6. Which of the following is *not* a feature of type 2 diabetes mellitus?
   A. Those with it have increased insulin resistance.
   B. It typically occurs at 40 years of age or older.
   C. Autoimmunity is the key to its development.
   D. Glucose control can be achieved without daily insulin injections in many cases.

7. Which of the following oral complications is *not* typically associated with diabetes mellitus?
   A. Candidiasis
   B. Xerostomia
   C. Excessive periodontal bone loss
   D. Multilocular radiolucencies with pathologic fracture

8. Which one of the following is *false* concerning Addison disease?
   A. It is also known as primary adrenal cortical insufficiency.
   B. There may be bronzing of the skin.
   C. It may be caused by a malignant tumor that destroys the adrenal gland.
   D. The patient may experience pathologic fracture.

9. Which of the following statements is *false* regarding diabetes mellitus?
   A. Candidiasis may be indicative of compromised immunity in a patient with diabetes.
   B. Hypoglycemic agents are more commonly used in the treatment of type 2 diabetes than in type 1 diabetes.
   C. Microvascular disease typically affects eyes, kidneys, and nerves.
   D. Diabetes mellitus is not considered a syndrome.

10. Which of the following statements is *false*?
    A. Primary immunodeficiencies are less common than secondary immunodeficiencies.
    B. Persons with T-lymphocyte deficiencies are susceptible to viral and fungal infections.
    C. All primary immunodeficiencies are combined B-lymphocyte and T-lymphocyte deficiencies.
    D. Secondary immunodeficiency can result from corticosteroid medication.

11. Which one of the following is *not* a cause of iron deficiency anemia?
    A. Chronic blood loss
    B. A deficiency of iron intake
    C. An increased requirement for iron
    D. Normal bone marrow function

12. Thalassemia major is:
    A. Caused by a nutritional deficiency
    B. The same as celiac sprue
    C. An autoimmune condition
    D. Associated with a severe hemolytic anemia

13. Achlorhydria, failure to absorb vitamin B_{12}, and megaloblastic anemia are characteristic features of which of the following?
    A. Pernicious anemia
    B. Thalassemia
    C. Sickle cell anemia
    D. Thrombocytopenic purpura

Continued

CHAPTER 9 *Synopsis—cont'd*

CONDITION/ DISEASE	CAUSE	AGE/RACE/SEX	LOCATION
Cyclic neutropenia	Autosomal dominant gene ELA-2, 19p13.3	From birth M=F	Oral mucosa and periodontium
Leukemias	Neoplastic Oncogenic viruses suggested	Children (acute lymphoblastic) Adolescents and young adults (acute myelogenous) Adults (chronic)	Systemic disease
Celiac disease	Sensitivity to dietary gluten resulting in injury to the intestinal mucosa and subsequent anemia	N/A	Systemic disease
Thrombocytopenic purpura: • Idiopathic (primary and autoimmune) types • Secondary type	Severe reduction in circulating platelets Idiopathic: cause unknown Autoimmune: drugs, often chemotherapeutic agents	Primary and autoimmune types: usually children and young adults No age predilection for secondary type	Systemic disease
Hemophilia: • Type A • Type B (Christmas disease)	Inherited (X-linked) • Type A: factor VIII deficiency • Type B: factor IX deficiency	Identified in childhood Affects boys	Systemic disease
Bisphosphonate-associated osteonecrosis	Bisphosphonate therapy for osteoporosis, multiple myeloma, metastatic carcinoma of the breast and prostate, and Paget disease	N/A	Maxilla and mandible

N/A, Not applicable.
*Not covered in text.

CLINICAL FEATURES	RADIOGRAPHIC FEATURES	MICROSCOPIC FEATURES	TREATMENT	DIAGNOSTIC PROCESS
Gingivitis, periodontitis, ulcers, hemorrhage	Alveolar bone loss, pocket formation	Cyclic diminished neutrophils in peripheral blood	Root planing, scaling, antibiotics G-CSF	Clinical and blood studies
Acute: sudden onset of symptoms; weakness, fever, lymph node enlargement, bleeding, enlarged liver and spleen; gingival enlargement because of infiltration of leukemic cells, oral infections, spontaneous gingival bleeding, petechiae, and ecchymoses Chronic: slow onset of symptoms; easy fatigability, weakness, weight loss, anorexia; pallor of the lips and gingiva, gingival enlargement, petechiae, ecchymoses, gingival bleeding, and atypical periodontal disease	N/A	*	Acute: chemotherapy, bone marrow transplantation Chronic: induction and maintenance chemotherapy, bone marrow transplantation	Laboratory
Same clinical features as for anemias; diarrhea, nervousness, and paresthesia of the extremities	N/A	*	Adherence to gluten-free diet	*
Spontaneous hemorrhagic lesions of the skin and/or mucosa Gingival bleeding Frequent nosebleeds Blood in urine (hematuria)	N/A	N/A	Transfusions, systemic corticosteroids, splenectomy Discontinuation of causative agent	Laboratory
Spontaneous bleeding, petechiae, ecchymoses Risk of hemorrhage after oral surgery and dental hygiene procedures	N/A	N/A	Replacement of missing clotting factors	Laboratory
Exposed bone persisting more than 8 wk in a patient taking bisphosphonate medication	*	*	*	Clinical Microscopic (rule out metastatic disease)

Chapter 10

Diseases Affecting the Temporomandibular Joint

Kenneth E. Fleisher

OBJECTIVES

After studying this chapter, the student will be able to:

1. Label the following on a diagram of the temporomandibular joint: glenoid fossa of the temporal bone, articular disk, mandibular condyle, joint capsule, and superior belly of the lateral pterygoid muscle.
2. State the function of the muscles of mastication.
3. List at least five causes of orofacial pain *not* including dental conditions and temporomandibular disorders.
4. State three factors that have been implicated in the cause of temporomandibular disorders and three questions that would be appropriate to ask of a patient suspected of having a temporomandibular disorder.
5. List at least two symptoms that are suggestive of temporomandibular dysfunction.
6. List three imaging techniques useful for evaluating the temporomandibular joint and describe the rationale for each one.
7. List five types of temporomandibular disorders.
8. List and describe the two main categories of treatment of temporomandibular disorders.
9. State the names of one benign tumor and one malignant tumor that may affect the temporomandibular joint area.

VOCABULARY

Arthrocentesis (ahr″thro-sen-te′sis) Surgical puncture of a joint followed by lavage of the joint space.

Arthrography (ahr-throg′rə-fe) Radiography of a joint after injection of opaque contrast material.

Arthroscopy (ahr-thros′kə-pe) Method for evaluating and manipulating a joint via the insertion of a camera and instruments.

Articulation (ahr-tik″u-la′shən) Joint.

Auscultation (aws″kəl-ta′shən) Listening to sounds within the body, using a stethoscope.

Crepitus (krep′ĭ-təs) Dry, crackling sound.

Iatrogenic (i-at″ro-jen′ik) Induced inadvertently by a medical or dental care provider or by medical treatment or a diagnostic procedure.

Magnetic resonance imaging (mag-net′ik rez′o-nəns im′ə-jing) MRI; noninvasive diagnostic technique that uses radio waves to produce computerized images of internal body tissues.

Palpation (pal-pa′shən) Physical examination, using pressure of the hand or fingers.

Sign (sīn) Objective evidence of disease that can be observed by a health care provider rather than by the patient.

Symptom (simp′təm) Subjective evidence of disease or a physical disorder that is observed by the patient.

Trismus (triz′məs) Inability to fully open the mouth.

Knowledge of the anatomy and function of the temporomandibular joint (TMJ) enables the dental hygienist to understand the diseases that affect the joint. Disorders of the TMJ include myofascial pain and dysfunction (MPD), internal derangements, osteoarthritis, and rheumatoid arthritis (Box 10-1). Benign and malignant tumors can also affect the TMJ.

ANATOMY OF THE TEMPOROMANDIBULAR JOINT

The TMJ is the **articulation** between the condyle of the mandible and the glenoid fossa of the temporal bone (Figure 10-1). It is a highly specialized joint that differs from other joints because of the fibrocartilage that covers the bony articulating surfaces, its ginglymoarthrodial (rotational and

---

BOX 10-1

Commonly Used Abbreviations

MPD: Myofascial pain and dysfunction
TMD: Temporomandibular disorder
TMJ: Temporomandibular joint
ID: Internal derangement

---

translational) movement, the fact that its function and overall health are dictated by jaw movement, and its dependence on the contralateral joint. An articular disk is interposed in the space between the temporal bone and the mandible. This disk divides the space into an upper compartment (superior joint space) and a lower compartment (inferior joint space) (Figure 10-1).

Translational movements occur in the upper compartment, whereas the lower compartment functions primarily as the hinge or rotational component. The superior and inferior spaces contain **synovial fluid,** which is produced by the **synovial membrane** that lines the joint. The synovial fluid provides nourishment and lubrication of the avascular structures. The articular disk is attached to the lateral and medial aspects of the condyle, to the superior belly of the lateral pterygoid muscle, and to the joint capsule (Figure 10-1). The articular disk and the bony surfaces are avascular (i.e., they do not contain blood vessels) and devoid of nerve fibers. The joint is further surrounded and protected by the fibrous connective tissue joint capsule. The primary innervation of the TMJ capsule and disk attachments is from the auriculotemporal nerve with secondary innervation from the deep temporal and masseteric nerves. The function of the disk is to separate the forces resulting from rotation

A

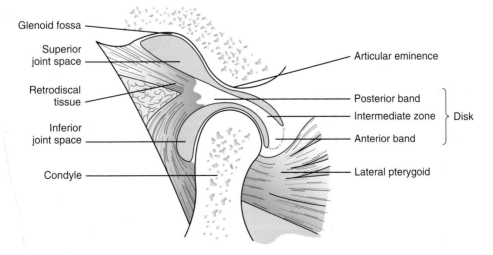

FIGURE 10-1 ■ Lateral views of the temporomandibular joint. **A,** Jaw closed. **B,** Jaw open. (From Kaplan AS, Assael LA: *Temporomandibular disorders,* Philadelphia, 1991, Saunders.)

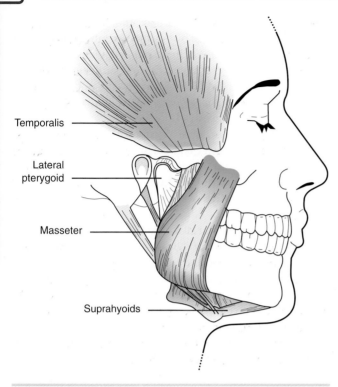

FIGURE 10-2 ■ Muscles of mastication: the temporalis, lateral pterygoid, masseter, and suprahyoid. (From Kaplan AS, Assael LA: *Temporomandibular disorders*, Philadelphia, 1991, Saunders.)

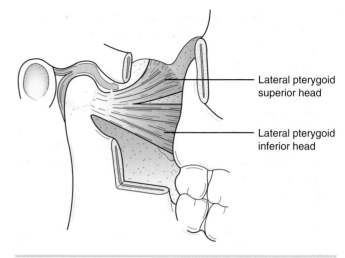

FIGURE 10-3 ■ Muscles of mastication. The two distinct heads of the lateral pterygoid muscle are illustrated. (From Kaplan AS, Assael LA: *Temporomandibular disorders*, Philadelphia, 1991, Saunders.)

and translation, absorb shock, improve the fit between bony surfaces, protect the edges of the articulating surfaces, distribute weight over a larger area, and spread the lubricating synovial fluid.

Understanding the location and action of the **muscles of mastication** is important in the evaluation of disorders affecting the TMJ. **Palpation** of these muscles during a clinical evaluation is done to determine whether muscle spasm or dysfunctional muscle activity is occurring. The muscles of mastication comprise major muscles about the facial region that govern the movement of the mandible. They include the masseter, temporalis, medial pterygoid, lateral pterygoid, anterior digastric, and mylohyoid (suprahyoids) (Figures 10-2 to 10-4). The function of these muscles is to create the mandibular envelope of motion. Three of these muscles, the masseter, medial pterygoid, and temporalis, are elevator muscles that, when activated, close the mandible. The opening, or depressor, function is accomplished mainly by the lateral pterygoid muscle with some help from the anterior digastric muscle. Studies have shown that the two components of the lateral pterygoid muscle are active at different times in the functioning of the mandible (Figure 10-4). The superior portion of the muscle seats the articular disk on the eminence of the articulating surface. The inferior belly is attached to the mandibular condyle and functions during mouth opening.

NORMAL JOINT FUNCTION

The harmonious function of the TMJ depends on various factors. The anatomic relationship of the condyle-disk

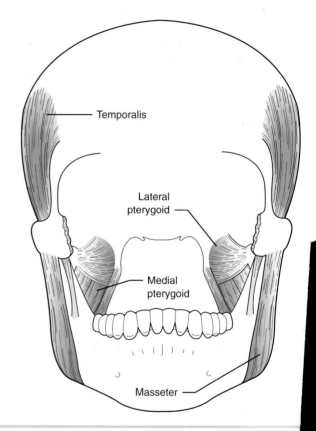

FIGURE 10-4 ■ Muscles of mastication. Illustrated are the four p[ ] muscles of mastication: the masseter, temporalis, medial ptery[ ] and lateral pterygoid. (From Kaplan AS, Assael LA: *Temporomandi[ ] disorders*, Philadelphia, 1991, Saunders.)

complex governs the smooth functioning of the man[ ] This articulation, along with the muscles of mastica[ ] provides the movement of the mandible. The muscl[ ] mastication are the machinery that powers mandi[ ] movement; the anatomic joint structures such a[ ] condyle, articular eminence, and disk act as the ge[ ] bearings of the jaw.

In **normal joint function** the jaw begins at a rest position of maximal occlusal contact. In this position the mandibular condyle rests within the glenoid fossa, with the articular disk situated between the condyle, roof of the glenoid fossa, and articular eminence (see Figure 10-1, *A* and *B*). The first phase of opening is characterized by rotational (hinge) movement of the condyle, followed by anterior translation (sliding movement) to approximately the anterior peak of the articular eminence. During translation the disk assumes a more posterior position in relation to the condyle. The inferior and superior joint spaces assume different configurations during each of these movements.

TEMPOROMANDIBULAR DISORDERS

EPIDEMIOLOGY

Temporomandibular disorders (TMDs) are caused by abnormalities in the functioning of the TMJ or associated structures. TMDs, which have been a clinical and diagnostic challenge in dentistry for many years, are reported to affect up to 36 million adults in the United States. Hippocrates documented jaw dysfunction problems as early as the fifth century BCE. However, it was not until 1934 that James Costen, an otolaryngologist, described a group of symptoms centered around the jaw and ear. Costen syndrome included such symptoms as impaired hearing, ear pain, tinnitus, dizziness, burning in the throat and tongue, headache, and trismus. Although most if not all of Costen's explanations have been refuted, the dental profession's interest was stimulated by his view that malocclusion plays a pivotal role in this condition. The 1980s were marked by a growing interest in TMDs facilitated by advances in pain neurophysiology, multicenter research, the American Academy of Craniomandibular Disorders (later to become the American Academy of Orofacial Pain), the American Dental Association, and pivotal work published in 1986 by Sanders for the treatment of closed lock by arthroscopy.

Although up to 75% of the adult population has at least one sign, with 33% having at least one symptom, most studies suggest that clinically significant TMD-related jaw pain, dysfunction, or both affects 10% to 16% of the adult population. The majority of patients with TMDs are female aged between 20 and 40 years, and some researchers suggest that female sex hormones may have a role in the pathogenesis. Furthermore, TMDs are often associated with comorbid conditions such as depression, rheumatoid arthritis, chronic fatigue syndrome, chronic headache, fibromyalgia, sleep disturbances, and irritable bowel syndrome.

PATHOPHYSIOLOGY

The precise cause of TMDs remains controversial and is often considered multifactorial. Trauma, which overloads the masticatory system, has been suggested as the most likely cause of TMDs. Trauma affecting the TMJ is classified as *direct* (assault), *indirect* (whiplash injury), or secondary to *parafunctional habits* (clenching, bruxism). In addition,

psychosocial factors such as stress have been implicated in masticatory muscle pain. The relationship between TMDs and dentofacial deformity is controversial. Numerous studies continue to dispute the significance of occlusal relationships, and there is little evidence that malocclusion, loss of teeth, loss of vertical dimension, or occlusal instability is the primary cause of TMDs; although these conditions should be addressed to achieve optimal dental occlusion and masticatory function. Nor is there sufficient evidence to suggest that oral surgery procedures (e.g., extraction of third molars) can cause TMDs. TMJ disorders may also be the result of disorders in growth and development as seen in condylar hyperplasia or hypoplasia. The most common systemic conditions that may affect the TMJ are rheumatoid arthritis and juvenile rheumatoid arthritis; less common systemic diseases include Sjögren syndrome, ankylosing spondylitis, psoriatic arthritis, reactive arthritis (Reiter syndrome), systemic lupus erythematosus, scleroderma, mixed connective tissue disease, calcium pyrophosphate deposition disease, and gout. **Iatrogenic** causes (resulting from the action of a health care provider) of TMDs include the indiscriminate use of corticosteroid injection into the joint.

PATIENT EVALUATION

Temporomandibular dysfunction can be caused by disorders of the muscles of mastication or internal derangements of the components of the joint. The "gold standard" for evaluating patients with potential TMDs and establishing a differential diagnosis involves a comprehensive history (i.e., chief complaint, history of the chief complaint, dental and medical history), a thorough clinical examination, and a panoramic radiograph to detect dental, periodontal, or other potential problems. Although dental hygienists do not generally perform comprehensive TMD examinations, they may participate in diagnostic procedures and should recognize risk factors, signs, and symptoms of TMDs to facilitate the appropriate referral. Understanding TMDs is clinically significant for the dental hygienist, as these conditions may impact patient management (e.g., reduced mouth opening, shorter appointment times, pain control). Three cardinal features suggest a TMD: orofacial pain, joint noise, and restricted jaw function.

HISTORY

A history of aberrant growth, previous injuries, illnesses, musculoskeletal complaints, and possible emotional disturbances is an important consideration in the evaluation of patients with TMDs. The patient history specific to TMDs includes questions regarding the following:
- Medical/dental history
- Precipitating events (mastication, spontaneous, yawning, trauma)
- Circumstances that exacerbate or diminish symptoms
- Onset of symptoms (sudden, gradual)
- Joint symptoms (clicking, popping)
- Pain (localized or diffuse; quality such as sharp, dull, burning, aching)

- Problems with mastication
- Trismus
- Malocclusion
- Parafunctional habits (bruxing, clenching, chronic gum chewing)
- Dental symptoms
- Extensive dental or orthodontic treatment
- History of surgical treatment of the jaws

Clicking and popping most commonly reflect disk displacement with reduction and occur in approximately 33% of asymptomatic patients. They are of little clinical consequence in the absence of pain or other symptoms relating to the TMJ, as there is controversy concerning whether these noises represent an adaptive response (i.e., normal variant) or an early symptom of progression to disk displacement without reduction. The incidence of orofacial pain among the adult population has been reported to be 26% and the differential diagnosis includes TMDs, odontogenic pain (e.g., pericoronitis, caries, cracked tooth syndrome, infection, pulpalgia), mucosal disorders, burning mouth syndrome, headache, neuralgia (e.g., trigeminal neuralgia), fibromyalgia, otitis media, sinus infection, cervical spine pain, salivary gland pathology, and tumor (e.g., TMJ, intracranial). Therefore, referral to a medical specialist (e.g., otolaryngologist, neurologist) may be necessary if the patient's signs and/or symptoms are unclear or suggest the presence of other pathology or conditions. Etiologies of **trismus** other than TMDs include odontogenic infection, oral surgery procedures, local anesthetic during dental treatment (e.g., inferior alveolar nerve block, posterior maxillary infiltration), tumors, facial bone fractures, radiation therapy, and medications (e.g., phenothiazine).

CLINICAL EXAMINATION

A comprehensive examination of a patient in relation to TMJ disorders includes an examination of the joint, muscles of mastication (e.g., masseter, temporalis, medial and lateral pterygoid muscles), oral cavity, and cervical spine. Joint examination involves **auscultation** (using a stethoscope) and palpation. The clinician relates joint noises such as clicking, **crepitus** (crackling), or popping to the mandibular movement cycle. Tenderness over the lateral pole of the condyle suggests **capsulitis**. The muscles of mastication are palpated to determine tenderness. The lateral pterygoid muscle cannot be reliably palpated and the superior head can be assessed by asking the patient to bite on tongue blades placed bilaterally over the posterior teeth. The inferior head of the lateral pterygoid muscle can be examined for symptoms by asking the patient to protrude and laterally move the mandible against resistance. In addition to a thorough oral examination, the patient is asked to move the mandible in a normal rotation (hinge) and translatory (forward slide) cycle. Although maximal mouth opening tends to decrease with age, it is generally considered restricted only if it is less than 40 mm. *Deviation* (shifting of the mandible to one side before returning to midline) and *deflection* (shifting of the mandible to one side, with no return to midline) to the right or left side are also observed on maximal interincisal opening. The patient's ability to manipulate the mandible into right and left lateral excursions is also noted. Assisted mouth opening beyond the patient's maximal opening should be attempted to determine additional range of motion and to palpate "end-feel." Muscle restrictions are associated with a soft end-feel, and the range of motion can be increased by 5 mm, unlike disk displacement without reduction, in which assisted opening is less than 5 mm with a firm end-feel. Finally, anesthetic injections (e.g., auriculotemporal nerve block, local infiltration) may be useful to distinguish between arthrogenous (joint-related), myogenous (muscle-related), and odontogenic (dental) pain. Signs of parafunctional habits such as ridging of the buccal mucosa on the inside of the cheeks or abnormal dental attrition should be documented.

IMAGING

Radiographic studies may be helpful in determining the cause of the patient's pain or dysfunction. Several different types of radiographs and views are obtained to determine the shape of the condyle and whether evidence of degenerative joint disease exists (Figures 10-5 and 10-6).

FIGURE 10-5 ■ Panoramic radiograph of a patient with temporomandibular dysfunction and normal anatomy of the mandibular condyles.

FIGURE 10-6 ■ Panoramic radiograph shows resorption of both the right and the left condyles. In this patient degenerative arthritis followed bilateral surgery of the temporomandibular joint. The left coronoid process was removed during surgery.

Radiographic evaluation of patients with TMDs typically includes panoramic or transcranial imaging. These radiographs are limited to identifying gross changes in bone, which are often not seen until a significant volume of destruction or alteration in bone mineral content has occurred. Tomography may provide greater accuracy in assessing condylar position and range of mobility.

Several specialized imaging studies that are useful in the diagnosis of TMDs have become available. Computerized tomography (CT) and cone-beam CT are most accurate for identifying bone abnormalities such as osteophytes, condylar erosion, fractures, ankylosis and condylar hyperplasia. In-office cone-beam CT is advantageous because of its accessibility, higher spatial resolution, reduced radiation exposure, and faster imaging, and it is less expensive compared with conventional CT (Figure 10-7). **Magnetic resonance imaging (MRI)** is mandatory for examining disk position, function, and morphology, and the presence of joint effusions (inflammatory changes) (Figure 10-8). MRI is advantageous because no ionizing radiation is used. **Arthrography,** which uses a radiopaque contrast agent that is injected into the joint, may be useful when MRI is not tolerated and information regarding the position and morphology of the disk is required.

TYPES OF TEMPOROMANDIBULAR DISORDERS

TMDs can be classified according to structural and functional changes (Box 10-2).

MYOFASCIAL PAIN AND DYSFUNCTION

MPD comprises at least 50% of all TMDs and most commonly involves the masseter muscle. Pain is frequently worse in the morning, particularly in patients who clench or grind their teeth during sleep. It is characterized as dysfunctional muscle hyperactivity with regional pain, tenderness of the affected muscles (i.e., trigger points), and variable amounts

---

BOX 10-2

TMD Classification

Masticatory muscle disorder:
- Myofascial pain and dysfunction

Internal derangement (disk derangement):
- Disk displacement with reduction
- Disk displacement without reduction
- Disk perforation

Arthritis:
- Inflammatory: rheumatoid arthritis
- Noninflammatory: osteoarthritis (degenerative joint disease)

TMJ mobility disorders:
- Hypermobility: subluxation, dislocation
- Hypomobility: ankylosis

Neoplasia:
- Benign
- Malignant

TMD, temporomandibular disease; TMJ, temporomandibular joint.

---

of reduced opening and complaints of malocclusion. The direction of deflection depends on the location of the involved muscle.

INTERNAL DERANGEMENT

Internal derangement or **disk derangement** is defined as an abnormal positional relationship of the disk (meniscus) relative to the mandibular condyle and the articular eminence. Patients often present with continuous pain localized to the TMJ and that is exacerbated by jaw movement. In some cases the disk is displaced anteriorly and returns to its normal position on opening of the mouth or movement away from the affected side (disk displacement with reduction). In another form of disk displacement the displaced disk acts as an obstacle to the sliding condyle. In this type of displacement patients complain of problems such as intermittent locking of the jaw; a sudden onset of limited mouth opening, usually associated with cessation of joint sounds; deflection of the mandible to the affected (ipsilateral) side;

TREATMENT OF TEMPOROMANDIBULAR JOINT DISORDERS

NONSURGICAL TREATMENT

Treatment goals for MPD, internal derangement, and arthritis of the TMJ include the following:

- Improving joint function (i.e., range of motion)
- Reducing pain
- Preventing further joint damage (i.e., reducing mechanical stress and inflammation)

Treatment typically begins with nonsurgical modalities. The first phase of nonsurgical treatment includes pharmacologic therapy, heat/ice packs, physical therapy, soft mechanical diet, stretch therapy, and exercise therapy. Passive jaw exercises are effective to improve pain and mobility for MPD but are contraindicated with severely displaced disks. The local application of heat or ice will increase circulation and relax muscles. It may seem paradoxical that both heat and ice can be used for the same purpose, but localized vasodilation occurs in response to both, in the body's attempt to return the area to its normal temperature. While patients may benefit from occlusal adjustment, this has not been found to prevent or improve TMD symptoms. Despite numerous studies that have demonstrated the usefulness of acupuncture, its efficacy is considered equivocal.

Medications are used to control pain and inflammation. Traditional nonsteroidal antiinflammatory drugs (NSAIDs) are often used in the acute stage. Cyclooxygenase-2 selective inhibitors (coxibs or COX-2 inhibitors) are the newest types of NSAIDs and may be considered for patients at high risk for gastrointestinal bleeding and who do not respond to traditional NSAIDs. Caution is recommended with the chronic use of either type of NSAID because of possible cardiovascular complications. Tramadol, when used with acetaminophen, is more effective than NSAIDs for reducing musculoskeletal pain but should be restricted to short-term use because of the potential for habituation and dependence. Tricyclic antidepressants (TCAs) and serotonin and norepinephrine reuptake inhibitors (SNRIs) have shown the greatest benefit in patients with chronic pain, probably due to their analgesic and antidepressant actions. Although these drugs may be considered for chronic muscle pain, side effects include nausea, sedation, psychomotor impairment, xerostomia, and constipation. Muscle relaxants, botulinum toxin, and antianxiety agents can be used to reduce muscle hypertonicity. Intramuscular botulinum toxin-A may also reduce stress on the TMJ and may be considered for patients with myofascial pain who cannot be treated effectively with conservative modalities. Data are emerging that intraarticular injection with sodium hyaluronate, which is normally produced by synovial cells, will facilitate joint lubrication and restore joint stabilization for patients with positional disk abnormalities.

If a patient fails to improve or worsens after approximately 1 to 2 months of conservative nonsurgical management, the second phase, which involves the use of occlusal appliances, may be initiated. **Stabilization appliances** function by relaxing muscles, protecting the dentition, stabilizing and protecting the joint, redistributing occlusal forces, providing biofeedback by making patients aware of bruxing habits, or relieving the load on the disk to allow repair of damaged retrodiskal tissues. Reduction of TMJ pain and not sounds (e.g., clicking, popping, crepitus) is the primary objective for oral appliance therapy. **Anterior repositioning appliances** are indicated for patients with painful clicking or frequent locking but should be carefully monitored and used part-time because of possible irreversible changes to the occlusion.

Psychosocial (e.g., stress, coping abilities) and environmental factors (e.g., ethnicity, culture) may negatively impact the prognosis for orofacial muscle pain, and early cognitive-behavioral intervention (e.g., education, biofeedback, relaxation training, stress management) may improve outcomes.

SURGICAL TREATMENT

Patients with TMDs other than MPD may be considered for surgical treatment if they do not respond to nonsurgical therapy and continue to suffer from pain and functional impairment because of interferences in TMJ function. Various surgical techniques are used to treat TMDs. **Arthrocentesis** is a minimally invasive procedure that involves lavaging the joint through a needle to address three common symptoms of the TMJ associated with closed lock: limited opening, pain, and dysfunction. The rationale is to release the disk and adhesions, reduce the viscosity of the synovial fluid, and wash out inflammatory mediators. The success rate for arthrocentesis has been reported to be 83%. **Arthroscopy** is a minimally invasive closed joint procedure that allows direct visualization and manipulation of the joint. **Open joint surgery** (i.e., arthrotomy) is a broad term encompassing all procedures allowing direct assess to the TMJ and generally used to improve the disk-condyle relationship. Such procedures include disk manipulation (i.e., diskoplasty, disk repositioning, disk replacement, diskectomy), condylar repositioning (i.e., condylotomy), recontouring of the articular surfaces of the condyle and glenoid fossa (i.e., gap arthroplasty), and total joint reconstruction using a prosthetic device or autogenous graft. Eminectomy is performed for recurrent mandibular hypermobility/subluxation and involves removal of the articular eminence of the temporal bone, which blocks the path of the condyle when closing. The chronic nature associated with rheumatoid arthritis is especially challenging and management strategies are focused on prevention and repair.

MULTIDISCIPLINARY MANAGEMENT

Temporomandibular disorders remain a frequent cause of visits to primary care physicians and general dentists. Additional considerations for patients with oral, facial, and head and neck pain may necessitate referral to medical and dental specialists. This management strategy is especially relevant for patients with headaches, which may be exacerbated by TMDs.

SELECTED REFERENCES

Books

Greenberg M, Glick M, Ship J: *Burket's oral medicine*, ed 11, Hamilton, 2008, BC Decker.

Hupp J, Ellis E, Tucker M: *Contemporary oral and maxillofacial surgery*, ed 6, St. Louis, 2014, Elsevier.

Okeson J: *Management of temporomandibular disorders and occlusion*, ed 7, St. Louis, 2013, Elsevier.

Journal Articles

Aggarwal V, Tickle M, Javidi H, et al: Reviewing the evidence: can cognitive behavioral therapy improve outcomes for patients with chronic orofacial pain? *J Orofac Pain* 24:163, 2010.

Al-Belasy F, Dolwick M: Arthrocentesis for the treatment of temporomandibular joint closed lock: a review article, *Int J Oral Maxillofac Surg* 36:773, 2007.

Benoliel R, Sharav Y: Chronic orofacial pain, *Curr Pain Headache Rep* 14:33, 2010.

Clark G: Classification, causation and treatment of masticatory myogenous pain and dysfunction, *Oral Maxillfofac Surg Clin N Am* 20:147, 2008.

Conti P, dos Santos C, Kogawa E, et al: The treatment of painful temporomandibular joint clicking with oral splints: a randomized clinical trial, *J Am Dent Assoc* 137:1108, 2006.

de Bont L, Dijkgraaf L, Stegenga B: Epidemiology and natural progression of articular temporomandibular disorders, *Oral Surg Oral Med Oral Pathol Oral Radiol Endod* 83:72, 1997.

Dimitroulis G: Temporomandibular disorders: a clinical update, *BMJ* 317:190, 1998.

Dimitroulis G: The prevalence of osteoarthrosis in cases of advanced internal derangement of the temporomandibular joint: a clinical, surgical and histologic study, *Int J Oral Maxillofac Surg* 34:345, 2005.

Dworkin S, Huggins K, LeResche L, et al: Epidemiology of signs and symptoms in temporomandibular disorders: clinical signs in cases and controls, *J Am Dent Assoc* 120:273, 1990.

Gatchel R, Wright-Stowell A, Wildenstein L, et al: Efficacy of an early intervention for patients with acute temporomandibular disorder–related pain, *J Am Dent Assoc* 137:339, 2006.

Hoffman R, Kotchen J, Kotchen T, et al: Temporomandibular disorders and associated clinical comorbidities, *Clin J Pain* 27:268, 2011.

Humphrey S, Lindroth J, Carlson C: Routine dental care in patients with temporomandibular disorders, *J Orofac Pain* 16:129, 2002.

Ingawale S, Goswami T: Temporomandibular joint: disorders, treatments, and biomechanics, *Ann Biomed Eng* 37:976, 2009.

Israel H, Syrop S: The important role of motion in the rehabilitation of patients with mandibular hypomobility: a review of the literature, *J Craniomandibular Pract* 15:74, 1993.

LeResche L: Epidemiology of temporomandibular disorders: implications for the investigation of etiologic factors, *Crit Rev Oral Biol Med* 8:291, 1997.

McNeill C: History of evolution of TMD concepts, *Oral Surg Oral Med Oral Pathol Oral Radiol Endod* 83:51, 1997.

Sanders B: Arthroscopic surgery of the temporomandibular joint: treatment of internal derangement with persistent closed lock, *Oral Surg Oral Med Oral Pathol* 62:361, 1986.

Scrivani SJ, Keith DA, Kaban LB: Temporomandibular disorders, *N Engl J Med* 359:2693, 2008.

Wilkes C: Internal derangement of the temporomandibular joint: pathological variations, *Arch Otolaryngol Head Neck Surg* 115:469, 1989.

Review Questions

1. Disorders of the articulation between the mandible and maxilla are called:
   A. Synovial hyperplasias
   B. Mandibulomaxillary dysfunction
   C. Temporomandibular disorders
   D. Mandibular dysfunction

2. Using a stethoscope to listen to abnormal noises in the temporomandibular joint is called:
   A. Audiology
   B. Auscultation
   C. Arthrography
   D. Crepitus

3. Which of the following is the most important aspect of the management of temporomandibular diseases?
   A. Palpation of the muscles of mastication
   B. Using a nonsurgical approach
   C. Adjusting the occlusion
   D. Establishing an accurate diagnosis

4. Translational movements of the temporomandibular movements are:
   A. Hinge movements
   B. Sliding movements
   C. Rotational movements
   D. Used only for diagnosis

5. Which of the following is considered a parafunctional habit?
   A. Palpation
   B. Mastication
   C. Bruxing
   D. Trauma

6. All of the following are considered functions of the articular disk *except*:
   A. Shock absorption
   B. Sensory innervation
   C. Dissipation of synovial fluid
   D. Facilitation of rotation and translation

7. Which of the following is a symptom of a temporomandibular disorder?
   A. Pain
   B. Malocclusion
   C. A history of surgical treatment of the jaws
   D. Occlusal adjustment

8. Which of the following comprises at least 50% of all temporomandibular disorders?
   A. Hypermobility
   B. Myofascial pain and dysfunction
   C. Internal disk derangements
   D. Osteoarthritis

Continued

Review Questions—cont'd

9. Immobility of the temporomandibular joint because of fibrous or bony union between the articulating structures of the joint is called:
   A. Hypermobility
   B. Ankylosis
   C. Disk displacement
   D. Osteoarthritis

10. Which of the following is *not* a form of surgical treatment used for temporomandibular joint disorders?
    A. Arthrocentesis
    B. Condylotomy
    C. Joint reconstruction
    D. Occlusal appliance

11. Which of the following is the most common benign tumor of the synovium of the temporomandibular joint?
    A. Osteoblastoma
    B. Osteochondroma
    C. Chondroblastoma
    D. Synovial chondromatosis

12. Which of the following diagnostic modalities should be used for patients suspected of osteoarthritis of the temporomandibular joint?
    A. Cone-beam computed tomography
    B. Magnetic resonance tomography
    C. Local anesthesia injected into the joint
    D. Arthrography

13. Which of the following muscles *cannot* be palpated on clinical examination?
    A. Medial pterygoid
    B. Lateral pterygoid
    C. Masseter
    D. Temporalis

14. The primary goals for management of temporomandibular disorders include all of the following *except*:
    A. Improving oral function
    B. Reducing pain
    C. Preventing further joint damage
    D. Improving oral health

15. Which management would you recommend to a patient who complains of chronic subluxation?
    A. Arthrocentesis
    B. Eminectomy
    C. Appliance therapy
    D. Nonsteroidal antiinflammatory drugs (NSAIDs)

16. How may dental hygiene management be modified for a patient with myofascial pain and dysfunction?
    A. Shorter appointments
    B. Jaw exercises before and after the appointment
    C. Pain management with nitrous oxide analgesia
    D. All of the above

17. Which of the following therapies would you recommend to a patient diagnosed with myofascial pain and dysfunction and who did not respond to a 2-month course of soft diet, oral appliance therapy, and hot/cold compresses?
    A. Continue the present therapy for another 2 months
    B. Occlusal adjustment
    C. TMJ arthrotomy
    D. Physical therapy

18. Which condition is associated with crepitus?
    A. Disk displacement with reduction
    B. Disk displacement without reduction
    C. Degenerative joint disease
    D. Myofascial pain and dysfunction

19. Which nerve is primarily responsible for innervating the temporomandibular joint?
    A. Deep temporal nerve
    B. Great occipital nerve
    C. Masseteric nerve
    D. Auriculotemporal nerve

20. All of the following are mandatory for evaluating a patient suspected of disk displacement without reduction *except*:
    A. Panoramic radiographic examination
    B. Medical history
    C. History of symptoms
    D. Medical consultation

Chapter 1

1. C
2. D
3. C
4. B
5. D
6. A
7. B
8. C
9. A
10. C
11. A
12. B
13. D
14. B
15. A
16. A
17. D
18. A
19. C
20. C
21. A
22. D
23. B
24. D
25. B
26. D
27. D
28. A

Chapter 2

1. B
2. B
3. D
4. B
5. C
6. C
7. D
8. D
9. A
10. A
11. D
12. C
13. A
14. C
15. D
16. B
17. D
18. B
19. B
20. A
21. B
22. B
23. C
24. B
25. C
26. D
27. D
28. A
29. A
30. A
31. D
32. A
33. D
34. B
35. A
36. D
37. C
38. B
39. C
40. B
41. B
42. A
43. C
44. C
45. B
46. D
47. D
48. C
49. D

50. B
51. B
52. C
53. C
54. C
55. B
56. A
57. B
58. B

Chapter 3

1. C
2. B
3. D
4. A
5. D
6. C
7. D
8. A
9. B
10. A
11. A
12. C
13. B
14. C
15. B
16. D
17. B
18. D
19. A
20. C
21. D
22. D
23. A
24. D
25. B
26. C
27. B
28. B
29. A

30. D
31. C
32. D
33. D
34. D
35. B
36. B
37. C
38. D
39. C
40. C
41. C
42. B
43. B
44. B
45. C

Chapter 4

1. B
2. B
3. B
4. B
5. B
6. C
7. B
8. C
9. D
10. B
11. B
12. D
13. C
14. C
15. D
16. B
17. D
18. D
19. B
20. B
21. C
22. C
23. D
24. B
25. A
26. D
27. C
28. C
29. D
30. D

Chapter 5

1. C
2. A
3. D
4. C
5. A
6. B
7. B
8. C
9. D
10. C
11. A
12. B
13. A

14. B
15. D
16. C
17. D
18. C
19. C
20. A
21. B
22. B
23. C
24. D
25. D
26. A
27. D
28. A
29. B
30. B
31. B
32. A
33. D
34. A
35. B
36. D
37. C
38. C
39. A
40. B
41. D
42. C
43. C
44. C
45. D
46. C
47. B
48. B

Chapter 6

1. D
2. D
3. C
4. B
5. C
6. D
7. A
8. B
9. B
10. C
11. A
12. D
13. D
14. B
15. C
16. A
17. C
18. A
19. C
20. D
21. B
22. A
23. D
24. A
25. D
26. B

27. C
28. B
29. A
30. B
31. B
32. C
33. D
34. C
35. A

Chapter 7

1. C
2. A
3. C
4. C
5. D
6. B
7. C
8. D
9. A
10. C
11. D
12. C
13. A
14. D
15. B
16. B
17. A
18. B
19. C
20. A
21. B
22. A
23. C
24. C
25. A
26. C
27. B
28. B
29. D
30. B
31. D
32. A
33. C
34. B
35. C
36. B
37. A
38. C
39. B
40. C
41. A
42. A
43. C
44. B
45. D
46. B
47. D
48. A
49. A
50. D
51. B
52. D

Glossary

A

Aberrant Deviating from the usual or natural type; atypical.

Abfraction A wedge-shaped area that typically occurs on the cervicofacial areas of teeth.

Abrasion The pathologic wearing away of tooth structure that results from repetitive mechanical habit.

Abscess A collection of pus that has accumulated in a cavity formed in the tissue.

Acantholysis Dissolution of the intercellular bridges of the prickle cell layer of the epithelium.

Acantholytic cells Cells detached from the epithelium that appear rounded. This process is caused by a loss of attachment between the epithelial cells. These cells are present with pemphigus vulgaris. Also known as *Tzanck cells*.

Acanthosis nigricans A skin condition characterized by hyperpigmented, velvety-textured plaques that appear symmetrically distributed in folds and creases of the body. It has been reported to be associated with type 2 diabetes mellitus and has been used as a clinical indicator when screening for it.

Acquired immune response A response by the body generated by the memory of past exposure to a foreign substance; this response is quicker when encountered a second time.

Acquired immunodeficiency syndrome A syndrome involving a defect in cell-mediated immunity that has a long incubation period, follows a protracted and debilitating course, manifests as opportunistic infections, and has a poor prognosis without treatment. It is caused by the retrovirus human immunodeficiency virus.

Acromegaly A condition caused by hyperfunction of the pituitary gland in adults.

Actinic Relating to or exhibiting chemical changes produced by radiant energy, especially the visible and ultraviolet parts of the spectrum; relating to exposure to the ultraviolet rays of sunlight.

Actinic cheilitis Degeneration of the tissue of the lips caused by sun exposure. Also called *solar cheilitis*.

Actinomycosis An infection caused by a filamentous bacterium called *Actinomyces israelii*. The most characteristic manifestation of the disease is the formation of abscesses that drain through fistulas.

Active immunity Immunity acquired naturally or artificially. It occurs naturally when a microorganism infects a person, causing disease to which immunity is then developed. It occurs artificially when a person is injected with or ingests either altered pathogenic microorganisms or products of those microorganisms.

Acute Of short duration or of short and relatively severe course.

Acute inflammation The initial phase of inflammation that is of short duration, lasting only a few days.

Acute lymphonodular pharyngitis An infectious disease caused by the coxsackieviruses. It is characterized by fever, sore throat, and mild headache. Hyperplastic lymphoid tissue of the soft palate or tonsillar pillars appears as yellowish or dark pink nodules.

Acute necrotizing ulcerative gingivitis (ANUG) A painful erythematous gingivitis with necrosis and cratering of the interdental papillae. Presently called *necrotizing ulcerative gingivitis (NUG)* because it is not an acute condition.

Acute osteomyelitis An acute inflammation of the bone and bone marrow. Acute osteomyelitis of the jaws is most commonly a result of the extension of a periapical abscess. Other potential causes include fracture of the bone, surgery, and bacteremia.

Addison disease A condition characterized by insufficient production of adrenal steroids. Also known as *primary adrenal cortical insufficiency*.

Adenocarcinoma A nonspecific name for malignant tumors of glandular origin.

Adenoid cystic carcinoma A slow-growing malignant tumor of salivary gland origin that can originate from either the major or minor salivary gland tissue. It is unencapsulated and infiltrates surrounding tissue.

Adenoma A benign tumor that originates from glandular epithelium.

Adenomatoid Glandlike.

Adenomatoid odontogenic tumor An encapsulated, benign epithelial odontogenic tumor that has a distinctive age,

53. C
54. D
55. A
56. B
57. A
58. C
59. C

Chapter 8

1. B
2. D
3. C
4. D
5. A
6. A
7. C
8. A
9. C
10. D
11. B
12. A
13. B
14. B
15. D
16. A
17. B
18. A
19. B
20. D
21. B
22. D

23. D
24. D
25. A

Chapter 9

1. A
2. D
3. C
4. B
5. C
6. C
7. D
8. D
9. D
10. C
11. D
12. D
13. A
14. D
15. B
16. A
17. D
18. B
19. A
20. D
21. A
22. B
23. D
24. D
25. C
26. D

27. A
28. D
29. B
30. D
31. A
32. A
33. B
34. C

Chapter 10

1. C
2. B
3. D
4. B
5. C
6. B
7. A
8. B
9. B
10. D
11. B
12. B
13. B
14. D
15. B
16. D
17. D
18. C
19. D
20. D

sex, and site distribution. Seventy percent occur in females less than 20 years of age; 70% involve the anterior part of the jaws. May be associated with impacted teeth. Also known as an *odontogenic adenomatoid tumor*.

Agammaglobulinemia Lack of immunoglobulins.

Agranulocytosis A marked decrease in the number of granulocytes, particularly neutrophils.

Alleles Genes that are located at the same level or locus in the two chromosomes of a pair and that determine the same functions or characteristics.

Allergen Antigen producing a hypersensitivity or an allergic reaction.

Allergy A hypersensitive state acquired through exposure to a particular allergen. Reexposure to the same allergen elicits an exaggerated reaction.

Alveolar osteitis A postoperative complication of tooth extraction in which after extraction the blood clot breaks down and is lost before healing occurs. The socket appears empty, and the bone surface is exposed. Also known as *dry socket*.

Amalgam tattoo A flat, bluish-gray lesion of the oral mucosa resulting from the introduction of amalgam particles into the tissue.

Ameloblastic fibroma A nonencapsulated, benign odontogenic tumor of mixed tissue origin that is composed of strands and small islands of ameloblast-like epithelial cells and mesenchymal cells that resemble the dental papilla. It occurs in young children and adults, and the most common location is the mandibular bicuspid and molar region. Most patients are asymptomatic, but bone expansion or swelling may be noted.

Ameloblastic fibro-odontoma A benign odontogenic tumor that has features of both an ameloblastic fibroma and an odontoma. It typically arises in the posterior jaws and is often asymptomatic.

Ameloblastoma A benign, slow-growing but locally aggressive epithelial odontogenic tumor that may arise in either the maxilla or the mandible. It is an unencapsulated tumor that infiltrates into surrounding tissue and can cause extensive destruction.

Amelogenesis The formation of enamel.

Amelogenesis imperfecta A broad group of conditions that affect the structural formation of enamel. The disease is divided into four main types: type I, hypoplastic; type II, hypocalcified; type III, hypomaturation; type IV, hypoplastic-hypomaturation.

Amenorrhea Abnormal temporary or permanent cessation of menstrual cycles.

Amino acid An organic compound containing the amino group NH_2. Amino acids are the main component of proteins.

Anaphylaxis A type of hypersensitivity or allergic reaction in which the exaggerated immunologic response results from the release of vasoactive substances such as histamine. The reaction occurs on reexposure to a foreign protein or other substance after sensitization.

Anaplastic A loss of differentiation of cells and their orientation to one another; a characteristic of malignant tumor tissue.

Anemia Reduction to less than the normal number of red blood cells, quantity of hemoglobin, or volume of packed red blood cells in the blood.

Aneuploid Any extra number of chromosomes that do not represent an exact multiple of the total chromosome complement (e.g., trisomy [a pair with an identical extra chromosome] and monosomy [a missing chromosome from a pair]).

Aneurysmal bone cyst A pseudocyst that consists of blood-filled spaces surrounded by multinucleated giant cells and fibrous connective tissue. The radiolucent lesion has a multilocular appearance that is often described as "honeycomb" or "soap bubbles."

Angioedema A lesion that appears as a diffuse swelling of tissue caused by increased permeability of deeper blood vessels. The skin covering the swelling appears normal.

Angiogenesis The formation and differentiation of blood vessels.

Angular cheilitis Erythema or fissuring at the labial commissures. Angular cheilitis may be caused by factors such as nutritional deficiency; however, it most commonly results from *Candida* infection.

Ankyloglossia Extensive adhesion of the tongue to the floor of the mouth or the lingual aspect of the anterior portion of the mandible; caused by a short lingual frenum.

Ankylosed teeth Teeth in which bone has fused to cementum and dentin, preventing exfoliation of deciduous teeth and eruption of the underlying permanent tooth; ankylosed teeth typically appear submerged clinically.

Ankylosis Immobility of a joint because of fibrous or bony union between the articulating structures of the joint. Ankylosis can be classified by tissue type, location, and extent of fusion.

Anodontia Complete or almost complete congenital lack of teeth.

Anomaly Marked deviation from normal, especially as a result of a congenital or hereditary defects.

Anorexia nervosa An eating disorder characterized by a distorted perception of body image, in addition to depression, intense fear of weight gain, and self-imposed starvation.

Anterior repositioning appliances Indicated for patients with TMJD who have painful clicking or frequent locking; should be carefully monitored to prevent irreversible changes to occlusion.

Antibody A protein molecule, also called an *immunoglobulin*, which is produced by plasma cells and reacts with a specific antigen.

Antibody titer The specific level of an antibody in the blood. It can be measured by a laboratory test.

Antigen Any substance that is able to induce a specific immune response.

Antigenic determinate The portion of an antibody that recognizes and binds to the antigen.

Antigens Foreign substances against which the immune system defends the body.

Apertognathia Anterior open bite.

Aphthous ulcer Painful oral ulcers that frequently recur in episodes. There are three types of aphthous ulcers: minor, major, and herpetiform. Also known as *canker sore* or *aphthous stomatitis*.

Aplasia Lack of development.

Aplastic anemia A type of anemia in which patients experience a dramatic decrease in all the circulating blood cells (pancytopenia) because of a severe depression of bone marrow activity. Can be primary (cause unknown) or secondary (caused by a drug or chemical agent).

Arthralgia Severe pain in a joint.

Arthritis Inflammation of a joint. It is classified as either osteoarthritis or rheumatoid arthritis.

Arthrocentesis Surgical puncture of a joint, usually for the withdrawal of fluid, followed by lavage of the joint space.

Arthrography Radiography of a joint after injection of an opaque contrast material.

Arthroscopy A method for evaluating and manipulating a joint by the insertion of a camera and instruments.

Articular disk A pad of fibrocartilage or dense fibrous tissue present in some synovial joints (e.g., the temporomandibular joint).

Articulation A Joint.

Aspirin burn A type of chemical injury that occurs when a patient places an aspirin tablet directly on mucosal tissue instead of swallowing it. The soft tissue becomes necrotic and appears white.

Atherosclerosis The process by which lipid accumulates within the walls of large and medium-sized arteries. It leads to reduced blood flow to and death of vital organs.

Atrophy The decrease in size and function of a cell, tissue, organ, or whole body.

Attenuate To reduce the severity of a disease or the virulence of a pathogenic agent, as is done in the development of certain vaccines.

Attrition The wearing away of tooth structure during mastication. Attrition occurs normally but may also be accelerated by teeth grinding.

Auscultation The act of listening to sounds within the body using a stethoscope.

Autoantibody An antibody that reacts against an antigenic constituent of the person's own tissues.

Autoimmune disease A disease characterized by tissue injury caused by a humoral or cell-mediated immune response against constituents of the body's own tissues.

Autoimmunity Immune-mediated destruction of the body's own cells and tissues; immunity against self.

Autosomal Related to nonsex chromosomes that are identical for males and females.

Autosomes (adjective, autosomal) The nonsex chromosomes that are identical for men and women.

B

B-cell lymphocyte A lymphocyte, also called a *B cell*, that matures without passing through the thymus and later can develop into a plasma cell that produces antibodies.

Barr body Condensed chromatin of the inactivated X chromosome, which is found at the periphery of the nucleus of cells in women.

Basal cell carcinoma A malignant skin tumor associated with excessive sun exposure that appears as a nonhealing ulcer with characteristic rolled borders. It does not occur in the oral cavity.

Behçet syndrome A chronic, recurrent, autoimmune disease consisting primarily of oral ulcers, genital ulcers, and ocular inflammation. The oral ulcers that appear are similar to aphthous ulcers.

Bence Jones proteins Fragments of immunoglobulins found in the urine of patients with multiple myeloma.

Benign A condition that, if untreated or treated symptomatically, will not become life-threatening.

Benign cementoblastoma A cementum-producing tumor that is fused to the root or roots of a vital tooth. It typically occurs in young adults, and pain is a frequent symptom.

Benign cystic teratoma A lesion with a cystic component that resembles the dermoid cyst. In addition, teeth, bone, muscle, and nerve tissue may be found in the wall of this lesion.

Benign fibro-osseous lesion A benign lesion of bone characterized histologically by cellular fibrous connective tissue mixed with irregularly shaped bone trabeculae or cementoid material.

Benign mixed tumor The most common of the benign salivary gland tumors. Also known as a *pleomorphic adenoma*.

Benign mucous membrane pemphigoid A chronic autoimmune disease that affects the oral mucosa, conjunctiva, genital mucosa, and skin. It is also known as *mucous membrane pemphigoid* and *cicatricial pemphigoid*.

Benign tumor A tumor that is not malignant; favorable for treatment and recovery.

Bleeding time A test that provides an assessment of the adequacy of platelet function. It measures how long it takes a standardized skin incision to stop bleeding by the formation of a temporary hemostatic plug or clot.

Botryoid odontogenic cyst When a lateral periodontal cyst is multilocular, it is called a botryoid cyst; microscopically, they are the same. A botryoid cyst has a greater potential for recurrence.

Brachydactyly Short fingers or toes or both.

Branchial arch One of a series of mesodermal bars located between the branchial clefts. During embryonic stages the arch contributes to the formation of the face, jaws, and neck.

Brittle diabetes A term used to describe diabetes in patients who have blood glucose levels that are unstable or are not well controlled.

Brown tumor A lesion of bone identical to the central giant cell granuloma that occurs in patients with hyperparathyroidism.

Brush test A technique used to obtain information from oral mucosal epithelium. This technique uses a circular brush to obtain cells from the full thickness of the epithelium, including cells from the keratin layer through the basal layer.

Bruton disease A type of primary immunodeficiency in which B cells do not mature. Plasma cells are deficient throughout the body; T cells are normal. Also called *X-linked congenital agammaglobulinemia*.

Bruxism The habit of grinding and clenching of the teeth together for nonfunctional purposes.

Bulimia An eating disorder characterized by food binges, usually of high caloric intake, followed by self-induced vomiting. (Erosion is seen on the lingual aspects of maxillary anterior teeth.)

Bulla (adjective, *bullous*; plural, *bullae*) A circumscribed, elevated, fluid-filled lesion within or below the skin or mucous membranes that is greater than 5 mm in diameter and usually contains serous fluid.

Bullous lichen planus The type of lichen planus in which the epithelium separates from the connective tissue and erosions, bullae, or ulcers form.

C

Café au lait Refers to a macular skin pigmentation that is the color of coffee with milk.

Café au lait spots Light brown skin lesions.

Calcifying epithelial odontogenic tumor A benign epithelial odontogenic tumor in which the proliferating cells do not resemble odontogenic epithelium. The tumor is composed of islands and sheets of polyhedral (multisided) epithelial cells. It is also known as a *Pindborg tumor*.

Calcifying odontogenic cyst A nonaggressive cystic lesion lined by odontogenic epithelium with associated ghost cell keratinization.

Calcitonin A polypeptide secreted by the C cells of the thyroid gland.

Cancer Malignancy

Candidal leukoplakia A type of candidiasis that appears as a white lesion that does not wipe off the mucosa. An important diagnostic feature of this type of candidiasis is that it responds to treatment with antifungal medication. Also called *chronic hyperplastic candidiasis* and *hypertrophic candidiasis*.

Candidiasis An overgrowth of the yeastlike fungus *Candida albicans*. It is the most common oral fungal infection. It can result from many different conditions, including antibiotic use, cancer, corticosteroid therapy, dentures, diabetes mellitus, and HIV infection. Also called *moniliasis* and *thrush*.

Capillary hemangioma A hemangioma that contains numerous small capillaries.

Capsulitis Inflammation; tenderness over the lateral pole of the condyle.

Carcinoma A malignant tumor of epithelial tissue origin.

Carcinoma arising in a pleomorphic adenoma Occurs when a pleomorphic adenoma undergoes malignant transformation.

Carrier In genetics a heterozygous individual who is clinically normal but who can transmit a recessive trait or characteristic; also, a person who is homozygous for an autosomal-dominant condition with low penetrance.

Catabolism Component of metabolism that involves the breakdown of molecules with the concomitant release of energy.

Cavernous hemangioma A hemangioma containing large blood vessels.

Celiac disease A chronic disorder associated with sensitivity to dietary gluten, a protein found in wheat and wheat products. When gluten is ingested, injury to the intestinal mucosa results. Also called *celiac sprue* and *gluten-sensitive enteropathy*.

Cell-mediated immunity Immunity in which the predominant role is played by T lymphocytes.

Cementogenesis The formation of cementum.

Cementoma An apical lesion associated with the apices of teeth. It may present as a mass of fibrous connective tissue, fibrous connective tissue with spicules of cementum, or calcified mass resembling cementum and having few cellular elements. Also known as *periapical cemento-osseous dysplasia*.

Cemento-ossifying fibroma A tumor that has a mixture of globular calcifications resembling cementum and bone trabeculae that results from the potential of periodontal ligament cells to produce either cementum or bone.

Cementum Outermost layer of the root of the tooth.

Centimeter (cm) One hundredth of a meter. Equivalent to a little less than ½ inch (0.393 of an inch).

Central Occurring within the bone. In oral pathology, a lesion occurring within the maxilla or mandible.

Central cementifying fibroma A benign, well-circumscribed tumor classified as a fibro-osseous lesion. The calcifications are rounded and globular, resembling cementum. Affected patients may be asymptomatic or demonstrate bone expansion or facial asymmetry.

Central ossifying fibroma A benign, well-circumscribed tumor classified as a fibro-osseous lesion. The calcifications resemble bone trabeculae. Affected patients may be asymptomatic or demonstrate bone expansion or facial asymmetry.

Centromere The constricted portion of the chromosome that divides the short arms from the long arms.

Cervical lymphoepithelial cyst Located on the lateral neck at the anterior border of the sternocleidomastoid muscle. Also called *Branchial cleft cyst*.

Chancre Lesion of the primary stage of syphilis. It is highly infectious and forms at the site at which the spirochete enters the body.

Chemotaxis The movement of white blood cells, directed by chemical mediators, to the area of injury.

Chemotherapy Cancer treatment that uses chemical agents to modify or destroy cancer cells.

Cherubism A disorder beginning in childhood characterized by progressive bilateral facial swelling that can occur in either the maxilla or mandible, with involvement of the mandible being most common. The swollen jaws and raised eyes give a "cherublike" appearance, and radiographs show multilocular radiolucent lesions.

Chiasmata The intercrossing of chromatids of the same or homologous chromosomes that takes place at metaphase of first meiosis for the purpose of genetic recombination.

Chickenpox A highly contagious disease caused by the varicella-zoster virus. It is characterized by vesicular and pustular eruptions of the skin and/or mucous membranes, along with systemic symptoms such as headache, fever, and malaise. It usually occurs in children.

Chondroma A benign tumor of cartilage.

Chondrosarcoma A malignant tumor of cartilage that can occur in either the maxilla or mandible.

Chromatid Either of the two vertical halves of a chromosome that are joined at the centromere.

Chromatin A general term used to refer to the material (DNA) that forms the chromosomes.

Chromosomes The small bodies in the nucleus of a cell that carry the chemical instructions for reproduction of the cell in addition to other cellular functions.

Chronic Persisting over a long time.

Chronic apical periodontitis A localized mass of chronically inflamed granulation tissue that forms at the opening of the pulp canal generally at the apex of a nonvital tooth. Also called *periapical granuloma* and *dental granuloma*.

Chronic atrophic candidiasis The most common type of candidiasis affecting the oral mucosa. This type of candidiasis presents as erythematous mucosa, but the erythematous change is limited to mucosa that is covered by a full or partial denture. Also called *denture stomatitis*.

Chronic hyperplastic candidiasis A type of candidiasis that appears as a white lesion that does not wipe off the mucosa. An important diagnostic feature of this type of candidiasis is that it responds to treatment with antifungal medication. Also called *candidal leukoplakia* and *hypertrophic candidiasis*.

Chronic hyperplastic pulpitis An excessive proliferation of chronically inflamed dental pulp tissue within the crown of a carious tooth. Also called *pulp polyp*.

Chronic inflammation Inflammation that may last weeks, months, or indefinitely.

Chronic mucocutaneous candidiasis A severe form of candidiasis that usually occurs in patients who are severely immunocompromised. Oral involvement may appear as pseudomembranous, erythematous, or hyperplastic candidiasis.

Chronic neutropenia A type of neutropenia in which the intraoral manifestations are similar to those of cyclic neutropenia but are constant. Also known as *Kostmann syndrome.*

Chronic osteomyelitis A long-standing inflammation of bone.

Chronic sclerosing osteomyelitis A condition that is characterized by an inflamed bone that has developed dense calcifications.

Cicatricial pemphigoid A chronic autoimmune disease that affects the oral mucosa, conjunctiva, genital mucosa, and skin. It is also known as *mucous membrane pemphigoid* and *benign mucous membrane pemphigoid.*

Cleft lip Congenital anomaly of the face caused by the failure of fusion between the embryonic maxillary and medial nasal processes.

Cleft palate Congenital anomaly of the oral cavity caused by the failure of fusion between the embryonic palatal shelves.

Cleidocranial dysplasia An inherited disease or congenital disorder characterized by slow or failed formation of the clavicles; delayed closure of the sutures and fontanels of the skull; and delayed eruption of teeth, with formation of supernumerary teeth. Characterized by underdevelopment of the maxillae, agenesis or aplasia of the clavicle, abnormalities in other skeletal bones and muscles, and irregularities of the dentition.

Clotting factors A cascade of circulating plasma proteins (made almost exclusively in the liver) that are necessary to convert precursor fibrinogen to fibrin. Also called *coagulation factors.*

Coagulation Formation of a clot.

Coagulation factors A cascade of circulating plasma proteins (made almost exclusively in the liver) that are necessary to convert precursor fibrinogen to fibrin. Also called *clotting factors.*

Coalescence The process by which parts of a whole join together, or fuse, to make one.

Codominance The full expression in a heterozygote of both alleles of a pair of chromosomes, with neither influenced by the other. A good example is the AB blood group.

Codon The sequence of three bases in DNA that encodes one amino acid.

Cold sore The most common type of recurrent oral herpes simplex infection that occurs on the vermilion border of the lips. Also called *herpes labialis* or *fever blister.*

Coloboma A cleft generally seen on the iris or the eyelids.

Colors Red, pink, salmon, white, blue-black, gray, brown, and black are the words used most frequently to describe the colors of oral lesions; they can be used to identify the specific lesions and may also be incorporated into general descriptions.

Commissural lip pits Epithelium-lined blind tracts located at the corners of the mouth. This is a relatively common developmental anomaly.

Commissure The site of union of corresponding parts (e.g., the corners of the lips).

Complete blood count A series of tests that examines the red blood cells, white blood cells, and platelets.

Complex odontoma An odontogenic tumor that radiographically consists of a mass of enamel, dentin, cementum, and pulp, which does not resemble a normal tooth. It commonly occurs in the posterior mandible.

Compound odontoma An odontogenic tumor that consists of a collection of numerous small teeth. They do not exhibit unlimited growth potential and therefore are more accurately classified as developmental lesions rather than true tumors. They are usually located in the anterior maxilla.

Concrescence A condition in dentistry in which two adjacent teeth are united by cementum.

Condensing osteitis A change in bone near the apices of teeth seen as a radiopacity; thought to be a reaction to low-grade infection.

Condyloma acuminatum A benign papillary lesion caused by human papillomavirus. Oral condylomas appear as papillary bulbous masses and can occur anywhere in the oral mucosa. They are considered a sexually transmitted disease.

Congenital Present at and existing from the time of birth.

Congenital disorder A disorder that is present at birth. It can be either inherited or developmental.

Congenital epulis A benign neoplasm composed of cells that closely resemble those seen in a granular cell tumor. The neoplasm most likely arises from a primitive mesenchymal cell. This tumor is present at birth and appears as a sessile or pedunculated mass on the gingiva and is seen predominantly in girls. Also known as *congenital epulis of the newborn.*

Congenital lip pit Congenital depression on the vermilion portion of the lower lip that may appear either unilaterally or bilaterally.

Congenital syphilis The type of syphilis that is transmitted from an infected mother to the fetus because the organism can cross the placenta and enter the fetal circulation.

Connective tissue disease Diseases in which the body's recognition mechanism breaks down and certain body cells are no longer tolerated. The immune system treats body cells as antigens. Some conditions can also be known as *autoimmune diseases.*

Consanguinity Blood relationship. In genetics the term is generally used to describe matings or marriages among close relatives.

Contact dermatitis Lesions resulting from the direct contact of an allergen with the skin.

Contact mucositis Lesions resulting from the direct contact of an allergen with the mucosa.

Cooley anemia The name of a group of inherited disorders of hemoglobin. Also called *thalassemia.*

Corrugated Having a surface that appears wrinkled.

Coxsackieviruses A group of viruses named for the town in New York where they were first discovered. Coxsackieviruses cause several different infectious diseases. Three of these diseases have distinctive oral lesions: herpangina, hand-foot-and-mouth disease, and acute lymphonodular pharyngitis.

C-reactive protein (CRP) A protein produced in the liver that becomes elevated during episodes of acute inflammation or infection.

Crepitus A dry, crackling sound.

Cretinism The presence of hypothyroidism during infancy and childhood.

Crossing over The exchange of segments between chromatids of the same or homologous chromosomes that takes place at metaphase of first meiosis. Crossing over results from the formation of chiasmata.

Cyclic neutropenia A hereditary disease characterized by a cyclic decrease in the number of circulating neutrophils. The cycles occur in intervals of 21-27 days, and the episodes of neutropenia persist for 2-3 days.

Cylindroma Another name for adenoid cystic carcinoma; so-called because of its microscopic appearance, which shows round and oval islands that represent cylinders of tumor.

Cyst An abnormal pathologic sac or cavity that is lined with epithelium and enclosed in a connective tissue capsule.

Cyst of the palatine papilla A cyst found in the incisive papilla.

Cytokines Chemical mediators produced by cells involved in the immune response.

Cytolysis The dissolution or destruction of a cell.

D

Dark-field microscopy Examination of a specimen by microscopy, in which illumination causes the specimen to appear to glow against a dark background. Used to identify the syphilis spirochete.

Delayed hypersensitivity The type of hypersensitivity in which there is a latent period between the antigen introduction and the reaction. Cellular reactions are mediated by T lymphocytes. It can be used to test for tuberculosis and is responsible for rejection of tissue grafts and transplanted organs.

Deletion In genetics the loss of part of a chromosome.

Dendritic cell A type of white blood cell that acts as an antigen-presenting cell in the skin and mucosa.

Dens evaginatus An accessory enamel cusp found on the occlusal tooth surface. This developmental anomaly occurs most often on the mandibular premolars.

Dens in dente "A tooth within a tooth"; a developmental anomaly that results when the enamel organ invaginates into the crown of a tooth before mineralization. It is most commonly seen in the maxillary lateral incisor. Also called *dens invaginatus.*

Dens invaginatus "A tooth within a tooth"; a developmental anomaly that results when the enamel organ invaginates into the crown of a tooth before mineralization. Also called *dens in dente.*

Dental fluorosis A condition resulting from the ingestion of high concentrations of fluoride, causing the affected teeth to have a mottled discoloration of the enamel.

Dental granuloma A localized mass of chronically inflamed granulation tissue that forms at the opening of the pulp canal generally at the apex of a nonvital tooth. Also known as *periapical granuloma and chronic apical periodontitis.*

Dental papilla The mesenchymal tissue within a tooth germ. After dentin is produced, the dental papilla is called the dental pulp.

Dentigerous cyst A cyst that forms around the crown of an unerupted or developing tooth. Also called a *follicular cyst.*

Dentin Body of the tooth. It surrounds the pulp and underlies the enamel on the crown and the cementum on the root of teeth.

Dentin dysplasia A genetic disturbance of the dentin characterized by early calcification of the pulp chambers and root canals and root resorption. It is subdivided into radicular dentin dysplasia and coronal dentin dysplasia.

Dentinogenesis The formation of dentin.

Dentinogenesis imperfecta A disturbance of the dentin, of genetic origin; characterized by early calcification of the pulp chambers and root canals, marked attrition, and an opalescent hue to the teeth. It is hereditary and associated with osteogenesis imperfecta, or it may occur in isolation.

Denture-associated inflammatory hyperplasia A lesion caused by an ill-fitting denture and generally located in the vestibule along the denture flange. Also called *denture-induced fibrous hyperplasia* and *epulis fissuratum.*

Denture-induced fibrous hyperplasia A lesion caused by an ill-fitting denture. It is located in the vestibule adjacent to the denture border. It is composed of dense fibrous connective tissue surfaced by stratified squamous epithelium. Commonly called *epulis fissuratum* or *inflammatory hyperplasia.*

Denture stomatitis The most common type of candidiasis affecting the oral mucosa. This type of candidiasis presents as erythematous mucosa, but the erythematous change is limited to the mucosa covered by a full or partial denture. Also called *chronic atrophic candidiasis.*

Deoxyribonucleic acid (DNA) A substance composed of a double chain of polynucleotides; both chains, coiled around a central axis, form a double helix. DNA is the basic genetic code or template for polypeptide formation.

Dermoid cyst A developmental cyst that is often present at birth or noted in young children. It is uncommon in the head and neck, but occurs in the anterior floor of the mouth. It is lined by orthokeratinized, stratified squamous epithelium surrounded by a connective tissue wall. The lumen is usually filled with keratin.

Desquamative gingivitis A clinical and descriptive term for gingival lesions that may be seen in lichen planus, pemphigus vulgaris, and mucous membrane pemphigoid. The gingival margin is ulcerated or eroded and shows loss of normal stippling.

Development The process by which an individual reaches maturity.

Developmental anomalies A failure or disturbance that occurs during the process of prenatal development that may result in a lack, excess, or deformity of a body part. Also known as *developmental disorder.*

Developmental disorder A failure or disturbance that occurs during the process of prenatal development that can result in a lack, excess, or deformity of a body part. Also called *developmental anomaly.*

Diabetes mellitus A chronic disorder of carbohydrate (glucose) metabolism that is characterized by abnormally high blood glucose levels (hyperglycemia). This is caused by either a lack of the hormone insulin, defective insulin that does not work properly, or increased insulin resistance.

Differentiation The distinguishing of one thing from another.

Diffuse In the description of a lesion, the borders of the lesion are not well defined, and it is not possible to detect the exact parameters of the lesion.

DiGeorge syndrome A type of primary immunodeficiency in which the thymus is deficient or lacking; therefore T lymphocytes do not mature. Also called *thymic hypoplasia.*

Dilaceration An abnormal bend or curve in the root of a tooth.

Diploid Having two sets of chromosomes; the normal constitution of somatic cells.

Disk displacements Problems in which the disk of the temporomandibular joint (meniscus) is displaced.

Dislocation Referring to the mandible, when one or both of the condyles translates anterior to the articular eminence, resulting in an open lock that the patient cannot reduce.

Disorder Derangement of function.

Distomolar A maxillary fourth molar; the second most common supernumerary tooth.

Dominant In genetics, a trait or characteristic that is manifested when it is carried by only one of a pair of homologous chromosomes.

Double helix The coiled structure of double-stranded DNA in which strands linked by hydrogen bonds form a spiral configuration.

Down syndrome A type of abnormality in which three of chromosome 21 are found instead of two. This results in abnormal physical characteristics and mental impairment. Also called *trisomy 21*.

Dry socket A postoperative complication of tooth extraction. After extraction the blood clot breaks down and is lost before healing occurs. The socket appears empty, and the bone surface is exposed. Also known as *alveolar osteitis*.

Duplication A chromosome that is larger than normal; the extra segment is identical to a segment of the normal chromosome.

Dysplasia Disordered growth; alteration in size, shape, and organization of adult cells or structures.

E

Ecchymosis A small, flat, hemorrhagic patch larger than a petechia on the skin or mucous membrane.

Ectopic geographic tongue A term used to described the condition of geographic tongue when it is found on mucosal surfaces other than the tongue.

Ectopic lingual thyroid nodule A mass of thyroid tissue located on the tongue, distant from the normal anatomic location of the thyroid gland. It is an uncommon developmental anomaly that results from the failure of the primitive thyroid tissue to migrate from its developmental location in the area of the foramen cecum on the posterior portion of the tongue to its normal position in the neck. Also called *lingual thyroid*.

Edema Excess plasma or exudate in the interstitial space of the tissues that causes swelling.

Ellis–Van Creveld syndrome A syndrome characterized by dwarfism, polydactyly, and possible retardation and congenital heart defects. Oral manifestations include fusion of the anterior portion of the maxillary gingiva to the upper lip from canine to canine. Most teeth have a conical shape and exhibit enamel hypoplasia.

Embedded teeth Teeth that do not erupt because of a lack of eruptive force.

Emigration The passage of white blood cells through the endothelium and wall of the microcirculation into an area of injured tissue.

Enamel Hard outer layer of the crown of a tooth.

Enamel hypocalcification A developmental anomaly that results in a disturbance of the maturation of the enamel matrix. It usually appears as a localized, chalky white spot on the middle third of smooth crowns, and the underlying enamel may be soft and susceptible to caries.

Enamel hypoplasia The incomplete or defective formation of enamel, resulting in the alteration of tooth form or color.

Enamel pearl A small, spherical enamel projection located on a root surface. Also called an *enameloma*.

Enameloma A small, spherical enamel projection located on a root surface. Also called an *enamel pearl*.

Encapsulated Surrounded by a capsule of fibrous connective tissue.

Endogenous Originating or produced within an organism or one of its parts.

Enucleation Surgical removal without cutting into the lesion; involves "scooping" out of a lesion along its peripheral borders.

Enzyme-linked immunosorbent assay (ELISA) A serologic laboratory procedure used to identify circulating antibodies. It is routinely used in HIV testing.

Eosinophilic granuloma of bone A solitary or chronic localized form of Langerhans cell disease. This form primarily affects older children and young adults. The skull and mandible are commonly involved with eosinophilic granuloma. The radiographic appearance varies, and the lesion may resemble periodontal disease or periapical inflammatory disease; or it may appear as a well-circumscribed radiolucency with or without a sclerotic border.

Epidemic parotitis A viral infection of the salivary glands caused by a paramyxovirus. The disease most commonly occurs in children and is characterized by painful swelling of the salivary glands, most commonly bilateral swelling of the parotid glands. Also called *mumps*.

Epidermal cyst A raised nodule in the skin. It is lined by keratinizing epithelium that resembles the epithelium of skin (epidermis). The cyst lumen is usually filled with keratin scales.

Epidermoid carcinoma A malignant tumor of the squamous epithelium. It is the most common primary malignancy of the oral cavity and, like other malignant tumors, can infiltrate adjacent tissues and metastasize to distant sites. Also known as *squamous cell carcinoma*.

Epidermoid cells Squamouslike epithelial cells

Epilepsy A group of neurologic disorders characterized by recurrent episodes of convulsive seizures, sensory disturbances, abnormal behavior, and loss of consciousness.

Epistaxis Nosebleed.

Epithelial Pertaining to the epithelium.

Epithelialization The process of being covered with epithelium.

Epithelial dysplasia A histologic diagnosis that indicates disordered growth. It is considered a premalignant condition.

Epithelial tumor A tumor that develops from the epithelium. There are three types: (1) tumors derived from squamous epithelium, (2) tumors derived from glandular epithelium, and (3) tumors derived from odontogenic epithelium.

Epithelium The layer of cells that lines a body cavity.

Epstein-Barr virus A herpesvirus associated with several diseases that occur in the oral region, including infectious mononucleosis, nasopharyngeal carcinoma, Burkitt lymphoma, and hairy leukoplakia.

Epulis fissuratum A lesion caused by an ill-fitting denture located in the vestibule along the dental border. Also called *redundant tissue* and *denture-induced fibrous hyperplasia*.

Erosion The loss of tooth structure resulting from chemical action.

Erosive lichen planus The type of lichen planus in which the epithelium separates from the connective tissue and erosions or ulcers form.

Eruption cyst A cyst that forms in the soft tissue around the crown of an erupting tooth.

Erythema An abnormal redness of the skin or mucosa.

Erythema multiforme An acute, self-limited disease that affects the skin and mucous membranes. The cause is not clear, but some evidence exists that it is a hypersensitivity reaction.

Erythematous candidiasis A type of candidiasis characterized by an erythematous, often painful, mucosa. It may be localized to one area of the oral mucosa or be more generalized.

Erythroplakia A clinical term that is used to describe an oral mucosal lesion that appears as a smooth red patch or a granular red and velvety patch.

Euploid A cell or organism that has an integral multiple of the monoploid number of chromosomes.

Excision Surgical removal.

Exopthalmus Bulging eyes; an abnormal protrusion (bulging) of one or both eyeballs.

Exostosis (plural, *exostoses*) A small nodular excrescence of normal compact bone. Exostoses present as asymptomatic, bony hard nodules on the buccal aspect of the maxillary or mandibular alveolar ridges.

Expressivity In genetics, the degree of clinical manifestation of a trait or characteristic.

External tooth resorption Resorption of a tooth structure beginning at the outside of the tooth. It usually involves the root of the tooth but may involve the crown of an impacted tooth.

Extramedullary plasmacytoma A localized tumor of plasma cells located in soft tissue.

Extraosseous cyst A cyst that occurs in the soft tissue.

Exudate Inflammatory fluid formed as a reaction to injury of tissues and blood vessels.

F

Facial hemihypertrophy Localized enlargement affecting one side of the orofacial structures.

Facies The appearance of the face.

Factor IX A factor that is active in the formation of intrinsic blood thromboplastin. A deficiency results in Christmas disease (hemophilia B), which is caused by a decrease in the amount of thromboplastin formed. Also called *plasma thromboplastin*.

Familial In genetics, something that affects more members of a family than would be expected by chance.

Fever An elevation of body temperature to greater than normal (98.6° F, or 37° C).

Fever blister The most common type of recurrent oral herpes simplex infection that occurs on the vermilion border of the lips. Also called *cold sore* or *herpes labialis*.

Fibrin An insoluble protein that is essential to the clotting of blood.

Fibroma A broad-based, persistent exophytic benign lesion composed of dense, scarlike connective tissue containing few blood vessels. It occurs as a result of chronic trauma or an episode of trauma. It is also known as an *irritation fibroma* or *traumatic fibroma*.

Fibroplasia The formation of fibrous tissue, as normally occurs in healing.

Fibrous dysplasia A benign fibro-osseous lesion composed of vascularized, cellular fibrous connective tissue interspersed with irregular trabeculae of bone emerging from the connective tissue. It is characterized by the replacement of bone with abnormal fibrous connective tissue interspersed with varying amounts of calcification.

First meiosis Step one to reduce and then maintain the normal number of human chromosomes. The new embryo must have 46 chromosomes per cell as did its parents.

Fissure A cleft or groove, normal or otherwise, showing prominent depth.

Fissured Having surface clefting or grooves.

Fissured tongue Characterized by the dorsal surface of the tongue having deep fissures or grooves.

Fistula Formation of a drainage passage that bores through tissue, allowing drainage to the outside. It is formed at the expense of healthy, functioning tissue as the area that is lost becomes necrotic.

Fixed drug eruption A lesion that recurs at the same site with each exposure to a particular drug.

Flare Redness of the skin or mucosa around the area of exposure to an irritant.

Florid cemento-osseous dysplasia A fibro-osseous lesion characterized by disordered cementum and bone development. This lesion characteristically involves multiple quadrants in the maxilla and mandible. It is most common in middle-aged black women.

Focal cemento-osseous dysplasia An asymptomatic fibro-osseous lesion that typically arises in the posterior mandible. A characteristic feature is that it is composed of numerous gritty pieces of soft and hard tissue.

Focal epithelial hyperplasia A disease caused by a human papillomavirus (HPV) that is characterized by the presence of multiple whitish–to–pale-pink nodules distributed throughout the oral mucosa. Also known as *Heck disease*.

Focal palmoplantar and gingival hyperkeratosis A syndrome characterized by areas of hyperkeratinization of the palms and soles and marked hyperkeratinization of the labial and lingual gingiva.

Folic acid A member of the vitamin B complex necessary for the normal production of red blood cells.

Follicular cyst A cyst that forms around the crown of an unerupted or developing tooth. Also called a *dentigerous cyst*.

Fordyce granules Clusters of ectopic sebaceous glands. They are most commonly seen on the lips and buccal mucosa. They are considered a variant of normal.

Frenectomy Surgical removal of a portion of the lingual frenum.

Frontal process Covering of the brain from which the forehead and other facial structures develops; located just above the stomodeum.

Fusion The union of two adjoining tooth germs.

G

Gamete Spermatozoon or ovum.

Gap 1 (G₁) phase The phase the cell enters after each cell division is completed and before the next division can occur.

Gap 2 (G₂) phase The phase that follows the S phase; it ends when mitotic division begins.

Gardner syndrome An inherited syndrome characterized by the presence of osteomas in various bones, especially in the frontal bones, mandible, and maxilla. Osteomas of the facial skeleton expand, obliterate the sinuses, and cause facial asymmetry. Intestinal polyps are also present, which become malignant after age 30 years. Also known as *familial colorectal polyposis*.

Gemination "Twinning"; when a single tooth germ attempts to divide, resulting in the incomplete formation of two teeth; the tooth usually has a single root and root canal.

Genes The hereditary units that are transmitted from one generation to another.

Genetic heterogeneity Having more than one inheritance pattern.

Geographic tongue A condition characterized by diffuse areas devoid of filiform papillae that develop on the dorsal and lateral borders of the tongue. These areas appear as erythematous patches surrounded by a white or yellow perimeter. The fungiform papillae are distinct within the erythematous patch.

Ghost cells Characteristic of a calcifying odontogenic cyst; exhibits a clear central area; thought to represent degenerating epithelial cells.

Ghost teeth A developmental anomaly in which one or several teeth in the same quadrant radiographically exhibit a marked reduction in radiodensity and a characteristic ghostlike appearance. Very thin enamel and dentin are present. Also called *regional odontodysplasia*.

Giant cell granuloma A lesion that contains many multinucleated giant cells and well-vascularized connective tissue. It occurs only in the jaws.

Gigantism Excessive growth caused by hyperpituitarism resulting in a stature larger than the range that is normal for age and race.

Gingival cyst A small bulge or swelling of the attached gingiva or interdental papillae. It exhibits the same type of epithelial lining as a lateral periodontal cyst and is located in the soft tissue of the same area.

Gingival fibromatosis An enlargement of the gingiva that results from the marked collagenization of the fibrous connective tissue. It is a component of many different inherited syndromes, caused by certain drugs or is idiopathic.

Gingival fibromatosis with hypertrichosis An inherited syndrome characterized by gingival fibromatosis and excessive growth of hair (hypertrichosis), especially of the eyebrows, extremities, genitals, and sacral region.

Gingival fibromatosis with multiple hyaline fibromas An inherited syndrome characterized by gingival fibromatosis; hypertrophy of the nail beds; and multiple hyaline fibrous tumors developing on the nose, chin, head, back, fingers, thighs, and legs. Also known as *Murray-Puretic-Drescher syndrome*.

Gingival hyperkeratosis A syndrome characterized by areas of hyperkeratinization of the palms and soles and marked hyperkeratinization of the labial and lingual gingiva.

Gingival hyperplasia Enlargement of the gingiva.

Globular process A pair of bulges formed from the median nasal process that grow downward, forming a portion of the upper lip.

Globulomaxillary cyst A cyst found between the roots of the maxillary lateral incisor and cuspid. It is characterized by well-defined, pear-shaped radiolucency and is believed to be of odontogenic epithelial origin. When it is large enough, divergence of the roots of adjacent teeth can result.

Gluten-sensitive enteropathy Hypersensitivity to gluten. Also called *celiac sprue* and *celiac disease*.

Granular cell tumor A benign tumor composed of large cells with a granular cytoplasm. It likely arises from a neural or primitive mesenchymal cell. It most often occurs on the tongue or buccal mucosa. The tumor appears as a painless, nonulcerated nodule.

Granulation tissue The initial tissue formed in the connective tissue portion of the injury. It is immature tissue with many capillaries and fibroblasts.

Granuloma A tumorlike mass of inflammatory tissue consisting of a central collection of macrophages, often with multinucleated giant cells, surrounded by lymphocytes.

Granulomatous disease A disease characterized by the formation of granulomas.

Granulomatous inflammation A distinctive form of chronic inflammation characterized by the formation of granulomas.

Gumma A localized, noninfectious, destructive lesion that occurs during the tertiary stage of syphilis. The most common oral sites are the tongue and palate. The lesion appears as a firm mass that eventually becomes an ulcer.

H

Hairy leukoplakia An irregular, corrugated, white lesion that occurs almost exclusively on the lateral border of the tongue. Epstein-Barr virus has been identified in the epithelial cells of hairy leukoplakia and is considered to be the cause of the lesion.

Hairy tongue A condition in which the patient has elongated filiform papillae due to an increased accumulation of keratin. This results in either a light or dark "hairy" appearance.

Hand-foot-and-mouth disease An infectious disease caused by a coxsackievirus, characterized by painful vesicles and ulcers that can occur anywhere in the mouth. Multiple macules or papules occur on the skin, typically on the feet, toes, hands, and fingers. Usually occurs in epidemics in children less than 5 years of age.

Hand-Schüller-Christian disease A chronic disseminated or multifocal form of Langerhans cell disease. This form occurs in children, usually less than 5 years of age. All changes are caused by localized collections of Langerhans cells. The triad includes single to multiple well-defined or "punched-out" radiolucent areas in the skull (may also occur in the jawbones), unilateral or bilateral exophthalmos, and diabetes insipidus that is caused by collections of macrophages in the sella turcica area, affecting the pituitary gland.

Haploid A cell with a single set of chromosomes. A gamete is haploid.

Hemangioma A benign proliferation of capillaries. It is a common vascular lesion considered by many to represent a developmental lesion rather than a tumor. It may also occur in adults as a result of trauma.

Hematocrit The volume percentage of red blood cells in whole blood.

Hematoma A lesion that results from the accumulation of blood within tissue as a result of trauma.

Hemolysis The release of hemoglobin from red blood cells by destruction of the cells.

Hemophilia A disorder of blood coagulation that results in severely prolonged clotting time. The problem results from a deficiency of one of the plasma proteins involved in the coagulation cascade that is necessary for the conversion of fibrinogen to fibrin.

Hemostasis The stoppage or cessation of bleeding.

Hepatomegaly Enlargement of the liver.

Hereditary hemorrhagic telangiectasia A syndrome characterized by multiple capillary dilations of the skin and mucous membranes. The skin of the face shows numerous pinpoint and spiderlike telangiectasias, especially on the lips, eyelids, and around the nose. Telangiectasias of the oral mucosa are prominent on the tip and anterior dorsum of the tongue; and the palate, gingiva, and buccal mucosa are often affected but to a lesser degree. Also known as *Osler-Rendu–Parkes Weber syndrome*.

Herpangina An infectious disease caused by a coxsackievirus, characterized by vesicles on the soft palate, along with fever, malaise, sore throat, and difficulty swallowing (dysphagia). An erythematous pharyngitis is also present.

Herpes labialis The most common type of recurrent oral herpes simplex infection that occurs on the vermilion border of the lips. Also called a *cold sore* or *fever blister*.

Herpes simplex Infections caused by herpes virus types 1 and 2.

Herpes zoster A disease caused by the varicella-zoster virus that occurs in adults. It is characterized by a unilateral, painful eruption of vesicles along the distribution of a sensory nerve. Also called *shingles*.

Herpetic whitlow A painful infection of the fingers caused by the herpes simplex virus.

Herpetiform aphthous ulcer Tiny aphthous ulcers (1 to 2 mm) that resemble ulcers caused by the herpes simplex virus.

Hertwig epithelial root sheath An epithelial structure that proliferates to shape the root of the tooth and induce the formation of the root dentin.

Heterozygote (adjective, heterozygous) Individual with two different genes at the allele loci.

Highly active antiretroviral therapy (HAART) A combination of various types of antiretroviral (anti-HIV) drugs used in the management of HIV infection.

Hives Multiple areas of well-demarcated swelling of the skin, usually accompanied by itching. The lesions are caused by localized areas of vascular permeability in the superficial connective tissue beneath the epithelium. Also known as *urticaria*.

hnRNA Heterogenous nuclear RNA; the fourth type of RNA. It is found within the nucleus and is the precursor of mRNA.

Homozygote (adjective, homozygous) An individual having identical genes at the allele loci.

Hormone A chemical substance produced in the body that has a specific regulatory effect on certain cells or a certain organ or organs.

Human immunodeficiency virus (HIV) A retrovirus that causes acquired immunodeficiency syndrome (AIDS). It is transmitted through contact with an infected individual's blood, semen, cervical secretions, cerebrospinal fluid, or synovial fluid. It infects T-helper cells, dendritic cells, and macrophages of the immune system.

Human papillomavirus (HPV) A group of more than 150 related viruses. The papillomaviruses are attracted to and are able to live only in squamous epithelial cells. Low-risk types cause warts and papillomas. High-risk types are associated with malignant transformation of squamous cells.

Humoral immunity Immunity in which antibodies play the predominant role.

Hutchinson incisor Malformed incisor that results from the presence of congenital syphilis during tooth development. It is shaped like a screwdriver; broad cervically and narrow incisally, with a notched incisal edge.

Hypercalcemia An excess of calcium in the blood.

Hyperchromic Staining more intensely than normal.

Hyperemia An excess of blood in a part of the body.

Hyperglycemia An excess of glucose in the blood.

Hypermobility An increase in the range of movement of a body part, especially a joint.

Hypermobility disorders Include **dislocation** and **subluxation.** See these terms elsewhere in this glossary.

Hyperparathyroidism A condition that results from excessive secretion of parathyroid hormone (parathormone or PTH), which is secreted by the parathyroid glands.

Hyperpituitarism Excess hormone production by the anterior pituitary gland.

Hyperplasia An abnormal increase in the number of normal cells in an organ or tissue.

Hypersensitivity A state of altered reactivity in which the body reacts to a foreign agent with an exaggerated immune response.

Hypertelorism A condition in which there is greater-than-normal distance between two paired organs. Orbital or ocular hypertelorism is a condition marked by a greater-than-normal distance between the eyes.

Hyperthermia Increased body temperature.

Hyperthyroidism A condition characterized by excessive production of thyroid hormone. Also called *thyrotoxicosis*.

Hypertrichosis The excessive growth of hair.

Hypertrophic candidiasis A type of candidiasis that appears as a white lesion that does not wipe off the mucosa. An important diagnostic feature of this type of candidiasis is that it responds to treatment with antifungal medication. Also called chronic *hyperplastic candidiasis* and *candidal leukoplakia*.

Hypertrophy An enlargement of a tissue or organ caused by an increase in size but not in the number of cells.

Hypochromic Staining less intensely than normal.

Hypodontia Partial anodontia. The lack of one or more teeth.

Hypoglycemia Low blood sugar.

Hypohidrosis Abnormally diminished secretion of sweat.

Hypohidrotic ectodermal dysplasia The most severe form of ectodermal dysplasia. Its major characteristics are hypodontia, hypotrichosis, and hypohidrosis.

Hypophosphatasia A syndrome characterized by a decrease in serum alkaline phosphatase levels with increased urinary and plasma levels of phosphoethanolamine. This can cause total or partial aplasia of the cementum, an abnormal periodontal ligament in the primary teeth, and a decreased phosphatase level that has been linked to premature loss of teeth.

Hypophosphatemia Deficiency of phosphates in the blood.

Hypophosphatemic vitamin D–resistant rickets A disorder characterized by low serum levels of phosphorus. This can be caused by low absorption of inorganic phosphate in the renal tubules, rickets, or osteomalacia. This condition demonstrates resistance to treatment with usual doses of vitamin D.

Hypoplasia The incomplete development of an organ or tissue.

Hypoplastic Underdeveloped.

Hyposalivation Decreased salivary flow.

Hypothyroidism A condition characterized by decreased output of thyroid hormone.

Hypotrichosis Presence of less than the normal amount of hair.

I

Iatrogenic Induced inadvertently by a medical/dental care provider or by medical treatment or a diagnostic procedure.

Icterus A condition characterized by an abnormal accumulation of bilirubin (red bile pigment) in the blood and manifested by a yellowish discoloration of the skin, mucous membranes, and cornea. Also called *jaundice*.

Idiopathic leukoplakia A term used to emphasize that the specific cause of leukoplakia is unknown. See also **Leukoplakia.**

Idiopathic thrombocytopenic purpura A condition in which spontaneous bleeding occurs for an unknown reason.

Idiopathic tooth resorption Resorption that can involve the crown of an impacted tooth or roots of teeth. The cause cannot be identified.

Immune complex A combination of antibody and antigen.

Immunity The ability of an organism to resist or not be susceptible to injury or infection.

Immunization A process by which resistance to an infectious disease is induced. It lowers the risk of a microorganism causing disease because it prepares the immune system to fight future attacks by the disease-causing microorganism.

Immunodeficiency A deficiency of the immune response caused by hypoactivity or decreased numbers of lymphoid cells.

Immunoglobulin A protein, also called an *antibody*, synthesized by plasma cells in response to a specific antigen.

Immunologic tolerance The recognition and nonresponsiveness of the immune system to the body's own cells and tissues.

Immunomodulator A substance that alters the immune response by augmenting or reducing the ability of the immune system to produce antibodies or sensitized cells that recognize and react with the antigen that initiated their production.

Immunopathology The study of immune reactions involved in disease.

Impacted teeth Teeth that cannot erupt into the oral cavity because of a physical obstruction.

Impetigo A bacterial skin infection caused primarily by *Staphylococcus aureus* and occasionally by *Streptococcus pyogenes*. Impetigo most commonly involves lesions on the skin of the face or extremities.

Incisive canal cyst A developmental cyst located within the incisive canal or incisive papilla. It appears as a heart-shaped radiolucency. Also known as *nasopalatine canal cyst*.

Incubation period The period between the infection of an individual by a pathogen and the manifestation of the disease it causes.

Infectious mononucleosis An infectious disease caused by the Epstein-Barr virus. It is characterized by sore throat, fever, generalized lymphadenopathy, enlarged spleen, malaise, and fatigue. Palatal petechiae occur in infectious mononucleosis, usually appearing early in the course of the disease.

Inflammatory response (inflammation) A nonspecific response to injury that involves the microcirculation and its blood cells.

Inherited disorder A disorder caused by an abnormality in the genetic makeup (genes and chromosomes) of an individual that is transmitted from parent to offspring through the egg or sperm.

Injury Tissue damage caused by trauma or an alteration in the environment.

In situ Confined to the site of origin without invasion of neighboring tissues.

Insulin A peptide hormone produced in the pancreas by the beta cells in the islets of Langerhans. Insulin regulates glucose metabolism and is the major fuel-regulating hormone.

Insulin-dependent diabetes mellitus The type of diabetes that requries the administration of insulin to prevent ketosis. The onset is abrupt and may be characterized by polydipsia, polyuria, and polyphagia. Also called *type 1 diabetes*.

Insulin shock Profound hypoglycemia, or low blood sugar, that necessitates emergency intervention.

Internal derangement Disk (meniscal) displacements, ankylosis, and hypermobility disorders related to the temporomandibular joint.

Internal tooth resorption Resorption usually involving a single tooth, often associated with an inflammatory response in the pulp. It can occur in any tooth.

International Normalized Ratio (INR) An expression of the ratio of prothrombin time to thromboplastin activity. It is a more accurate determination of prothrombin time (PT).

Intraosseous cyst A cyst that occurs within bone.

Intrinsic Naturally occurring within; essential.

Intrinsic staining Tooth discoloration that occurs as a result of the deposition of substances circulating systemically during tooth development.

Invagination The infolding of one portion of a structure into another portion of the same structure.

Invasion The infiltration and active destruction of surrounding tissues.

Inversion In genetics, a portion of a chromosome arranged upside-down.

Iron deficiency anemia A condition that occurs when an insufficient amount of iron is supplied to the bone marrow for red blood cell development.

J

Jaundice A condition characterized by an abnormal accumulation of bilirubin (bile pigment) in the blood and manifested by a yellowish discoloration of the skin, mucous membranes, and cornea. Also called *icterus*.

K

Kaposi sarcoma A malignant vascular tumor that may arise in multiple sites, including the skin and oral cavity. In HIV-positive patients these lesions are often seen on the hard palate and gingiva, where they present as purple macules, plaques, or exophytic tumors.

Karyotype A photomicrographic representation of a person's chromosomal constitution arranged according to the Denver classification.

Keloid Excessive skin scarring that appears raised and extends beyond its original boundaries.

Keratin pearl Rounded concentric masses of epithelial cells and keratin found in some squamous cell carcinomas.

Keratoconjunctivitis sicca The eye damage that occurs in Sjögren syndrome caused by lack of tears.

Ketoacidosis A metabolic acidosis resulting from the accumulation of ketone bodies. It is most commonly a consequence of untreated type 1 diabetes mellitus.

Koplik spots Small erythematous macules with white necrotic centers seen intraorally in patients with macules.

L

Laband syndrome An inherited syndrome characterized by gingival fibromatosis, dysplastic or absent nails, malformed nose and ears, hepatosplenomegaly, and hypoplasia of terminal phalanges of the fingers and toes.

Labial melanotic macule A flat, well-circumscribed, brown lesion that occurs on the vermilion of the lip that darkens with exposure to sunlight.

Lack of penetrance The ability to carry a gene with a dominant effect without presenting any clinical manifestations.

Langerhans cell Specialized dendritic cell found in the skin and mucosa that is involved in the immune response.

Langerhans cell disease A disease formerly called histiocytosis X. Three entities traditionally grouped under the category of histiocytosis X are (1) Letterer-Siwe disease, (2) Hand-Schüller-Christian disease, and (3) solitary eosinophilic granuloma.

Lateral nasal processes The processes that form the sides of the nose.

Lateral palatine processes The processes that develop from the maxillary tissues laterally and grow to the midline to form the palate.

Lateral periodontal cyst A cyst named for its location. It is most often seen in the mandibular cuspid and premolar area and presents as an asymptomatic, unilocular or multilocular radiolucent lesion located on the lateral aspect of a tooth root. A thin band of stratified squamous epithelium that exhibits focal epithelial thickenings lines the cyst.

LE cell A cell that is a characteristic of lupus erythematosus and other autoimmune diseases. It is a mature neutrophil that has phagocytized a spherical inclusion derived from another neutrophil.

Leiomyoma A benign tumor of smooth muscle. When associated with blood vessels, it is called a vascular leiomyoma.

Letterer-Siwe disease An acute disseminated form of Langerhans cell disease that usually affects children younger than 3 years of age. The disease resembles a lymphoma in that it generally has a rapidly fatal course that sometimes responds to chemotherapy.

Leukemia A form of cancer characterized by an overproduction of atypical white blood cells. Can be acute or chronic.

Leukocytosis A temporary increase in the number of white blood cells circulating in the blood.

Leukoedema A condition that is a variant of normal and characterized by generalized opalescence of the buccal mucosa.

Leukopenia A decrease in white blood cells.

Leukoplakia A clinical term used to identify a white, plaquelike lesion of the oral mucosa that cannot be wiped off and cannot be diagnosed as any other disease on a clinical basis.

Lichen planus A benign, chronic disease affecting the skin and oral mucosa. The lesions have a characteristic pattern of interconnecting lines called Wickham striae.

Linea alba A white raised line that forms commonly on the buccal mucosa at the occlusal plane and is usually considered a variant of normal.

Linear gingival erythema A type of gingival disease that develops in patients with HIV infection. It has three characteristic features: (1) spontaneous bleeding, (2) punctate or petechia-like lesions on the attached gingiva and alveolar mucosa, and (3) a bandlike erythema of the gingiva that does not respond to therapy.

Lingual mandibular bone concavity A well-defined cystlike radiolucency in the posterior region of the mandible inferior to the mandibular canal that is caused by a lingual depression in the mandible, which contains normal salivary gland tissue. Also known as a *static bone cyst* or *Stafne bone cyst*. Often referred to as a pseudocyst because it is not a pathologic cavity and is not lined with epithelium.

Lingual thyroid Mass of thyroid tissue found on dorsal tongue posterior to circumvallate papillae.

Lingual thyroid nodule A mass of thyroid tissue located on the tongue away from the normal anatomic location of the thyroid gland. It is an uncommon developmental anomaly that results from the failure of the primitive thyroid tissue to migrate from its developmental location in the area of the foramen cecum on the posterior portion of the tongue to its normal position in the neck. Also called *ectopic lingual thyroid nodule*.

Lingual varicosities Prominent lingual veins usually observed on the ventral and lateral surfaces of the tongue.

Lipoma A benign tumor of fat.

Lobule (adjective, lobulated) A segment or lobe that is part of a whole. Lobules sometimes appear fused together.

Local Confined to a limited part; not general or systemic.

Locus In genetics the position occupied by a gene on a chromosome.

Lymphadenopathy Any disease process that affects lymph nodes such that they become enlarged and palpable.

Lymphangioma A benign tumor of lymphatic vessels. The most common intraoral location is the tongue, where a lymphangioma presents as an ill-defined mass with a pebbly surface.

Lymphoepithelial cyst A cyst that is composed of a stratified squamous epithelial lining surrounded by a well-circumscribed component of lymphoid tissue. Also known as a *branchial cleft cyst* when located in the neck. The lymphoepithelial cyst occurs in the parotid gland and oral mucosa.

Lymphoid tissue Tissue composed of lymphocytes supported by a meshwork of connective tissue.

Lymphokines Cytokines produced by B-cell or T-cell lymphocytes in contact with antigens; mediators in an immune response.

Lymphoma A malignant tumor of lymphoid tissue.

Lyon hypothesis The hypothesis, postulated by Mary Lyon, that during the early period of embryonic development the genetic activity of one of the X chromosomes in each cell of a female embryo is inactivated.

Lysosomal enzyme An enzyme found in the granular cytoplasm of a neutrophil. Lysosomal enzymes destroy substances after the cell has engulfed them.

M

Macrodontia Abnormally large teeth.

Macrophage A large, mononuclear phagocyte derived from monocytes. Macrophages become mobile when stimulated by inflammation and interact with lymphocytes in an immune response.

Macrovascular disease Atherosclerosis of large- and medium-sized blood vessels.

Macule An area that is usually distinguished by a color different from that of the surrounding tissue; it is flat and does not protrude above the surface of the normal tissue. A freckle is an example of a macule.

Magnetic resonance imaging (MRI) A noninvasive diagnostic technique that uses radio waves to produce computerized images of internal body tissues.

Major aphthous ulcer A nonspecific aphthous ulcer that is greater than 1 cm in diameter, is deeper, and lasts longer than a minor aphthous ulcer. The presence of multiple major aphthous ulcers is known as *Sutton disease* or *periadenitis mucosa necrotica recurrens*.

Major histocompatibility complex Unique cell surface molecules that help T cells to recognize antigen fragments.

Malaise A vague, indefinite feeling of discomfort, debilitation, or lack of health.

Malignant Resistant to treatment; able to metastasize and kill the host; describing cancer.

Malignant melanoma Malignant tumor of melanocytes that commonly arises on the skin as a result of exposure to sunlight.

Malignant tumor Cancer; a tumor that is resistant to treatment and may cause death; a tumor that has the potential for uncontrolled growth and dissemination or recurrence or both.

Mandibular process The first branchial arch divides into two maxillary processes and the mandibular process (or mandibular arch). It forms the lower part of the cheeks, the mandible, and part of the tongue.

Mandibular tori (singular, *torus*) Outgrowths of normal dense bone found on the lingual aspect of the mandible in the area of the premolars above the mylohyoid ridge. Also known as *torus mandibularis.*

Mandibulofacial dysostosis A syndrome characterized by developmental disturbance of the cranial bones and hypoplasia of the lower part of the face. The mandibular body is underdeveloped, and the eyes slant downward. The teeth are crowded and malposed. A high vaulted palate and deafness are other characteristic features. Also known as *Treacher Collins syndrome.*

Margination A process during inflammation in which white blood cells tend to move to the blood vessel walls.

Maxillary processes The first branchial arch divides into two maxillary processes and the mandibular process. The maxillary processes give rise to the upper part of the cheeks, the lateral portions of the upper lip, and part of the palate.

Measles A highly contagious disease, caused by paramyxovirus, with systemic symptoms and a skin rash . The disease occurs most commonly in childhood. Early in the disease, Koplik spots, which are small erythematous macules by white necrotic centers, may occur in the oral cavity.

Median mandibular cyst A rare cyst located in the midline of the mandible. It is characterized by a well-defined radiolucency that is seen below the apices of the mandibular incisors and is lined with squamous epithelium.

Median nasal process The process that forms the center and tip of the nose.

Median palatine cyst A cyst located in the midline of the hard palate. It is characterized by a well-defined unilocular radiolucency and is lined with stratified squamous epithelium that is surrounded by dense fibrous connective tissue.

Median rhomboid glossitis A flat or slightly raised oval or rectangular erythematous area in the midline of the dorsal surface of the tongue, beginning at the junction of the anterior and middle thirds and extending posterior to the circumvallate papillae. It is devoid of filiform papillae; therefore its texture is smooth. It may be associated with *Candida albicans.*

Megaloblastic anemia A type of anemia characterized by hyperplastic bone marrow changes and maturation arrest resulting from a dietary deficiency, impaired absorption, impaired storage and modification, or impaired use of one or more hematopoietic factors.

Megaloblasts Red blood cells that are immature, abnormally large, and have nuclei. Megaloblasts are seen in high numbers in the bone marrow in megaloblastic anemia.

Meiosis The two-step cellular division of the original germ cells, which reduces the chromosomes from 4nDNA to 1nDNA. The two steps are called *first meiosis* and *second meiosis.*

Melanin The pigment that gives color to the skin, eyes, hair, mucosa, and gingiva.

Melanin pigmentation Discoloration of the oral tissues produced by the deposition of melanin.

Melanocytes Pigment-producing cells in the skin, hair, and eye that determine their color. The pigment that melanocytes make is called *melanin.*

Mesiodens The most common supernumerary tooth; found between the maxillary central incisors. It can be unerupted or erupted. The crown has a conical shape.

Mental retardation A disorder characterized by certain limitations in a person's mental functioning and in skills such as communicating, taking care of himself or herself, and social skills.

Metaphase The phase of cellular division in which the chromosomes are lined up evenly along the equatorial plate of the cell; during this time the chromosomes are most visible.

Metastasis (plural, metastases) The transport of neoplastic cells to parts of the body remote from the primary tumor and the establishment of new tumors in those sites.

Metastatic tumor A tumor formed by cells that have been transported from the primary tumor to a site not connected with the original tumor.

Methamphetamine A sympathomimetic amine related to amphetamine and ephedrine that stimulates central nervous system activity. It is used to treat obesity, minimal brain dysfunction, and attention deficit hyperactivity disorder. It is also used illicitly as a recreational drug.

Meth mouth The extensive and rapid destruction of teeth due to methamphetamine abuse.

Microcirculation Small blood vessels, including arterioles, capillaries, and venules.

Microcyte A red blood cell that is smaller than normal.

Microdontia Abnormally small teeth.

Microvascular disease Damage to small blood vessels.

Miliary tuberculosis The type of tuberculosis in which the bacteria are carried to widespread areas of the body and cause involvement of organs such as the kidneys and liver.

Millimeter (mm) One thousandth of a meter (1 m is equivalent to 39.3 inches). A periodontal probe is of great assistance in documenting the size or diameter of a lesion that can be measured in millimeters.

Minor aphthous ulcer The most commonly occurring type of aphthous ulcer. It appears as a discrete, round-to-oval ulcer that is up to 1 cm in diameter and exhibits a yellowish-white fibrin surface surrounded by a halo of erythema.

Mitochondria Cytoplasmic energy-producing organelles that have their own DNA in a circular chromosome.

Mitochondrial DNA DNA located in the mitochondria, and needed for mitochondrial function; inherited maternally.

Mitosis The way in which somatic cells divide so that the two daughter cells receive the same number of identical chromosomes.

Mitotic cycle The part of the life span of a somatic cell when cellular division is achieved by mitosis.

Mitotic figures The microscopic appearance of cells during mitosis.

Moniliasis An overgrowth of the yeastlike fungus *Candida albicans.* It is the most common oral fungal infection. It can result from many different conditions, including antibiotic use, cancer, corticosteroid therapy, dentures, diabetes mellitus, and HIV infection. Also called *candidiasis* and *thrush.*

Monoclonal spike An elevation of a single type of immunoglobulin detected by immunoelectrophoresis; seen in patients with multiple myeloma.

Monokines Cytokines produced by monocytes or macrophages; mediators in an immune response.

Monomorphic adenoma A benign encapsulated salivary gland tumor composed of a uniform pattern of epithelial cells. It occurs most commonly in adult females, with a predilection for the upper lip and buccal mucosa.

Monostotic fibrous dysplasia The most common type of fibrous dysplasia. It is characterized by involvement of a single bone. The mandible and maxilla are commonly affected; the maxilla is more frequently involved than the mandible.

Mosaic bone A microscopic pattern seen in the involved bone of a patient with Paget disease of bone. It demonstrates prominent reversal lines that result from the resorption and deposition of bone.

mRNA Messenger RNA; the first type of RNA. It carries the message from the DNA to the ribosomes, where proteins are produced.

Mucocele A lesion that forms when a salivary gland duct is severed and the mucous salivary gland secretion spills into the adjacent connective tissue.

Mucoepidermoid carcinoma An unencapsulated and infiltrating malignant salivary gland tumor composed of a combination of mucous cells interspersed with squamouslike epithelial cells. Major gland tumors occur most often in the parotid gland. Minor gland tumors occur most commonly on the palate.

Mucormycosis A rare fungal infection caused by an organism that is a common inhabitant of soil and is usually nonpathogenic. Infection occurs in diabetic and debilitated patients and often involves the nasal cavity, maxillary sinus, and hard palate; it can present as a proliferating or destructive mass in the maxilla. Also called *phycomycosis*.

Mucositis Mucosal inflammation.

Mucous cyst (mucous retention cyst) An epithelium-lined cystic structure that occurs in association with a salivary gland duct. Most are not true cysts but dilated salivary gland ducts that develop as a result of obstruction.

Mucous membrane pemphigoid A chronic autoimmune disease that affects the oral mucosa, conjunctiva, genital mucosa, and skin. It is also known as *cicatricial pemphigoid* and *benign mucous membrane pemphigoid*.

Mucous patches Oral lesions that appear in the secondary stage of syphilis. They are characterized by multiple, painless, grayish-white plaques covering ulcerated mucosa. They are very infectious.

Mucous retention cyst A mucosal swelling due to a dilated salivary gland duct that is caused by salivary duct obstruction; a form of mucocele.

Mulberry molar First molar with an irregularly shaped crown made up of multiple tiny globules of enamel instead of cusps, which imparts a berrylike appearance. Can be a manifestation of congenital syphilis.

Multifactorial conditions Conditions in which the phenotype results from a combination of genetic factors and environmental influences.

Multifactorial inheritance The type of hereditary pattern seen when there is more than one genetic factor involved and, sometimes, when there are also environmental factors participating in the causation of a condition.

Multilocular A term used to describe the radiographic appearance of multiple rounded compartments or locules. These can appear "soap bubble–like" or "honeycomb-like."

Multiple mucosal neuroma syndrome A syndrome composed of multiple mucosal neuromas, medullary carcinoma of the thyroid gland, and pheochromocytoma. Also termed *multiple endocrine neoplasia syndrome (MEN syndrome)*.

Multiple myeloma A systemic, malignant proliferation of plasma cells that causes destructive lesions in bone.

Mumps A viral infection of the salivary glands caused by a paramyxovirus. The disease most commonly occurs in children and is characterized by painful swelling of the salivary glands, most commonly bilateral swelling of the parotid glands. Also called *epidemic parotitis*.

Muscles of mastication The major muscles about the facial region that govern the movement of the mandible and chewing motions.

Mutation A permanent transmissible change in the genetic material, usually in a single gene.

Myalgia Muscle pain.

Myoepithelial cell A specific type of salivary gland cell with contractile properties.

Myofibroblasts A fibroblast that has some of the characteristics of smooth muscle cells, such as the ability to contract.

Myxedema The presence of hypothyroidism in older children and adults.

N

Nasolabial cyst A soft tissue cyst of the midlateral face with no alveolar bone involvement. It is lined with pseudostratified, ciliated columnar epithelium with multiple goblet cells. There is usually no associated radiographic change.

Nasopalatine canal cyst A cyst located within the nasopalatine canal or the incisive papilla. It arises from epithelial remnants of the embryonal nasopalatine ducts. Also known as an *incisive canal cyst*.

Natural killer cell (NK cell) A lymphocyte that is part of the body's initial innate immunity, which by unknown mechanisms is able to destroy cells recognized as foreign.

Natural passive immunity Passive immunity acquired by a developing fetus or newborn from its mother via the transfer of antibodies. These antibodies protect a newborn infant from disease while the infant's own immune system matures.

Necrosis The pathologic death of one or more cells or a portion of tissue or organ, resulting from irreversible damage.

Necrotizing sialometaplasia A benign condition of the minor salivary glands characterized by moderately painful swelling and ulceration in the area due to necrosis of the minor glands. Most common on the hard palate.

Necrotizing stomatitis A condition characterized by extensive focal areas of bone loss along with the features of necrotizing ulcerative periodontitis.

Necrotizing ulcerative gingivitis (NUG) A painful erythematous gingivitis with necrosis of the interdental papillae. Also formerly called *acute necrotizing ulcerative gingivitis (ANUG)*.

Necrotizing ulcerative periodontitis A condition that resembles necrotizing ulcerative gingivitis in which patients experience pain, spontaneous gingival bleeding, interproximal necrosis, and interproximal cratering along with intense erythema and, most characteristically, extremely rapid bone loss.

Neoplasia New growth; the process of the formation of tumors by the uncontrolled proliferation of cells.

Neoplasm Tumor; a new growth of tissue in which the growth is uncontrolled and progressive.

Neoplastic Pertaining to the formation of tumors by the uncontrolled proliferation of cells.

Neurofibroma A benign tumor derived from Schwann cells and perineural fibroblasts, which are components of the connective tissue surrounding a nerve. The tongue is the most common intraoral location.

Neurofibromatosis of von Recklinghausen A syndrome characterized by multiple neurofibromas on the skin. Oral involvement is characterized by single or multiple tumors at any location in the oral mucosa. Café au lait skin pigmentation is common. Also called *von Recklinghausen disease*.

Neutropenia A diminished number of circulating neutrophils in the blood.

Neutrophil The first type of white blood cell to arrive at the site of injury and the primary cell involved in acute inflammation. The nucleus of this cell is multilobed. Also called a *polymorphonuclear leukocyte*.

Nevoid basal cell carcinoma syndrome A syndrome characterized by mild hypertelorism and mild prognathism, the appearance of basal cell carcinomas early in life, and multiple cysts of the jaws characterized histologically as odontogenic keratocysts. A variety of skeletal abnormalities may occur, including bifurcation of one or more ribs. Also known as *Gorlin syndrome*.

Nevus (plural, nevi) (1) A tumor of melanocytes (melanin-producing cells). (2) A pigmented congenital lesion (a lesion present at birth).

Nevus cells Melanocytes (melanin-producing cells).

Nicotine stomatitis A benign lesion on the hard palate typically associated with pipe and cigar smoking. It may also occur with cigarette smoking.

Nikolsky sign Seen in some bullous diseases such as pemphigus vulgaris and bullous pemphigoid; the superficial epithelium separates easily from the basal layer on exertion of firm sliding manual pressure.

Nodule A palpable, solid lesion in soft tissue that is up to 1 cm in diameter and may be above, level with, or beneath the skin or mucosal surface.

Nondisjunction In genetics, when chromosomes that are crossing over do not separate; therefore, both migrate to the same cell.

Non–insulin-dependent diabetes mellitus The type of diabetes that is characterized by increased insulin resistance. It includes patients who can maintain proper blood sugar levels without the administration of insulin. However, insulin administration may be required. Also called *type 2 diabetes*.

Non-neoplasitic Not neoplastic.

Nonodontogenic Not related to tooth development.

Nonthrombocytopenic purpuras Bleeding disorders that can result from either a defect in the capillary walls or disorders of platelet function.

Normal joint function The harmonious function of the temporomandibular joint and jaws.

Nucleotide A hydrolytic product of nucleic acid formed by a nitrogen-containing base, a five-carbon sugar (deoxyribose), and a phosphate.

O

Ocular hypertelorism A condition marked by a greater-than-normal distance between the eyes.

Odontogenesis Tooth development.

Odontogenic adenomatoid tumor An encapsulated, benign epithelial odontogenic tumor that has a distinctive age, sex, and site distribution. Seventy percent occur in females less than 20 years of age; 70% involve the anterior part of the jaws. May be associated with impacted teeth. Also known as an *adenomatoid odontogenic tumor*.

Odontogenic keratocyst An odontogenic developmental cyst with a unique histologic appearance. The lumen is lined by epithelium that is 8 to 10 cell layers thick and surfaced by parakeratin. The basal cell layer is palisaded and prominent; the interface between the epithelium and the connective tissue is flat. This cyst has a higher recurrence rate than many other odontogenic cysts.

Odontogenic myxoma A benign mesenchymal odontogenic tumor that occurs anywhere in the maxilla or mandible, with the mandible being more common. It may displace teeth and spread to other locations.

Odontogenic Arising from tooth-forming tissues.

Odontogenic tumor A tumor derived from tooth-forming tissues. It is most often benign.

Odontoma An odontogenic tumor composed of mature enamel, dentin, cementum, and pulp tissue. The odontoma is the most common of the odontogenic tumors, and there are two types: compound and complex.

Olfactory pits Two pits that mark the future openings of the nose that develop on the surface of the frontal process.

Oligodontia A subcategory of hypodontia in which six or more teeth are congenitally missing.

Oligogenic inheritance Characteristics or traits that are inherited by the participation of several genes.

Oncology The study of tumors or neoplasms.

Oogenesis The process of formation of female germ cells (ova).

Opacification The process of becoming opaque.

Open joint surgery Surgery used to perform disk repositioning, replacement or excision, and total joint reconstruction using a prosthetic device or autogenous graft.

Opportunistic infection A disease caused by a microorganism that does not ordinarily cause disease but becomes pathogenic under certain circumstances.

Opsonization The enhancement of phagocytosis.

Oral melanotic macule A flat, well-circumscribed brown lesion of unknown cause. They are usually small and may require biopsy and histologic examination for diagnosis.

Osteoarthritis Characterized by degenerative changes of the articular cartilage with associated remodeling. It is the most common disease affecting the temporomandibular joint. It is also referred to as *degenerative joint disease*.

Osteogenesis imperfecta A congenital disorder characterized by abnormally formed bones that fracture easily. Other abnormalities include blue sclerae (mild cases), bowing of the legs, curvature of the spine, deformity of the skull, and shortening of arms and legs (severe cases). The oral manifestation of this syndrome is a dentinogenesis imperfecta–like condition.

Osteoma Benign tumor of normal compact bone.

Osteomalacia A disease of bone that develops over a long period of time as the result of a deficiency of calcium. When this disease occurs in young children, it is usually caused by a nutritional deficiency of vitamin D, and the associated disease is termed *rickets*.

Osteoporosis A hereditary disease marked by abnormally porous bone lacking normal density.

Osteoradionecrosis Necrosis of bone associated with radiation therapy.

Osteosarcoma A malignant tumor of the bone-forming tissue. Also known as *osteogenic sarcoma.*

Ovum (plural, ova) The mature female germ cell.

P

Paget disease of bone A chronic metabolic bone disease characterized by resorption, osteoblastic repair, and remineralization of the involved bone. It typically involves the pelvis and spinal column. Also called *osteitis deformans* and *leontiasis ossea.*

Palatal papillomatosis A form of denture stomatitis. Also called *papillary hyperplasia of the palate.*

Palatal torus An inherited exophytic growth of normal compact bone in the midline of the hard palate. Also known as *torus palatinus.*

Palatine processes Processes formed during development from the maxillary processes that fuse with the premaxilla to form the palate.

Palisaded encapsulated neuroma (PEN) A benign lesion that presents as a mucosal nodule. It appears microscopically as a well-circumscribed lesion composed of nerve tissue partially surrounded by a fibrous tissue capsule.

Pallor Paleness of the skin or mucosal tissues.

Palpation The evaluation of a lesion by feeling it with the fingers to determine the texture of the area; the descriptive terms for palpation are *soft, firm, semifirm,* and *fluid-filled;* these terms also describe the consistency of a lesion.

Pancytopenia A dramatic decrease in all the circulating blood cells.

Papillary Describing a small nipple-shaped projection or elevation; usually found in clusters.

Papillary cystadenoma lymphomatosum A unique type of monomorphic adenoma characterized by an encapsulated tumor composed of two types of tissue: epithelial and lymphoid. It presents as a painless, soft, compressible, or fluctuant mass, usually located in the parotid gland. It is also called a *Warthin tumor.*

Papillary hyperplasia of the palate A form of denture stomatitis. Also called *palatal papillomatosis.*

Papilloma A benign tumor of squamous epithelium that presents as a small, exophytic, pedunculated, or sessile growth. It is often described as cauliflower-like in appearance and occurs most often on the soft palate or tongue.

Papillon-Lefèvre syndrome An inherited disease characterized by marked destruction of the periodontal tissues of both dentitions, with premature loss of teeth and hyperkeratosis of the palms of the hands and soles of the feet.

Papule A small circumscribed lesion usually less than 1 cm in diameter that protrudes above the surface of normal surrounding tissue.

Paramedian lip pit A congenital lip pit that occurs near the midline of the vermilion border of the lower lip.

Paramyxovirus A member of a family of viruses that include the organisms that cause influenza, mumps, and some respiratory infections.

Parathormone Parathyroid hormone.

Parenteral Administered by injection.

Paresthesia An abnormal alteration of touch sensation often perceived as numbness, prickling, or tingling.

Partial thromboplastin time A test that measures the effectiveness of clot formation. It is performed by measuring the time it takes for a clot to form after the addition of kaolin, a surface-activating factor, and cephalin, a substitute platelet factor, to the patient's plasma.

Passive immunity The type of immunity in which antibodies produced by another person are used to protect an individual against infectious disease. This type of immunity can occur naturally or be acquired.

Pathogenic microorganism A microorganism that causes disease.

Pavementing Adherence of white blood cells to the walls of a blood vessel during inflammation.

Pedunculated Attached by a stemlike or stalklike base.

Pegged Resembling a small peg.

Pegged/absent maxillary lateral incisors A condition characterized by a lateral incisor that is small and peg-shaped or congenitally lacking, either unilaterally or bilaterally. Both primary and secondary dentitions can be affected, but mostly the latter.

Pemphigus vulgaris A severe, progressive autoimmune disease that affects the skin and mucous membranes. It is characterized by intraepithelial blister formation that results from breakdown of the cellular adhesion between epithelial cells (acantholysis).

Penetrance In genetics, the prevalence of individuals with a given genotype who manifest clinically the phenotype associated with that trait.

Periapical abscess An abscess composed of pus and surrounded by connective tissue containing neutrophils and lymphocytes. The abscess may develop directly from the inflammation in the pulp or in an area of previously existing chronic inflammation.

Periapical cemento-osseous dysplasia A relatively common disease of unknown cause that affects periapical bone. It is commonly seen in the anterior mandible.

Periapical cyst A true cyst that is associated with the root of a nonvital tooth and consists of a pathologic cavity lined by squamous epithelium that is surrounded by inflamed fibrous connective tissue.

Periapical granuloma A localized mass of chronically inflamed granulation tissue that forms at the opening of a pulp canal, generally at the apex of a nonvital tooth root.

Periapical inflammation Inflammation at or around the root of a tooth.

Pericoronitis An inflammation of the mucosa around the crown of a partially erupted tooth. Usually the result of infection by bacteria that are part of the normal oral flora.

Peripheral Occurring outside of bone.

Peripheral ameloblastoma Ameloblastoma that occurs solely in the gingiva and not in the bone.

Peripheral giant cell granuloma A reactive lesion that occurs on the gingival or alveolar mucosa, typically anterior to the molars. It is usually a result of local irritating factors.

Peripheral ossifying fibroma A well-demarcated sessile or pedunculated lesion that appears to originate from the gingival interdental papilla and is most likely derived from cells of the periodontal ligament.

Pernicious anemia Anemia caused by impaired vitamin B_{12} absorption, resulting from a deficiency of intrinsic factor, a substance secreted by the parietal cells of the stomach.

Petechia (plural, *petechiae*) A minute red spot on the skin or mucous membranes resulting from escape of a small amount of blood.

Peutz-Jeghers syndrome Syndrome characterized by multiple melanotic macular pigmentations of the skin and mucosa, which are associated with gastrointestinal polyposis. The polyps are usually benign.

Phagocytosis A process of ingestion and digestion by cells.

Pharyngitis Inflammatory condition of the tonsils and pharyngeal mucosa caused by many different organisms. Clinical features include sore throat, fever, tonsillar hyperplasia, and erythema of the oropharyngeal mucosa and tonsils.

Phenotype The physical and clinical visible characteristics of an individual. Genotype is the genetic composition; phenotype is its observable appearance.

Pheochromocytoma A benign neoplasm that generally develops in ganglia around the adrenal glands. The tumor is often bilateral and is responsible for night sweats, high blood pressure, and episodes of severe diarrhea.

Philtrum The vertical groove in the midline of the upper lip.

Phycomycosis A rare fungal infection caused by an organism that is a common inhabitant of soil and is usually nonpathogenic. Infection occurs in diabetic and debilitated patients. It often involves the nasal cavity, maxillary sinus, and hard palate and can present as a proliferating or destructive mass in the maxilla. Also called *mucormycosis*.

Pituitary adenoma A benign tumor of the pituitary gland. Often causes hyperpituitarism.

Plasma cell A lymphoid or lymphocyte-like cell found in the bone marrow, connective tissue, and sometimes blood. It has the ability to produce immunoglobulins and is derived from B cells.

Plasma thromboplastin A factor that is active in the formation of intrinsic blood thromboplastin. A deficiency results in Christmas disease (hemophilia B), which is caused by a decrease in the amount of thromboplastin formed. Also called *factor IX*.

Platelet A disk-shaped structure, also called a *thrombocyte*, found in the blood, which plays an important role in blood coagulation.

Platelet count A quantitative or numeric evaluation of platelets.

Pleomorphic Occurring in various forms.

Pleomorphic adenoma The most common of the benign salivary gland tumors. It is also called a *benign mixed tumor*.

Polycythemia An increase in the total red blood cell mass in the blood.

Polydactyly The presence of extra fingers or toes or both.

Polydipsia Chronic excessive thirst and intake of fluid. A possible sign of type 1 diabetes.

Polymorphonuclear leukocyte The most prevalent of the white blood cells containing a multilobed nucleus; also called a *neutrophil*.

Polyostotic fibrous dysplasia A type of fibrous dysplasia characterized by involvement of more than one bone. The skull, clavicles, and long bones are commonly affected.

Polyphagia Excessive appetite. A possible sign of type 1 diabetes.

Polyploid Three (triploid) or four (tetraploid) complete sets of chromosomes. This has been occasionally described in humans and is incompatible with life.

Polyuria Excessive urination. A possible sign of type 1 diabetes.

Post-inflammatory melanosis Melanin pigmentation of the oral mucosa that occurs after an inflammatory response.

Predilection A disposition in favor of something; preference.

Pregnancy tumor A pyogenic granuloma that may occur in pregnant women. They may be caused by changing hormonal levels and increased response to plaque.

Premaxilla The area of the palate that develops from the globular process. It forms the anterior part of the maxillae.

Primary adrenal cortical insufficiency A condition characterized by an insufficient production of adrenal steroids. Also known as *Addison disease*.

Primary dental lamina A band of ectoderm in each jaw on which proliferations of epithelial cells develop, which become the early enamel organs for each of the primary teeth.

Primary herpetic gingivostomatitis Oral disease caused by initial infection with the herpes simplex virus. It is characterized by painful, erythematous, and swollen gingiva and multiple tiny vesicles on the perioral skin, vermilion border of the lips, and oral mucosa. Patients also experience malaise and cervical lymphadenopathy.

Primary immunodeficiencies Immunodeficiencies of developmental or genetic origin that can involve B cells, T cells, or both. They provide information about the functions of the various immunologic responses and are extremely rare.

Primary Sjögren syndrome Lacrimal and salivary gland involvement without the presence of another autoimmune disease.

Primary tumor The original tumor; the source of metastasis.

Primordial cyst A cyst that develops in place of a tooth.

Proliferation The multiplication of cells.

Prothrombin time A test that measures the patient's ability to form a clot. It is performed by measuring the time it takes for a clot to form when calcium and a tissue factor are added to the patient's plasma.

Pruritus Itching.

Pseudoanodontia A condition in which normal teeth cannot erupt due to interference, such as in cleidocranial dysplasia.

Pseudocyst An abnormal cavity that resembles a true cyst but is not a pathologic cavity and is not lined with epithelium.

Pseudomembranous candidiasis A type of candidiasis in which a white curdlike material is present on the mucosal surface. When the material is wiped off, the underlying mucosa is erythematous.

Pulp polyp An excessive proliferation of chronically inflamed dental pulp tissue. Also called *chronic hyperplastic pulpitis*.

Purified protein derivative An antigen used to test whether an individual has been exposed to and infected with *Mycobacterium tuberculosis*.

Purpura A group of disorders characterized by purplish or brownish-red discolorations caused by bleeding into the skin or tissues.

Purulent Containing or forming pus.

Pustule A variably sized, circumscribed, pus-filled, elevated lesion.

Pyogenic granuloma A commonly occurring intraoral lesion characterized by a proliferation of connective tissue containing numerous blood vessels and inflammatory cells. It occurs in response to injury. The lesion does not produce pus and is not a true granuloma.

R

Radiation The process of emitting radiant energy in the form of waves or particles.

Radiation therapy The treatment of a disease or condition with a type of radiation.

Radicular Pertaining to the root of a tooth.

Radicular cyst A cyst with a wall of fibrous connective tissue and a lining of stratified squamous epithelium that is attached to the root apex of a tooth with a necrotic pulp or a defective root canal filling.

Radiolucent The black or dark areas in a radiograph that result from the ability of radiant energy to pass through the structure. Less dense structures (e.g., the pulp) are radiolucent.

Radiolucent and radiopaque Terms used to describe a mixture of light and dark areas within a lesion, usually denoting a stage in the development of the lesion; for example, in a stage I periapical cemento-osseous dysplasia (cementoma), the lesion is radiolucent; in stage II it is radiolucent and radiopaque.

Radiopaque The white or clear appearance in a radiograph that results from the inability of radiant energy to pass through a structure. The more dense the structure (e.g., amalgam restorations), the whiter it appears in a radiograph.

Ranula A large mucocele-like lesion that forms unilaterally on the floor of the mouth. It is associated with the sublingual and submandibular glands. It is caused by a sialolith or trauma to the major duct.

Raynaud phenomenon A disorder that affects the fingers and toes. Cold and emotional stress trigger a reaction, which is characterized by an initial pallor of the skin that results from vasoconstriction and reduced blood flow. The initial pallor is followed by cyanosis, which occurs because of the decreased blood flow.

Reactive connective tissue hyperplasia Proliferating exuberant granulation tissue and dense fibrous connective tissue resulting from overzealous repair.

Receptor A cell surface protein to which a molecule can bind; such binding leads to biochemical events.

Recessive In genetics a trait or characteristic manifested clinically with a double gene dose in autosomal chromosomes or with a single dose in males if the trait is X-linked.

Recurrent herpes simplex infection Herpes simplex virus that persists in a latent state, usually in the nerve tissue of the trigeminal ganglion, and causes localized recurrent infections. Recurrent infections are often produced by stimuli such as sunlight, menstruation, or stress.

Regeneration The process by which injured tissue is replaced with tissue identical to that present before the injury.

Regional odontodysplasia A developmental problem in which one or several teeth in the same quadrant radiographically exhibit a marked reduction in radiodensity and a characteristic ghostlike appearance. Very thin enamel and dentin are present. Also called *ghost teeth*.

Repair The restoration of damaged or diseased tissues.

Residual cyst A cyst that forms when a tooth is removed and all or part of a periapical cyst is left behind.

Reticular lichen planus The most common form of lichen planus. The lesions are composed of Wickham striae along with white, slightly raised plaquelike areas.

Retrocuspid papilla A sessile nodule on the gingival margin of the lingual aspect of the mandibular cuspids.

Rhabdomyoma A benign tumor of striated muscle that has been reported to occur on the tongue.

Rhabdomyosarcoma A malignant tumor of striated muscle that grows rapidly and is destructive. It is the most common malignant soft tissue tumor of the head and neck in children.

Rheumatic fever A childhood disease that follows a group A β-hemolytic streptococcal infection, usually tonsillitis and pharyngitis. Characterized by an inflammatory reaction involving the heart, joints, and central nervous system.

Rheumatoid arthritis An inflammatory autoimmune disorder of the joints.

Rheumatoid factor An antibody against IgG found in serum and detectable on laboratory tests. It is associated with rheumatoid arthritis and other autoimmune diseases.

Ribonucleic acid (RNA) Single strands of polynucleotides found in all cells; different types of RNA have different functions in the production of proteins by the cell.

Ribosome The cytoplasmic organelles in which proteins are formed on the basis of the genetic code provided by an RNA template.

Root resorption Observed radiographically when the apex of the tooth appears shortened or blunted and irregularly shaped. It occurs as a response to stimuli, which can result from a cyst, tumor, or trauma.

rRNA Ribosomal RNA; the third type of RNA. It combines with several polypeptides to form ribosomes.

S

S phase The phase in which the replication of DNA takes place.

Sarcoma A malignant tumor of connective tissue.

Scalloping around the roots The radiographic appearance of a radiolucent lesion that extends between the roots of multiple teeth, as seen in a traumatic bone cyst.

Scarlet fever Contagious childhood disease caused by group A β-hemolytic *Streptococcus*. Characterized by a red rash, strawberry tongue, sore throat, fever, enlarged lymph nodes, and prostration.

Schwannoma A benign tumor derived from Schwann cells, a component of the connective tissue surrounding nerves. The tongue is the most common intraoral location.

Scoliosis Lateral curvature of the spine.

Scrofula Pertaining to tuberculosis, the enlargement of the submandibular and cervical lymph nodes. Also known as *tuberculous lymphadenitis*.

Second meiosis Second stage of meiosis that is essentially a mitotic division in which each chromosome splits longitudinally. Replication of DNA occurs in second meiosis.

Secondary immunodeficiencies Immunodeficiencies that occur as a result of an underlying disorder. They are more common than the primary immunodeficiency disorders.

Secondary Sjögren syndrome The combination of another autoimmune disease with salivary and lacrimal gland involvement.

Secondary thrombocytopenic purpura The condition of thrombocytopenic purpura secondary to an existing disease or condition.

Serous A substance having a watery consistency; relating to serum.

Serum sickness A delayed allergic response after exposure to some antibiotics or antiserum. It is caused by an antibody reaction to an antigen in the donor serum. Symptoms include fever, painful swelling of the joints, renal disturbance or failure, edema around the eyes, carditis, and skin lesions.

Sessile Broad-based.

Severe combined immunodeficiency A genetic disorder in which both B cells and T cells of the immune system are crippled, leaving the patient extremely vulnerable to infectious diseases.

Shingles A disease, caused by the varicella-zoster virus, that occurs in adults. It is characterized by a unilateral, painful eruption of vesicles along the distribution of a sensory nerve. Also called *herpes zoster*.

Sialadenitis A painful swelling of a salivary gland that may be caused by obstruction or infection. It can be acute or chronic.

Sialolith A salivary gland stone.

Sicca syndrome A combination of dry mouth and dry eyes.

Sickle cell anemia An inherited disorder of the blood that is found predominantly in black individuals and those of Mediterranean origin. It occurs as a result of an abnormal type of hemoglobin in red blood cells that causes the cells to develop a sickle shape in the presence of decreased oxygen.

Sickle cell trait People who are heterozygous for sickle cell anemia.

Sign Objective evidence of disease that can be observed by a health care provider.

Simple bone cyst A pathologic cavity in bone that is not lined with epithelium. Also known as a *traumatic bone cyst*.

Single-gene inheritance Characteristics that are governed by the action of one gene.

Sjögren syndrome An autoimmune disease that affects the salivary and lacrimal glands, resulting in a decrease in saliva and tears.

Smokeless tobacco–associated keratosis A white lesion that develops in the oral mucosa in the area where smokeless tobacco is habitually placed. Also known as *smokeless tobacco keratosis* and *tobacco pouch keratosis*.

Smoker's melanosis (smoking-associated melanosis) A type of melanosis in which the melanin pigmentation is associated with smoking and the intensity is related to the amount and duration of smoking.

Solar cheilitis Degeneration of the tissue of the lips caused by sun exposure. Also called *actinic cheilitis*.

Somatic cells All the cells of the human body with the exception of the primitive germ cells (oogonia and spermatogonia).

Smooth, rough, folded Terms used to describe the surface of a lesion.

Speckled leukoplakia An oral mucosal lesion that shows a mixture of red and white areas.

Spermatogenesis The process of formation of spermatozoa (sperm).

Spermatozoon The mature masculine germ cell.

Spina bifida A defect in the spine caused by a lack of the vertebral arches through which the spinal cord protrudes.

Spina bifida occulta Similar to spina bifida, but with little or no protrusion of the spinal cord.

Splenomegaly Enlargement of the spleen.

Squamous cell carcinoma A malignant tumor of squamous epithelium. It is the most common primary malignancy of the oral cavity and, like other malignant tumors, can infiltrate adjacent tissues and metastasize to distant sites. Also known as *epidermoid carcinoma*.

Stabilization appliances A treatment modality used in the management of certain temporomandibular joint disorders that consists of the fabrication of occlusal appliances.

Stafne bone defect Often referred to as a pseudocyst because it is not a pathologic cavity and is not lined with epithelium. It is characterized by a well-defined radiolucency in the posterior region of the mandible inferior to the mandibular canal, which is caused by a lingual depression in the mandible containing normal salivary gland tissue. Also known as a *lingual mandibular bone concavity* or *static bone cyst*.

Static bone cyst Often referred to as a pseudocyst because it is not a pathologic cavity and is not lined with epithelium.

It is characterized by a well-defined radiolucency in the posterior region of the mandible inferior to the mandibular canal, which is caused by a lingual depression in the mandible containing normal salivary gland tissue. Also known as a *lingual mandibular bone concavity* or *Stafne bone cyst*.

Stevens-Johnson syndrome A severe form of erythema multiforme characterized by oral, ocular, and genital involvement.

Stomodeum The embryonic invagination that becomes the oral cavity.

Strawberry tongue Oral manifestation of scarlet fever in which the fungiform papillae are red and prominent, with the dorsal surface of tongue exhibiting either a white coating or erythema.

Striae Streaks or interconnecting lines.

Subclinical infection An infectious disease not detectable by the usual clinical signs.

Subluxation Hypermobility in which the patient is able to relocate the mandible back into the glenoid fossa.

Succedaneous Replacing or substituting for something else; often used when referring to the permanent teeth.

Supernumerary In excess of the normal or regular number, as in teeth or roots.

Supernumerary roots More than the normal number of roots. Supernumerary roots tend to occur in teeth in which roots form after birth.

Supernumerary teeth Extra teeth found in the dental arches.

Symptom Subjective evidence of disease or a physical disorder that is observed by the patient.

Syndactyly Soft tissue or bone fusion or both of fingers and toes.

Syndrome A set of signs or symptoms or both occurring together.

Synovial fluid The transparent viscous fluid that is secreted by the synovial membrane and found in joint cavities.

Synovial membrane Tissue that forms a portion of the lining of some joints; (e.g., the temporomandibular joint).

Syphilis A disease caused by the spirochete *Treponema pallidum*. The organism is transmitted from one person to another by direct contact. It occurs in three stages: (1) primary, (2) secondary, and (3) tertiary.

Systemic Pertaining to or affecting the body as a whole.

Systemic lupus erythematosus An acute and chronic inflammatory autoimmune disease of unknown cause. It includes a wide spectrum of disease activity and signs and symptoms.

T

T-cell lymphocyte A lymphocyte that passes through the thymus before migrating to tissues. The T lymphocyte, also called a *T-cell*, is responsible for cell-mediated immunity and may modulate the humoral immune response.

Talon cusp An accessory cusp located in the area of the cingulum of a maxillary or mandibular permanent incisor.

Taurodontism A condition characterized by very large pyramid-shaped molars with large pulp chambers and short roots.

Temporomandibular disorders (TMDs) Abnormalities in the functioning of the temporomandibular joint or associated structures.

Thalassemia A group of inherited disorders of hemoglobin synthesis. Also called *Mediterranean* or *Cooley anemia*.

Thalassemia major The homozygous form of thalassemia in which genes on both chromosomes are involved.

Thalassemia minor The heterozygous form of thalassemia in which only one gene locus is involved.

Thrombocyte A platelet.

Thrombocytopenia Decrease in the number of platelets in circulating blood. It is sometimes called immune thrombocytopenia because an autoimmune type of process has been identified.

Thrombocytopenic purpura A bleeding disorder that results from a severe reduction in circulating platelets.

Thrush An overgrowth of the yeastlike fungus *Candida albicans*. It is the most common oral fungal infection. It can result from many different conditions, including antibiotic use, cancer, corticosteroid therapy, dentures, diabetes mellitus, and HIV infection. Also called *candidiasis* and *moniliasis*.

Thymic hypoplasia A type of primary immunodeficiency in which the thymus is deficient or lacking; therefore T lymphocytes do not mature. Also called *DiGeorge syndrome*.

Thymus A lymphoid organ situated in the chest. It reaches maximal development at about puberty and then undergoes gradual involution.

Thyroglossal tract (duct) cyst A cyst that forms along the same tract that the thyroid gland follows in development, from the area of the foramen cecum to its permanent location in the neck. Most occur below the hyoid bone. The epithelial lining varies from stratified squamous to ciliated columnar epithelium.

Thyrotoxicosis A condition characterized by excessive production of thyroid hormone. Also called *hyperthyroidism*.

TNM staging system A staging and classification system of malignant tumors. T: tumor size; N: lymph nodes involved; M: presence of metastasis.

Tobacco pouch keratosis A lesion caused by tobacco chewing; typically located in the mucobuccal fold.

Tonsillitis Inflammatory condition of the tonsils and pharyngeal mucosa caused by many different organisms. Clinical features include sore throat, fever, tonsillar hyperplasia, and erythema of the oropharyngeal mucosa and tonsils.

Torus (plural, tori) A benign lesion composed of normal compact bone.

Torus mandibularis An exophytic growth of bone occurring on the lingual aspect of the mandible in the area of the premolars. Also known as *mandibular tori*.

Torus palatinus An exophytic growth of bone occurring in the midline of the hard palate. Also known as *palatal torus*.

Translocation In genetics, a portion of a chromosome attached to another chromosome.

Transudate The fluid component of blood that normally passes through the endothelial cell walls of the microcirculation.

Traumatic bone cyst A pathologic cavity in bone that is not lined with epithelium. Also known as a *simple bone cyst*.

Traumatic fibroma A broad-based, persistent, exophytic mucosal lesion that is composed of dense scarlike, fibrous connective tissue surfaced by stratified squamous epithelium. Also known as *irritation fibroma*, *fibroma*, and *focal fibrous hyperplasia*.

Traumatic granuloma A hard, raised ulcerated lesion resulting from persistent trauma.

Traumatic injury A disease process that results from injury that causes tissue damage.

Traumatic neuroma A lesion caused by injury to a peripheral nerve.

Traumatic ulcer An ulcer that occurs from some form or trauma such as biting the cheek, lip, or tongue; irritation from a denture; and injury from sharp edge of food.

Trismus Inability to open the mouth fully, due to one of many causes.

Trisomy A pair of chromosomes with an identical extra chromosome.

Trisomy 21 A type of abnormality in which three of chromosome 21 are found instead of two. This results in abnormal physical characteristics and mental impairment. Also called *Down syndrome*.

tRNA Transfer RNA; the second type of RNA. It transfers amino acids from the cytoplasm and matches them to the mRNA, positioning amino acids in the proper sequence to form polypeptides and proteins.

Tuberculosis An infectious chronic granulomatous disease usually caused by the organism *Mycobacterium tuberculosis*. The chief form of the disease is a primary infection of the lung.

Tuberculous lymphadenitis Pertaining to tuberculosis, the enlargement of the submandibular and cervical lymph nodes. Also known as *scrofula*.

Tumor A neoplasm; also a swelling or enlargement.

Turner tooth A permanent tooth showing enamel hypoplasia resulting from infection or trauma to the deciduous tooth.

Type 1 diabetes The type of diabetes that is characterized by profound insulin deficiency. It includes patients requiring the administration of insulin to prevent ketosis. The onset is abrupt and may be characterized by polydipsia, polyuria, and polyphagia. Also called *insulin-dependent diabetes mellitus*.

Type 2 diabetes The type of diabetes that is characterized by increased insulin resistance. It includes patients who can maintain proper blood sugar levels without the administration of insulin. Obesity is common finding. Also called *non–insulin-dependent diabetes mellitus*.

Tzanck cells (1) Detached rounded cells caused by a loss of attachment between epithelial cells. Also known as *acantholytic cells*. These cells are present with pemphigus vulgaris. (2) Enlarged multinucleated epithelial cells that occur as a result of infection with herpes simplex or varicella-zoster virus.

U

Undifferentiated Absence of normal differentiation; anaplasia; a characteristic of malignant tumor tissue.

Unilocular A term used to describe the radiographic appearance of a single rounded compartment or locule.

Urticaria Multiple areas of well-demarcated swelling of the skin, usually accompanied by itching. The lesions are caused by localized areas of vascular permeability in the superficial connective tissue beneath the epithelium. Also known as *hives*.

V

Varicella-zoster virus (VZV) The virus that causes both chickenpox (varicella) and shingles (herpes zoster).

Vascular leiomyoma A benign tumor of smooth muscle that may occur in association with blood vessels. They occur occasionally in the oral cavity.

Verruca vulgaris A white, papillary, exophytic lesion caused by a human papillomavirus. It is a common skin lesion. The lips are one of the most common intraoral sites for this lesion.

Verrucous carcinoma A specific type of squamous cell carcinoma that appears as a slow-growing exophytic tumor with a pebbly white and red surface, usually in the vestibule or buccal mucosa. Often associated with the use of smokeless tobacco.

Vesicle A small, elevated, fluid-filled lesion on the epithelium that is less than 1 cm in diameter.

Vitamin B$_{12}$ A vitamin that contains cobalt and is essential for the maturation of red blood cells.

von Willebrand disease An inherited disorder of platelet function. It is the most common hereditary coagulation anomaly in humans.

W

Waldeyer ring The ring of lymphatic tissue formed by the two palatine tonsils, the pharyngeal tonsil, the lingual tonsil, and intervening lymphoid tissue.

Well-circumscribed Used to describe the borders of a lesion that are specifically defined; the exact margins and extent of the lesion can be clearly seen.

Western blot test A confirmatory test for HIV infection that identifies antibodies to HIV proteins and glycoproteins.

Wheal A localized swelling of tissue caused by edema during inflammation; often accompanied by severe itching.

White sponge nevus An inherited disorder characterized by a white, corrugated, soft folding of the oral mucosa. The buccal mucosa is always affected, and in most patients the lesions are bilateral. A thick layer of keratin, which at times desquamates and leaves a raw mucosal surface, produces the whitening. Also called *Cannon disease* or *familial white folded mucosal dysplasia*.

Whitlow An infection involving the distal phalanx of a finger.

X

Xerophthalmia Abnormal dryness of the eyes caused by decreased lacrimal flow.

Xerostomia Dryness of the mouth caused by a decrease in salivary flow.

X-linked congenital agammaglobulinemia A type of primary immunodeficiency in which B cells do not mature. Plasma cells are deficient throughout the body; T-cells are normal. Also called *Bruton disease*.

Index

Page numbers followed by "f" indicate figures, "t" indicate tables, and "b" indicate boxes.